About the Authors

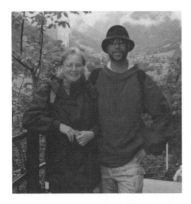

Patricia Barnes-Svarney is a science and science fiction writer. Over the past few decades, she has written or coauthored more than 30 books, including *When the Earth Moves: Rogue Earthquakes, Tremors, and Aftershocks* and *Why Do Women Crave More Sex in the Summer?: 112 Questions That Women Keep Asking—and Keep Everyone Else Guessing*; and she is the editor/author of the award-winning *New York Public Library Science Desk Reference*. In her spare time, she is a New York Master Gardener and teaches cooking classes at local shops.

Thomas E. Svarney is a scientist and researcher who has written extensively about the natural world. His books, with Patricia Barnes-Svarney, include Visible Ink Press' *The Handy Dinosaur Answer Book, The Handy Math Answer Book,* and *The Handy Biology Answer Book*, as well as *Skies of Fury: Weather Weirdness around the World* and *The Oryx Guide to Natural History.*

Also from Visible Ink Press

Please visit us at www.handyanswers.com

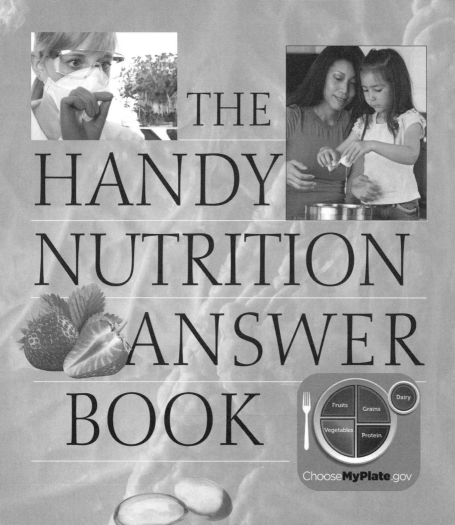

THE
HANDY
NUTRITION
ANSWER
BOOK

Fruits Grains Dairy
Vegetables Protein
Choose**MyPlate**.gov

Patricia Barnes-Svarney and Thomas E. Svarney

VISIBLE
INK
PRESS

Detroit

THE HANDY NUTRITION ANSWER BOOK

Visible Ink Press®
43311 Joy Rd., #414
Canton, MI 48187–2075

Visible Ink Press is a registered trademark of Visible Ink Press LLC.

Most Visible Ink Press books are available at special quantity discounts when purchased in bulk by corporations, organizations, or groups. Customized printings, special imprints, messages, and excerpts can be produced to meet your needs. For more information, contact Special Markets Director, Visible Ink Press, www.visibleink.com, or 734–667–3211.

Managing Editor: Kevin S. Hile
Art Director: Mary Claire Krzewinski
Typesetting: Marco Di Vita
Proofreaders: Nancy Crompton and Barbara Lyon
Indexer: Larry Baker

Cover images: Shutterstock.

Library of Congress Cataloging-in-Publication Data

Barnes-Svarney, Patricia L.
  The handy nutrition answer book / by Patricia Barnes-Svarney and Thomas E. Svarney.
    pages cm. – (The handy answer series)
    ISBN 978-1-57859-484-9 (pbk. : alk. paper)
    1. Nutrition–Miscellanea. I. Svarney, Thomas E. II. Title.
  TX355.B365 2015   363.8–dc23
  2014033781

Printed in the United States of America

10 9 8 7 6 5 4 3 2 1

A12006 443518

Contents

v

Acknowledgments

The authors would like to thank the many hard-working nutrition and food experts, health care providers, and our acquaintances and friends who helped us with this book—from the most recent scientific studies and some doctors' experiences to the simple to sometimes complex questions from the general public. We'd also like to acknowledge those people who struggle with the day-to-day balance of what they eat, especially those with a health concern—such as type 1 diabetes or celiac disease—who try to stay healthy. We also salute those of you who wish to eat better in order to live a healthier, happier, and longer life—and we hope this book will, in some way, help you and your family to maintain a nutritional balance.

As with all of our books in the "Handy Answer" series, there are many people behind the scenes: Above all, we'd like to thank Roger Jänecke once again for all his help, consideration, patience, and especially for asking us to write this book; also thanks to page and cover designer Mary Claire Krzewinski, typesetter Marco Di Vita, indexer Larry Baker, and proofreaders Nancy Crompton and Barbara Lyon. As always, an extra (huge) special thank you to Kevin Hile, our outstanding editor for many of our "Handy Answer" books. And to our wonderful agent, Agnes Birnbaum—thanks for your friendship … and for always being there for us.

Photo Credits

Jean-Paul Barbier: p. 142.

Friedrich Müller: p. 218.

Public domain: pp. 152, 229, 231.

U.S. Food and Drug Administration: p. 235.

U.S. Library of Congress: p. 11.

U.S. National Library of Medicine: p. 20.

All other photos were obtained from Shutterstock.

DISCLAIMER

In addition to facts about nutrition and the human body, *The Handy Nutrition Answer Book* contains information on diets, debates about certain foods and food supplements, information on food-related diseases, and text on other health issues. By including these entries in the book, the publisher and authors are in no way endorsing or recommending certain diets, foods, or medical treatments addressing any health issues that readers may have. Individuals who are experiencing medical problems should seek the advice and help of a qualified healthcare professional.

Introduction

"Tell me what you eat and I will tell you what you are," was spoken many years ago. The most recent work in science confirms the fact that the kind of food an individual eats has much to do with his ability to work. If you would be well, strong, happy, and full of vim choose your food carefully.

—*School and Home Cooking* by Carlotta C. Greer, 1920

Food is one topic humans never seem to mind discussing—the eating, cooking, and even harvesting of what we eat. The reason is obvious: everyone needs nutritious food to stay healthy; and without it, we have little or no chance of survival.

And food is not about what tastes good to us—it's truly about the many nutritious components of the foods that keep us alive. If we don't consume certain nutrients, we can suffer from many illnesses (scurvy from lack of vitamin C comes to mind); and without certain non-nutrients, the same would happen (water comes to mind). Thus, our overall health, and the health of every other organism on the planet, is irrevocably tied to nutrients found in food.

For many people, choosing the most nutritious foods to eat can be hard, especially in the fast-paced world in which we live. In addition, the answers to all our nutrition questions are not always easy—after all, we are all physically and chemically different—from how we process foods and their nutrients in our system to which foods taste best to us. And although most of us know that eating a greasy burger is not as good for us as eating a vegetable-rich salad, sometimes it's hard to stay on track to stay healthy.

There are other concerns about nutrition, too. For example, the "health" of our food is tied to *our* health; knowing where that burger meat came from, or where and how our vegetables are grown, can also impact our health. For instance, does that red pepper (grown in Argentina) you just ate carry the same nutritional value as the one you bought from the local farmer's market yesterday?

In these pages, we present to you many of these concerns—along with numerous other facts and data, such as:

- The basics behind nutrition and the consumption of food and beverages
- Both sides of several nutrition stories (for instance, why can't researchers decide if coffee is good or bad for you?)
- Examples of the chemistry behind nutrition and certain foods
- How our bodies process foods to obtain nutrients—and how our body uses those nutrients
- Food through the centuries, including some preservation techniques that help maintain a food's nutritional value (the "old" and "new" ways of preserving it)
- Some of the major nutrition and food controversies (for example, the pros and cons of Genetically Modified Organisms, or GMOs)
- Some of the more obscure notions about nutrition (for instance, can the lack of certain nutrients really affect our moods?)
- Several ways to keep track of your nutrition for a healthier body (for instance, calculating your Body Mass Index, something many doctors use to help you determine your health), and some basic nutrition guidelines you can use no matter what your phase of life
- The pros and cons of some of the most popular diets
- And, of course, the most up-to-date information and research on nutrition.

When we began writing this text, we asked a good friend what she wanted to see in a nutrition book. "I want a book about this size," she said, using her hands to measure about 8 by 11 inches, "with instructions telling me what I should eat every day so I'm never sick again."

We knew what she meant, but we broke it to her gently: it can't be done. And she knew what we meant, too.

Nutrition and the foods we consume are personal. Thus, there is no one book that can tell you everything about what you personally should or should not eat in order to stay healthy.

That being said, there are directions in which a book can lead you to make the best choices for you and your family's health. This, we hope, is a book that will help you make such choices.

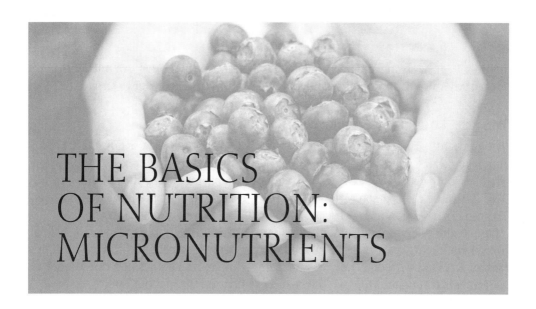

THE BASICS OF NUTRITION: MICRONUTRIENTS

NUTRIENT BASICS

What are nutrients?

A quick and basic definition of a nutrient is as follows: a chemical that any living organism needs to survive. These chemicals give organisms energy to perform all functions, provide fuel to build tissues, and help the organism to grow. Scientists usually divide nutrients into two main categories (although there are others who divide nutrients into several more groups depending on function): macronutrients and micronutrients. There are also compounds called non-nutrients that act like nutrients but are not classified as such (for more about macronutrients and non-nutrients, see the chapter titled "The Basics of Nutrition: Macronutrients and Non-nutrients").

Why are nutrients important to humans?

The main reason why nutrients are so important to humans (and to other animals, plants, fungi, etc.) is because these chemicals and compounds help us remain healthy and aid in our survival. Not all nutrients are the same, either—from vitamin A to zinc—and each one affects us in specific ways. Our foods contain these chemical substances, providing heat and energy, helping us to grow and repair our body's tissues, and assisting in regulating the body's overall processes.

What other organisms on Earth rely on nutrients?

Besides humans, all other organisms on Earth—from animals in the Amazon and plants in the Sahara Desert to bacteria on our skin and fungi on a tree—rely on nutrients. The biggest differences are the amounts and types of nutrients each organism needs. For example, plants need nutrients mostly in the form of nitrogen, potassium, and phosphorus

1

in order to grow strong and healthy, whereas a human needs even more nutrients in the form of vitamins and minerals—and many non-nutrients—in order to survive.

What are the nutritional requirements for human health?

The nutrients you take into your body—or what you eat—have a major effect on how much you weigh, your health, and your likelihood of developing or resisting a chronic disease. But in general, there is no one set of nutritional requirements for human health. This is because each person varies chemically, physically, and mentally; nutritional needs are also dependent on many other factors, including age, sex, and health condition. For example, the calcium requirements for a female teenager versus a menopausal woman are very different, as are nutritional food requirements for a person with type 1 diabetes versus a person who does not have diabetes. (For more about some nutritional requirements throughout life, see the chapter "Nutrition throughout Life.")

Is there a difference between plant and animal nutrients?

In general, the nutrients we obtain by ingesting plant and animal foods are relatively the same. In other words, the zinc you obtain from eating certain meats is really no different for your body from the zinc you obtain from ingesting whole grains. But there are differences in terms of plants and animals. For example (and the most obvious), there are differences in the cells that make up plants and animals. Another difference is that there are usually more essential nutrients found in animal foods, and that many of these nutrients are often more bioavailable (goes into our system better) than certain nutrients from plants; for example, zinc and iron in animal foods are usually more bioavailable to humans than from plants. Still another big difference is how your body absorbs or processes certain plant or animal nutrients. For example, people who have a dairy intolerance would turn to such plants as kale, cabbage, and broccoli for their natural calcium.

Does any single food supply all the nutrients humans need?

Although you may hear claims to the contrary, there is no single food that can supply all the nutrients in the amounts that humans need to survive. For example, lemons may supply vitamin C, but they offer no calcium. This is why nutritionists recommend a balanced diet of many kinds of foods to fill our daily nutritional needs.

Do Americans get enough nutrients from their daily diet?

According to studies at the University of Rochester, most Americans don't get enough nutrients—especially vitamins and minerals—in their daily diet. The researchers state that fewer than 5 percent of Americans follow all of the U.S. Department of Agriculture's Dietary Guidelines (for more about these guidelines, see the chapter "Nutrition throughout Life"). And it's also known that on average, one in three adults takes a multivitamin—often thought of as the "easy" way to obtain nutrients. In reality, the best and easiest way to be and stay healthy is to eat a well-balanced diet with nutrient-dense foods.

How do deficiencies in certain nutrients affect our health?

There are many problems that arise from deficiencies in certain nutrients—too many to mention here. But there are some common, well-known health problems and conditions caused by the lack of specific nutrients. For example, a person may be iron deficient because of a diet low in vitamins B_1, B_2, niacin, pantothenic acid, or choline; these nutrients help the stomach to secrete hydrochloric acid, essentially dissolving the iron so it's easily absorbed. Another example is excessive bruising—a condition that may mean that you are not consuming enough vitamin D, a natural blood-clotting agent; in addition,

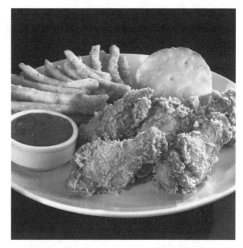

Many Americans do not eat a well-balanced diet, often indulging in meals that lack fruits, vegetables, and whole grains.

zinc, vitamin C, and bioflavonoid deficiencies can weaken small blood vessels, making it easier for you to bruise. (For more about the effects of nutritional deficiencies, see the chapter "Nutrition and Allergies, Illnesses, and Diseases.")

What are the six essential nutrients that cannot be synthesized by the human body?

The six essential nutrients (some are also classified as non-nutrients) are familiar to us all: carbohydrates, fats (lipids), proteins, vitamins, minerals, and water. Each has a specific function and relationship to the body—and not one of these nutrients can act independently of the others. In addition, scientists now know that each nutrient is equally valuable for human health. Thus, although factors can alter the amounts we ingest—based on factors such as our age, body volume, sex, and lifestyle—deficiencies in any of these nutrients can lead to a nutritional imbalance.

MICRONUTRIENTS

What are micronutrients?

Micronutrients (*micro* is Greek for "small") are defined as nutrients that humans need in smaller quantities, but are just as important as macronutrients (*macro* meaning "large-scale"). In particular, as the body uses oxygen, it undergoes aging, a process that can be destructive to our health—what some researchers have called a form of "biological rusting." The micronutrients we call vitamins and minerals help to keep us from aging more rapidly—especially our brains (some researchers also add two essential fatty

3

acids, omega-3 and omega-6, to the micronutrient list; for this text, specifics about these fatty acids are found in the chapter "The Basics of Nutrition—Macronutrients and Non-nutrients"). And because the body does not manufacture all of our needed vitamins and minerals, we have to obtain most of our micronutrients from our diet.

VITAMINS

How many vitamins do humans need?

All organisms need various vitamins; to date, there are thought to be 13 essential vitamins necessary for human health, although some researchers list 15 (or more) essential vitamins. There are many other vitamin-like substances that humans need, too, such as bioflavonoids and antioxidants—and although they are no doubt essential to health, no RDAs (Recommended Dietary Allowances) have been established for them. (For more about RDAs, see the chapter "Nutrition throughout Life.")

When were some of the various vitamins discovered?

After the discovery of vitamins—the first, called thiamine, around 1912 and vitamin C in 1928—many others were studied and synthesized in the early 1900s. For example, in 1935, riboflavin (vitamin B_2) was found; the same year, vitamin K was discovered; by 1937, vitamin A was found. (For more about vitamin discoveries, see the chapter "Nutrition throughout the Centuries.")

What are fat-soluble and water-soluble vitamins?

Vitamins are classified according to their ability to be absorbed or stored in the body. For example, vitamins A, D, E, and K are soluble only in fats, and thus are called fat soluble; vitamin C and the B vitamins are soluble in water, and thus are called water soluble. It is interesting to note that fat-soluble vitamins will not be lost when the foods that contain them are cooked; on the other hand, when water-soluble vitamin-rich foods are cooked, many (but not all) can lose their potency from the heat. (For more information about how certain nutrients respond to such actions as cooking, see the chapter "Food Chemistry and Nutrition.")

Which vitamins can the body store, and which ones do we barely store?

Because the human body does not need them every day, fat-soluble vitamins are most often stored in our fatty (adipose) tissues and liver. There are some problems; for example, because of this often long-term storage, the fat-soluble vitamins pose a greater risk for toxicity when consumed in excess (when compared to water-soluble vitamins). In addition, some health problems that decrease the absorption of fats (or even medications that cause this problem) may mean that a person can develop a mild deficiency in fat-soluble vitamins.

The water-soluble vitamins are not held in the body as long as fat-soluble vitamins. Excess amounts of these vitamins are excreted in the urine (which is why your urine is often a darker yellow if you take multivitamins, as most of the vitamins are not absorbed, but go right through your system). Thus, foods containing these nutrients must be eaten more frequently.

What is a provitamin?

The term *provitamin* is often used to describe a substance that the body can convert into a vitamin. For example, beta carotene, found in such food as carrots, pumpkins, and dark green leafy vegetables, is converted by the liver into vitamin A. Another example is vitamin D: A substance called 7-dehydrocholesterol forms from cholesterol in the wall of our intestines; the sun's ultraviolet radiation then converts the 7-dehydrocholesterol that reaches our skin's surface into cholecalciferol, or vitamin D_3.

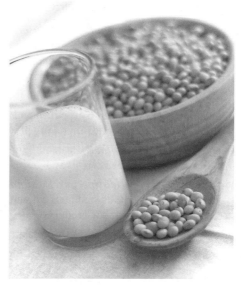

Soy milk and soybeans contain biotin, a water-soluble B vitamin that supports the intestinal tract, nervous system, and healthy skin.

What are the major known vitamins and their best-known food sources?

There are, to date, thought to be 13 essential vitamins our bodies need for good health (although some say there are up to 15). The following chart lists the 13 vitamins and some food sources that contain those vitamins. *Note*: Because of the many foods that contain certain vitamins, this is only a partial list of food sources.

Vitamin	Best Food Sources
FAT-SOLUBLE VITAMINS	
Vitamin A	*Beta carotene*: orange and yellow fruits and vegetables, such as carrots and squash; green leafy vegetables
	Retinols: found in liver, salmon, and many cold-water fish; egg yolks; and enriched and/or fortified soy; cow and other dairy products
Vitamin D	*Calciferol*: enriched and/or fortified dairy (cow, goat, sheep) and soy products; egg yolks; fish liver oils
Vitamin E	*Tocopherols, tocotrienols*: eggs, mayonnaise, nuts, seeds, and certain vegetable oils; fortified and/or enriched cereals
Vitamin K	Green leafy vegetables, such as spinach and cabbage; pork and liver; and green tea
WATER-SOLUBLE VITAMINS	
Biotin	Egg yolks, soybeans, certain cereals, soy milk, and yeast
Folate	*Folic acid, folacin, B_9*: liver; yeast; cruciferous vegetables, such as broccoli and cabbage, along with many raw vegetables and avocados

Vitamin	Best Food Sources
Niacin	*Vitamin B₃, nicotinic acid, nicotinamide*: lean meats, poultry and game meats, and certain seafood; milk (a source of tryptophan, a precursor to niacin), eggs, and fortified and/or enriched cereals, breads, and flours; certain legumes, such as black beans
Pantothenic acid	*Vitamin B₅*: almost all food
Riboflavin	*Vitamin B₂*: fortified and/or enriched cereals, grains, and flours; lean meats; milk and other dairy products; certain mushrooms
Thiamine	*Vitamin B₁*: lean pork; nuts and seeds; legumes; and fortified and/or enriched cereals and grains
Vitamin B₆	*Pyridoxine, pyridoxamine, pyridoxal*: lean meats, fish, and poultry; grains, cereals, and flours; green leafy vegetables, potatoes, and soybeans (and some soy products)
Vitamin B₁₂	*Cobalamin*: all animal products
Vitamin C	*Ascorbic acid*: citrus fruits, juices, and dried fruit; melons, berries, peppers, potatoes, broccoli, cabbage, and many other fruits and vegetables

Are there various forms of vitamins?

Yes, many vitamins come in various forms, usually depending on their source and if they affect humans in particular. For example, vitamin D comes in two forms that are important to humans—vitamin D_2 (synthesized by plants) and D_3 (synthesized by humans in their skin). And even though both are considered to be vitamin D, vitamin D_3 is the more potent form.

Why are the essential vitamins necessary for our health?

The essential vitamins are "essential" for many reasons. The following chart lists the vitamin and its role in human health (*note*: For this text, this list contains the 13 most-mentioned essential vitamins in the health research literature; other research papers can list up to 15 or more):

Vitamin	Essential for Health
FAT-SOLUBLE VITAMINS	
Vitamin A	*Beta carotene, retinols*: Needed for growth and cell development; prevents night blindness; helps fight some cancers; helps the cardiovascular system; needed to maintain healthy gums, glands, bones, teeth, nails, skin, and hair; beta carotene is also considered to be an antioxidant
Vitamin D	*Calciferol*: Needed for calcium absorption, and helps build strong bones and teeth; helps the brain, pancreas, and reproductive organs; also targets the kidneys and intestines
Vitamin E	*Tocopherols, tocotrienols*: Tocopherols help maintain muscles and red blood cells; both are antioxidants
Vitamin K	Necessary for efficient blood clotting

Vitamin	Essential for Health
WATER-SOLUBLE VITAMINS	
Biotin	Needed for energy and metabolism
Folate	*Folic acid, folacin (some call this vitamin F; it is more often thought of as B_9)*: Necessary to make DNA, RNA, and red blood cells, and to synthesize certain amino acids
Niacin	*Vitamin B_3, nicotinic acid, nicotinamide*: Necessary to metabolize energy and to promote normal growth; for some people, larger doses often help lower cholesterol
Pantothenic acid	*Vitamin B_5*: Helps to metabolize energy; normalizes blood sugar levels, and helps the body to synthesize antibodies, some hormones, cholesterol, and hemoglobin (in the blood)
Riboflavin	*Vitamin B_2*: Necessary to metabolize energy and helps the body's adrenal function
Thiamine (thiamin)	*Vitamin B_1*: Necessary to metabolize energy; needed for proper nerve function, normal digestion, and appetite
Vitamin B_6	*Pyridoxine, pyridoxamine, pyridoxal*: Helps to metabolize proteins and carbohydrates (for energy) in the body; good for proper nerve function and helps synthesize red blood cells
Vitamin B_{12}	*Cyanocobalamin*: Necessary to make DNA, RNA, red blood cells, and myelin (for the body's nerve fibers)
Vitamin C	*Ascorbic acid*: Helps to build blood vessel walls and promote wound healing; necessary for iron absorption; and is said to help prevent arthrosclerosis; it is also considered to be an antioxidant

What are free radicals and antioxidants?

Because your body's cells burn fuel for energy, they burn oxygen as well. And because of this, when the oxygen is "burned," it releases molecules called free radicals. These free radicals are called "incomplete," and carry a negative charge (they carry at lease one extra electron), and travel around the body "seeking" cells with which they can react. The potential damage to tissues, DNA, and other substances in the body's cells occurs when an incomplete free radical oxygen grabs a hydrogen ion from a nearby molecule, which in turn seizes one from another structure. This potentially causes a damaging chain reaction that puts stress on the body's defense system. And although many of the body's cells will repair themselves, some will not.

Thus, the antioxidants that enter your system when you ingest various nutritious foods. When these antioxidants—or molecules with a positive charge—meet up with a negatively charged free radical, they neutralize it so the free radical can do little harm to the body—and prevent or stop the chain reaction. Overall, antioxidants help to prevent damage by carcinogens (cancer-causing, such as the ultraviolet radiation from the sun), tobacco smoke, and environmental pollutants. But there is one caveat: Because the body's ability to repair itself decreases as we age, most nutritionists recommend that older adults eat even more foods containing antioxidants. (For more details about free radicals and antioxidants, see the chapter "The Basics of Nutrition: Macronutrients and Nonnutrients.")

What are some micronutrient antioxidants?

There are several major micronutrient antioxidants that can help protect the human body from free radicals—in other words, the byproducts of oxidation—all of which protect us by blocking the chemical reactions that damage both tissues and cells. These antioxidants include what are often

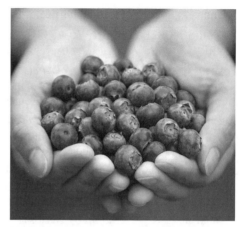

Blueberries are a great source of antioxidants.

called "the big three": vitamins C and E and beta carotene (which the body converts to vitamin A). All of them are easily ingested through food sources—for example, vitamin C by eating fresh fruits and vegetables, vitamin E by eating grains and seeds, and beta carotene by eating the more "colorful" vegetables and fruits, such as carrots, tomatoes (truly a fruit, not a vegetable), and dark leafy greens. Antioxidants are also tied to minerals—in particular, deficiencies of selenium, zinc, and copper can reduce antioxidant defenses—and even an excess of iron can encourage oxidation, thus increasing free radicals (for more about minerals, see below).

What is an ORAC score?

ORAC stands for Oxygen Radical Absorbance Capacity, a measurement of the total antioxidant power of certain foods and chemicals: the higher the number, the greater the antioxidant potential of the fruit, vegetable, or chemical; the lower the number, the less antioxidant potential. But more current research has shown that the ORAC scores are not reliable—and most nutritional sites no longer carry the information. (For more details about the ORAC score debate, see the chapter "Controversies with Food, Beverages, and Nutrition").

Why is beta carotene important to human health?

Vitamin A comes in several forms—including beta carotene, found only in plant foods, in a group called the carotenoids. When beta carotene (the most well-known food containing it being carrots) is ingested, the body converts the beta carotene to vitamin A. Overall, this carotenoid is one that helps the body's immune system by increasing the number of infection-fighting cells, and it is a powerful antioxidant that cleans up free radicals (in part responsible for accelerated aging). Beta carotene can also lower the risk for cardiovascular disease (it interferes with how fats and cholesterol oxidize in the bloodstream and form the plaque that often accompanies cardiovascular problems); pro-

What is the "nutrigenomic" effect of antioxidants?

Scientists are still debating how antioxidants are able to help keep us healthy. Overall, there are numerous types of these antioxidants found in whole plant foods as carotenes, such as in carrots, peppers, and squash, and in most plants as polyphenols, such as in berries, cocoa, onions, tea, beans, and whole grains. Some researchers now believe it may not be the direct result of the antioxidants that helps us, but an indirect effect: These compounds have what scientists call "nutrigenomic" influences—in other words, these antioxidants are able to help our gene switches and cellular signals that reduce levels of oxidation and inflammation in our bodies.

tects the body against cancer cells (by stimulating the body's immune cells to kill off cancer cells); and increases the production of T-cell lymphocytes and natural killer cells—both helpful cells that attack cancer cells in the body (for more about T-cells, see the chapter "Nutrition and Allergies, Illnesses, and Diseases").

Because too much vitamin A can be toxic to the body, most doctors recommend obtaining your beta carotene from foods, not supplements, thus allowing the body to "self-regulate" how much is converted to vitamin A. In this way, too, it is highly unlikely that a person could ingest a toxic amount of beta carotene—usually when the body has enough vitamin A, it stops making it.

What are some carotenoids?

It is estimated that there are more than 500 carotenoids, but only around 50 of them are actually converted into vitamin A. For example, alpha carotene is similar to beta carotene—it is one of many antioxidant carotenoids that is a precursor to vitamin A; it is found in vegetables such as carrots, pumpkins, and sweet potatoes, and in fruits such as apricots. Lutein is another carotenoid, and is found in brassicas, such as broccoli, Brussels sprouts, and cabbage.

What is a retinol?

Vitamin A comes in two forms in nature—the preformed vitamin A, and the precursor vitamin A, such as beta carotene. The preformed vitamin A groups are concentrated in animal tissues; it has already been metabolized from the carotene foods that the animal has eaten. For example, one of the richest natural sources is fish liver oil; others are milk, cheese, butter, eggs, and all meats. The term *retinol* (retinal or retinoic acid) is used to indicate the amount of usable vitamin A in a person's system—or the preformed vitamin A that has already been broken down and is now in the bloodstream—available for use by the body's many cells.

Can eating many carrots turn your skin yellow?

It depends on how many carrots you eat—but if you do eat large quantities of foods high in beta carotene (especially carrots), your skin can turn a bit yellow. This is not a harmful reaction (as long as you know it's definitely the beta carotene and not jaundice!); and it is totally reversible, although the time it takes to go away varies from person to person.

How much vitamin A is too much—or too little?

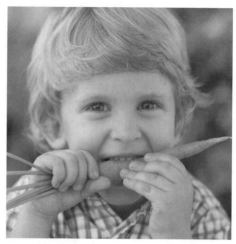

Carrots contain carotenoids, which help stave off heart disease and cancer.

There is such a thing as vitamin A toxicity—usually if a person takes over 10,000 international units (IU) of vitamin A (from supplements and/or food) per day. If more is ingested, toxic symptoms such as nausea, vomiting, headache, dizziness, muscle problems, and blurred vision may occur. In addition, if an excess amount of vitamin A is taken over a long period of time, it can increase the risk for liver problems and reduce the bones' mineral density (this is particularly important to older women who may be at risk for osteoporosis).

The average amount recommended for male adults is 3,000 IU of vitamin A per day, and for female adults, the recommended amount is 2,310 IU per day—numbers that are usually reached easily in the United States based on most people's diets. In contrast, especially in developing countries, vitamin A deficiency is common, often resulting in decreased vision, blindness, poor bone growth, and a depressed immune system. (For more about vitamin toxicity, see this chapter.)

Why is vitamin C important to human health?

Vitamin C (also called ascorbic acid) is probably the most well-known vitamin—mainly because of its connection to treating colds (thanks to Linus Pauling). It is known as one of the big three antioxidants; in addition, vitamin C is necessary to make and maintain collagen, the connective tissues that hold your body's cells together. It is also thought to lower the risk for certain cancers and heart disease, build teeth and bones, and even strengthen the walls of the body's blood vessels—from capillaries and veins to arteries.

Who was Linus Pauling?

American chemist Linus Carl Pauling (1901–1994) was a great proponent of ingesting vitamin C to treat the common cold; with his background in the study of chemical bonds and substances, he became interested in vitamins and micronutrients—especially in vitamin C. His most well-known book, with coauthor Ewan Cameron, is titled *Vitamin C and the Common Cold*.

Pauling was also involved in a plethora of other scientific works, including studying crystal structures and the properties of atoms; the structures of proteins, hemoglobin and related substances, and antibodies and the nature of serological reactions; and resonance phenomena in chemistry. He was also an inventor; for example, he helped develop an instrument for determining the partial pressure of oxygen in a gas. He received the Nobel Prize in Chemistry in 1954 for his "research into the nature of the chemical bond and its applications to the elucidation of the structure of complex substances"; and as an advocate of ending nuclear bomb testing and promoting peace (in 1958, he wrote the book *No More War!*), he was awarded the Nobel Peace Prize in 1962.

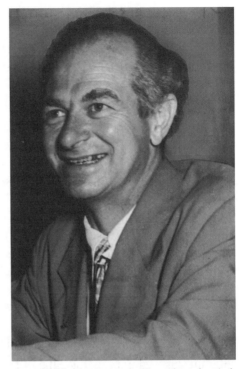

Linus Pauling, best known for his work on chemical bonds (he also won a Nobel Peace Prize), was an advocate for taking vitamin C supplements to treat the common cold.

Does vitamin C really prevent the common cold?

Since Linus Pauling and Ewan Cameron's book *Vitamin C and the Common Cold* came out, multiple studies have been conducted to test the vitamin's effectiveness. The consensus of opinion is that the vitamin does not stop a cold from striking us, but often helps to lessen its severity and shorten its duration.

Several recent studies have been conducted trying to discern the effects of vitamin C on colds and active people—but many of the studies are done on a small number of participants; thus, more research is needed. But some of the preliminary results are interesting: In one study, researchers found that people under heavy physical stress for short periods—such as soldiers during winter exercises or marathon runners—who took vitamin C seemed to halve their incidence of the common cold. Yet another study showed that adolescent male competitive swimmers taking vitamin C halved the duration of their colds—but the vitamin had no effect on female swimmers.

Does cooking a vitamin-C-rich vegetable destroy the vitamin?

Yes, if you cook vegetables rich in vitamin C, it can lower the levels of the vitamin—more so than other vitamins. The main reason is the vitamin itself: It is highly unstable and easily degrades through oxidation. For example, one study found that when tomatoes

11

were cooked at a temperature of 190.4 degrees Fahrenheit (88 degrees Celsius), vitamin C levels dropped by 10 percent after two minutes; after a half hour of cooking, the vitamin C levels dropped by 29 percent. (For more about cooking vegetables and nutrient retention, see the chapter "Food Chemistry and Nutrition.")

Why is vitamin D so important to human health?

Vitamin D is one of the more important vitamins for human health, as it plays a critical role in the body's use of calcium and phosphorus. For example, it increases the amount of calcium absorbed by the small intestines (which helps maintain strong bones). Vitamin D also helps the body's immune system; and it aids in the control of cellular growth, and thus is especially important for growing children.

Vitamin D is found in several forms, but two are important to humans: Vitamin D_2 (the synthetic form called ergocalciferol), usually obtained from supplements and fortified foods; and vitamin D_3 (called cholecalciferol). The latter type is produced when a certain cholesterol called 7-dehydrocholesterol forms in our intestines; from there, the sun's UVB (ultraviolet B) radiation converts the 7-dehydrocholesterol that reaches our skin's surface into cholecalciferol, or vitamin D_3.

How can humans get enough vitamin D?

Vitamin D is a vitamin that is difficult to get through foods alone because few are natural sources of the vitamin; but it can be found in fish-liver oils, in certain foods that are fortified with the vitamin (for example, vitamin D_2 is usually found in fortified milk products), and in supplements. Vitamin D (as vitamin D_3) also has a major natural source: When the sun's UVB rays shine on exposed parts of our bodies, they stimulate the cholesterol-like substance in the skin that makes vitamin D. Thus, for most of the general public, as little as 10 to 15 minutes of sunshine three times a week can produce sufficient vitamin D.

Do vitamin D levels change with the seasons?

Although most people can get their dose of vitamin D from the sun, there are exceptions. In one recent study, it was found that there is a correlation between the seasons and vitamin D levels—in particular, in the United States, vitamin D levels peak in August and bottom out in February (when the sun is not as high in the sky or as intense during the Northern Hemisphere's winter months). Thus, adults who have less exposure to the sun in the winter should probably have more vitamin D-fortified food (or in some cases, supplements); and because children need more vitamin D than adults—mainly because of their growing bones—being aware of their vitamin D intake is important during winter months.

What other factors influence a person's vitamin D levels?

Although the seasonal change in sunlight is one of the major reasons for fluctuations in a person's vitamin D levels, there are other reasons. For instance, wearing clothing that covers the arms and legs limits the sunlight that helps produce the body's vitamin D; and using sunscreen may affect vitamin D levels to a certain extent—although few people use enough sunscreen to block all of the UVB rays. Another influence is air quality: particles from the burning of wood, fossil fuels, and other industrial pollutants can scatter and/or absorb UVB rays in the atmosphere, thus limiting the amount of vitamin D our bodies can produce. And even our skin color can affect the absorption of sunlight. Because melanin—the substance in our skin that makes it darker or lighter—competes with the skin substance that produces vitamin D from UVB rays, most dark-skinned people will need more vitamin D than will light-skinned people.

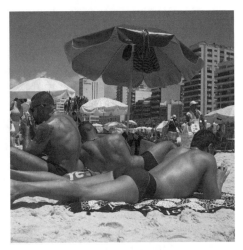

One way to get vitamin D is to get more sun exposure, but too much sun increases your likelihood of skin cancer.

But there are other reasons for changes in our vitamin D levels that have nothing to do with skin, clothing, melanin, or UVBs. For example, being overweight can affect vitamin D levels; body fat can "soak up" vitamin D, thus there may not be enough of the vitamin available to absorb. Age is also a factor in vitamin D levels, as research shows that older people are often less efficient vitamin D producers than younger people.

Who is at risk for vitamin D deficiencies?

In general, anyone who does not get enough sun—from people who live in areas with less sunshine in the winter to those who are housebound—can be vitamin D deficient. In addition, a person may need vitamin D if he or she has osteoporosis or a condition such as celiac disease (the disease can impair the body's ability to absorb fat soluble vitamins, such as vitamin D). But be careful not to take too much vitamin D—it can cause kidney damage, and toxic level symptoms can include confusion, nausea, and weakness.

What are the major members of the vitamin E family?

There are two major members of the vitamin E family—the tocopherols and the tocotrienols. They differ in their structure, but both function mostly as antioxidants that protect the body from free radicals. Vitamin E is made up of four tocopherols (alpha, beta, gamma, and delta) and four tocotrienols (alpha, beta, gamma, and delta). The tocopherols are found in such food sources as vegetable oil (soybean, corn, cottonseed, and safflower), fruits, vegetables, grains, nuts (almonds and hazelnuts), seeds (sunflowers), and fortified cereals; the tocotrienols are naturally found in certain vegetable oils, wheat germ, barley, and certain nuts and grains, although they are not found as much as tocopherols. In fact, because tocotrienols are not as readily found, there have been fewer studies done on this form of vitamin E.

Why is vitamin E so important to human health?

Vitamin E is considered to function as a powerful, nontoxic antioxidant because it has the ability to donate a hydrogen atom to a free radical in the body. In addition, it is thought that this vitamin contributes to a lower risk for heart disease, cancer, and several other diseases—especially if the vitamin is obtained from fruits, vegetables, and grains, and not supplements. Because it is often found in certain vegetable oils, people who excessively reduce their total dietary fat must be careful to get enough vitamin E from other food sources.

If your health-care provider recommends that you take a vitamin E supplement, remember that this vitamin is fat soluble. Thus, take the supplement with a meal, as it is best absorbed by the body when ingested with other foods. (As a supplement, vitamin E is most often found as d-alpha-tocopherol or d-alpha tocopheryl acetate.)

What is vitamin K and why is it such an important vitamin?

Not many people have heard about vitamin K, but research has determined that this vitamin is important to human health and nutrition. In particular, is it extremely necessary for proper blood clotting, and to help produce proteins needed for the blood, bones, and kidneys. For most people, a lack of vitamin K is not a problem—such a deficiency is rare, because certain bacteria most of us carry in our intestines make vitamin K for the body. In addition, it is easily digested and is found in green, leafy vegetables, such as kale, broccoli, cabbage, and spinach; and in certain vegetable oils, such as soybean, cottonseed, olive, and canola.

Can a person be deficient in vitamin K?

Yes, there are certain circumstances in which a person may have a deficiency in vitamin K, but it is rare. For example, newborn babies lack intestinal bacteria and are often given a vitamin K supplement during their first week of life. People who take anticoagulants, such as Coumadin (warfarin), or antibiotic drugs (because some intestinal bacteria are killed off, especially with the long-term use of antibiotics) may also have lower levels of vitamin K.

What are the B-complex vitamins?

Overall, to date, there are eight vitamins that make up the vitamin B complex: B_1 (thiamine or thiamin), B_2 (riboflavin), B_3 (niacin), B_5 (pantothenic acid), B_6 (pyridoxine, pyridoxal, pyridoxamine), B_9 (folate, folic acid, pteroylglutamic acid), B_{12} (cyanocobalamin), and biotin. The B-complex vitamins give the body energy by helping convert carbohydrates to glucose (the body burns glucose for energy) and helping metabolize fats and proteins; they are necessary for the nervous system to function (along with maintaining nerves) and they are important to the muscles that help food move along the gastrointestinal tract. They also help our skin, hair, eyes, mouth, and liver maintain good health.

Can B-complex vitamins be used to treat ailments?

Yes, the B-complex vitamins are essential to human health—and they also help to treat some human ailments. For example, they have been used to treat barbiturate overdose, alcoholic psychoses, and even drug-induced delirium. They have also been used to treat such ailments as migraine headaches; and some heart abnormalities have also responded to B-complex vitamins. These vitamins have also been used to improve the conditions of hypersensitive children who do not respond well to such drugs as Ritalin (methylphenidate); and it has even been shown to help some people with shingles. People also have been known to take B-complex vitamins when they are under stress; and for those who physically exert themselves more than most—such as people with more physical jobs—thiamine (B_1) and vitamin B_6 are known to help the body to recover faster.

Why do we need to eat plenty of foods with B-complex vitamins?

Because B-complex vitamins are water soluble, any excess is not stored in the body, but is excreted in the urine. Because of this, they must be continually replaced. Many drugs and other substances can interfere with the absorption of these vitamins; for example, some sleeping pills and sulfa drugs can cause a problem in the digestive tract, and actually destroy many of the B-complex vitamins. In addition, when you sweat, certain B vitamins are lost through perspiration. And long-term ingestion of large doses of B-complex vitamins can cause you to lose many of these vitamins through your urine.

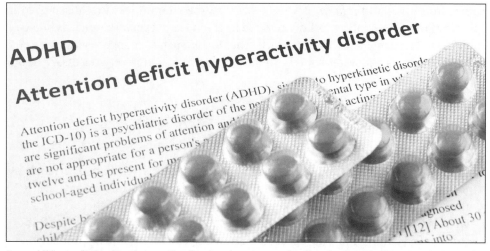

Some children suffering from hyperactive disorders do not respond well to the drug Ritalin; a vitamin B complex may help in such cases.

Since these vitamins are found in many foods, most healthy adults do not have to take B-complex vitamin supplements. In fact, recent research has shown that B vitamin supplementation—especially if the amount taken is over the Recommended Daily Allowance (RDA)—is probably not beneficial to your health. But, of course, if you cannot absorb enough of the vitamins in your system, supplementation of certain B vitamins is often suggested—but talk to your doctor about such measures.

What is important to remember when ingesting B-complex-rich foods?

Because they are so interrelated in function, if possible, B-complex vitamins should be ingested together—which is why most doctors recommend that you try to eat foods that contain the complete B complex rather than just foods that have a single B vitamin. You can find B complex vitamins in brewer's yeast, green vegetables, liver, whole grains, and other sources. And although supplements are available, they are synthetic—and obtaining the vitamins from foods makes it easier for your body to absorb them. But again, if you have to take supplements for health reasons, remember that many B vitamins taken singly are not as effective as a supplement that has the entire B complex of vitamins.

Why is biotin important to human health?

Biotin, one of the water-soluble vitamins and part of the B complex of vitamins, is found in many foods, including soybeans, egg yolks, beef, and yeast. It is also related to vitamins B_5, B_9, and B_{12}, all of which are needed for our bodies to metabolize carbohydrates, especially glucose, along with proteins and fats. Biotin is made by our intestines, so there are not many people who experience a deficiency in this vitamin.

Why is folic acid—or as some call it, vitamin F or B_9—so important to our health?

The name folic acid (also known as folate, folacin, or as some call it, vitamin F, or B_9) comes from the Latin *folium*, or "leaf," because the vitamin was first discovered in spinach leaves; in fact, it is most often found in green leafy vegetables, such as broccoli, spinach, and romaine lettuce (along with other foods, such as oranges, beans, rice, and liver). It is part of the water-soluble vitamin B complex, and is very necessary to our

What foods and drinks can interfere with the absorption of B-complex vitamins?

There are many foods and drinks that interfere with the absorption of certain B-complex vitamins. For example, eating excessive amounts of sugar will cause thiamine (B_1) depletion in the body (smoking will have the same effect). Some B vitamins are also destroyed by alcohol; in fact, alcohol can interfere with the absorption of all nutrients, but especially vitamins B_1 (thiamine) and B_2 (riboflavin).

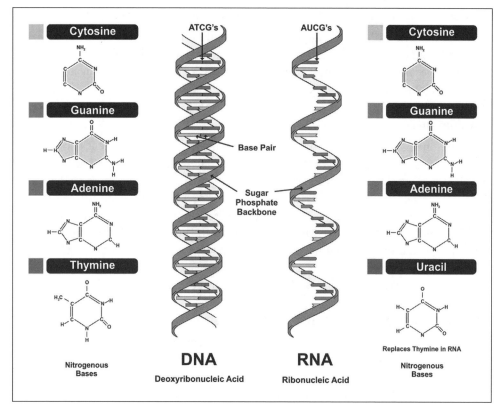

DNA and RNA are nucleic acids essential to life that are built on the molecules adenine, thymine, guanine, cytosine, and uracil.

overall health. For example, it is important to the body's cells, as the vitamin acts like a coenzyme (an organic molecule that helps enzymes function) that helps in the production of our body's nucleic acids, which carry our genetic characteristics: DNA, or deoxyribonucleic acid, and RNA, or ribonucleic acid. Folic acid is also necessary for the formation of red blood cells and for proper brain function; acts as a coenzyme along with vitamins B_{12} and C to break down and use proteins in the body; and, in a fetus, is important in forming the spinal bones.

What is the difference between DNA and RNA?

DNA and RNA are nucleic acids formed from a repetition of the simple building blocks of life called nucleotides—a combination of phosphate, sugar, and a nitrogen base (there are five types: adenine [A], thymine [T], guanine [G], cytosine [C], and uracil [U]). The DNA molecule is a double helix structure made from two chains of nucleotides linked between the bases; RNA consists of a single chain instead of a double. There are other differences, but in general, both are extremely necessary to our cells for reproduction—and for all of our life processes!

What are some health concerns associated with folic acid (folate)?

Most research shows that folic acid, or folate, should not be taken in large doses, as it may inhibit zinc absorption. Contrarily, certain people are more prone to folate deficiencies; for example, alcoholics usually have less folate, and the elderly may be deficient because of a poor diet or certain drug interactions.

How does niacin help our health?

Niacin (B_3) helps our health in many ways—and like many of the other B-complex vitamins, it helps assist the body's enzymes in the breakdown and use of proteins, fats, and carbohydrates. It also helps in the synthesis of fatty acids, DNA, and protein. Niacin is more stable than the B-complex vitamins thiamine or riboflavin—and it is very resistant to heat, light, and air, and is usually not affected by acid or basic liquids. The body actually makes niacin from protein (specifically from the amino acid tryptophan), but you can also ingest small amounts from certain foods, such as lean meats, poultry, fish, and peanuts. The synthetic forms of niacin include niacinamide, nicotinic acid (which is the one most used for its cholesterol-lowering properties), and nicotinamide.

Is it possible to lower cholesterol by taking niacin?

Yes, niacin (B_3, as nicotinic acid) has been used by some doctors to lower a patient's cholesterol—and even to improve circulation. But high doses are usually needed to lower cholesterol, so it must be done under medical supervision, with frequent blood checks for liver damage and high blood sugar. If you do take niacin, it can often lead to a flushing of the face, neck, and arms, although there are now time-released pills that lessen these effects.

Why is pantothenic acid necessary for our health?

Pantothenic acid (B_5) is from the Greek for "widespread," as it is found in almost all plant and animal foods. In fact, it is found in most (if not all) living organisms—including yeasts, molds, bacteria, and the individual cells of all animals and plants. Common food sources of pantothenic acid are organ meats, brewer's yeast, egg yolks, and whole-grain cereals.

The vitamin plays an important part in our cells' metabolism and acts like most of the other B-complex vitamins, as a coenzyme to help release energy from carbohydrates, fats, and proteins. It has many other claims, too—some of them still debated—such as boosting energy, improving athletic ability, speeding up wound healing, preventing loss and graying of hair, retarding aging, and even helping us to manage stress.

Why is vitamin B_2, or riboflavin, mentioned so often in the health literature?

Many of us have heard of riboflavin, particularly in terms of helping our health—from our eyes to our metabolism. For example, some research has shown that large amounts of riboflavin may help prevent cataracts from forming. In particular, the connection is

What are some interesting characteristics of riboflavin?

Riboflavin has some interesting characteristics. For example, it is stable when heated, oxidized, or even in an acid, but it will disintegrate in the presence of a basic solution or light (especially ultraviolet—UV—light). This is one reason why milk should not be stored in clear bottles, as light can destroy the riboflavin within only a few hours; but cooking a food that contains riboflavin does not destroy the vitamin. In fact, because you can get most of your needed riboflavin from a variety of foods, you probably don't need to take riboflavin as a supplement.

with antioxidants: the body uses riboflavin to manufacture glutathione, an antioxidant that attacks free radicals. If you don't have enough riboflavin in your diet, the free radicals have more time to cause damage to your eyes. Another possibility is oily skin: often people who are slightly deficient in riboflavin can have oily skin or hair (although there are also other reasons for this condition).

Why is thiamine (or thiamin) considered good for our health?

Thiamine, or thiamin or B_1, is found in both animal and plant sources. It acts as a coenzyme when glucose (blood sugar) is converted into energy. It is also vital to our metabolism, heart, and nervous systems; it stabilizes our appetites by allowing our bodies to assimilate and digest food better; and aids in the maintenance of red blood cells. Your body usually absorbs just the right amount of thiamine it needs—as long as you are ingesting enough thiamine-rich foods. It is also often called the "morale vitamin," as it has a healthy effect on our mental attitude.

What are some symptoms of thiamine deficiency?

There are many health problems connected to a thiamine deficiency. One of the more famous ones was recognized in the 1800s: An extreme deficiency of thiamine was to blame for the disease known as beriberi (for more about the discovery of beriberi's cause, see this chapter).

Today, milder deficiencies are found in people who get most of their "nutrients" from sugar or alcohol; in fact, some of the symptoms of thiamine deficiency mimic intoxication—from loss of coordination to a staggered walk and confusion. Some of the first signs of a mild deficiency are fatigue, loss of appetite, irritability, mental instability, and difficulty concentrating, which is why this deficiency is difficult to diagnose, as the symptoms often mimic so many other diseases. The more extreme deficiencies usually affect alcoholics, and people who are malnourished, especially the elderly or homeless. Such deficiencies can lead to problems with alertness, can damage the heart, and can cause confusion and loss of memory (which is why some recent research includes thiamine in relation to Alzheimer's disease).

Why is vitamin B_6 important to our health?

Vitamin B_6 (pyridoxine, pyridoxal, or pyridoxamine) has often been referred to as "the sleeping giant of vitamins"—mainly because it has not been mentioned as much in the health literature until recently. This vitamin needs to be taken daily with other B-complex vitamins because it is excreted in the urine within 8 hours of ingesting (it is not stored in the liver and can be found exclusively in the muscles). The best food sources are meats and whole grains.

Although it passes through our system relatively fast, this vitamin is still extremely important to our health. For example, like most B-complex vitamins, it acts as a coenzyme that is necessary for protein metabolism; it is often called a "woman's vitamin," as it is said to help many PMS (premenstrual syndrome) symptoms; it is responsible for the proper functioning of more than sixty enzymes,

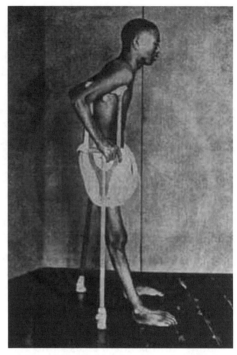

A U.S. government photo from the early twentieth century shows a Southeast Asia victim of beriberi, which is caused by a deficiency in thiamine.

and is necessary for normal DNA, RNA, and amino acid synthesis; it helps maintain our body's balance of sodium and potassium; it helps our nervous and immune systems to function; it aids in the manufacture of red blood cells; and it is necessary for the absorption of another B-complex vitamin—vitamin B_{12}.

Why is vitamin B_{12} necessary to our health?

Vitamin B_{12} is familiar to most of us—especially since it has been said to energize people who are under stress, fatigued, or recovering from an illness. It is also a vitamin containing an essential mineral element; in fact, it was the first cobalt-containing (a mineral) substance found to be essential for longevity. It also has a myriad of other functions, including the usual for a B-complex vitamin—for protein, fat, and carbohydrate metabolism; it helps iron function better in the body; aids in the growth and division of cells; helps folic acid to synthesize choline (for more about choline, see below); and aids in the production of the nucleic acids DNA and RNA, red blood cells, and even myelin, the fatty sheath that surrounds our nerve fibers.

The liver stores our extra vitamin B_{12} and the body has a recycling process for the vitamin; overall, it takes years to develop a deficiency once an adult stops taking the nutrient, but less time if the intake has been very low. But vitamin B_{12} is necessary for unborn ba-

What is choline and why is it important to our health?

Choline is not truly a vitamin, but in the latter part of the twentieth century, it was classified as an essential nutrient by the National Academy of Sciences. It was once thought that our bodies made enough of this nutrient, but research eventually revealed that our bodies needed to ingest additional choline, as it is important for fat metabolism and needed for healthy nerve function. It is also a precursor to acetylcholine, a brain neurotransmitter involved in memory, and is found most often in eggs, legumes, nuts, meats, and dairy products.

bies and infants—which is why this vitamin is also essential for pregnant and breastfeeding women—and for growing children; it is needed for physical and mental development.

How do you obtain vitamin B_{12}?

Substantial amounts of vitamin B_{12} are found in animal proteins, including liver (the best source), kidney, muscle meats, fish, and dairy products. It cannot be made synthetically, but must be grown (similar to penicillin) in bacteria or molds to use in supplements and fortified foods. This is why doctors often recommend that vegans (people who do not eat any animal products (including meat, dairy, and eggs) or those whose intestinal tract cannot absorb the vitamin (such absorption often declines with age) take supplements to obtain the vitamin, or eat foods fortified with B_{12}, such as most soy (not fermented) and rice products, some plant-based "meat" products, and cereals. (*Note*: Contrary to common knowledge, lacto-ovo vegetarians, those who eat milk, yogurt, cheese, and eggs, probably get enough vitamin B_{12}; ovo vegetarians, who eat eggs but not dairy products, also get vitamin B_{12}.)

What are some non-B vitamins often mistaken for B vitamins?

There are three compounds that are often mistaken for B vitamins: inositol, choline (this also gives lecithin part of its structure; see above for more about choline), and lipoic acid. Although they are not essential B-complex vitamins, they are useful coenzymes, or organic molecules that help enzymes function and help the body's metabolism. They are found in many foods, from beans to broccoli. In addition, substances such as para-aminobenzoic acid (PABA), bioflavonoids (for more about bioflavonoids, see this chapter), and ubiquinone are often mistaken for essential B nutrients.

There are also several B vitamins in the literature that are not the "true" B vitamins. One is called vitamin B_{15} (pangamic acid); according to some research, the chemical structure and the nature of this substance has not truly been determined, even though it has been promoted as a dietary supplement and a drug in the popular literature. In fact, no one has established its nutritional properties or even identified what happens if the body has a deficiency of this so-called vitamin—thus, most researchers believe that,

21

as a vitamin, it really doesn't exist. There is also B_{17} (laetrile), a chemically modified form of amygdalin, a naturally occurring substance that is found in almonds and peach and apricot kernels. But as to the claims of laetrile as a vitamin, there are none; in addition, although many claim that this substance is an alternative treatment for cancer (it was especially popular in the United States in the 1950s to 1970s), clinical trials showed it had no anticancer effect. Another nonvitamin is B_T—called carnitine (it was called vitamin B_T in the 1950s)—is derived from an amino acid and found in almost all of the body's cells, and plays a significant role in our energy production. It is considered the generic name for a number of compounds, including L-carnitine and acetyl-L-carnitine. In fact, healthy children and adults do not need to get carnitine from food or supplements because our liver and kidneys produce enough from the amino acids lysine and methionine to meet our daily needs.

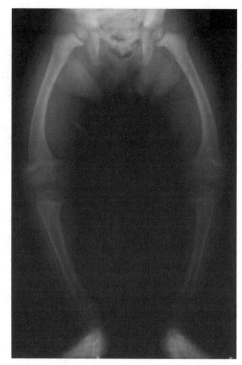

An X-ray of a young patient with rickets shows how the disease damages bones when one doesn't have enough vitamin D.

What are symptoms of deficiencies of the essential vitamins?

There are many symptoms if you are deficient in some of the essential vitamins. The following chart lists the vitamin and the symptoms if a human body lacks the vitamin (in alphabetical order):

Symptoms That Occur Because of Vitamin Deficiencies

Vitamin	Symptoms If the Body Is Deficient
FAT-SOLUBLE VITAMINS	
Vitamin A	*Beta carotene, retinols*: Night blindness; susceptibility to infections; dry skin and eyes; often stunted growth in children who are deficient
Vitamin D	*Calciferol*: Can lead to rickets in children who are deficient; lack of vitamin D can weaken bones
Vitamin E	*Tocopherols, tocotrienols*: Both rare; deficiencies of tocopherols usually only occur in premature infants and those unable to absorb fats; effects not as well known for tocotrienols
Vitamin K	Without sufficient amounts, hemorrhaging can occur; may interfere with anticlotting drugs

Symptoms That Occur Because of Vitamin Deficiencies

Vitamin	Symptoms If the Body Is Deficient
WATER-SOLUBLE VITAMINS	
Biotin	Because it is found in a wide variety of foods, there seem to be few people with deficiencies; lack of biotin mainly affects the skin and hair, including baldness, dermatitis, and grayish skin
Folate	*Folic acid, folacin, B₉*: Deficiencies result in poor growth, graying hair, gastrointestinal tract disturbances (because of inadequate dietary intake), anemia, and abnormal red blood cells
Niacin	*Vitamin B₃, nicotinic acid, nicotinamide*: Many symptoms mimic other diseases, the most common initially being muscle weakness, general fatigue, indigestion and lack of appetite, and skin eruptions; later it may lead to recurring headaches, mouth sores, diarrhea, insomnia, irritability, and deep depression—which is why a deficiency is often difficult to detect
Pantothenic acid	*Vitamin B₅*: Rare; detection of deficiencies is difficult, but some may include the slowing of metabolic processes, vomiting, restlessness, abdominal pains, burning feet, low blood sugar, skin disorders, and upper respiratory infections
Riboflavin	*Vitamin B₂*: Most symptoms are in the skin and mucous membranes, including sores or cracks in the nose and mouth, red, sore tongue, sensitivity to light, and eye fatigue
Thiamine	*Vitamin B₁*: Rare; deficiency often mimics intoxication; also mood swings and loss of appetite (for more, see above)
Vitamin B₆	*Pyridoxine, pyridoxamine, pyridoxal*: Results in low blood sugar and low glucose tolerance, and thus, a sensitivity to insulin in the blood; also loss of hair, weight loss, depression, numbness in arms and legs, slow learning, and many more symptoms
Vitamin B₁₂	*Cyanocobalamins* Nerve problems and weakness; impairs the growth of red blood cells in the bone marrow; changes in the nervous system, such as weakness in arms and legs and a diminished reflex response
Vitamin C	*Ascorbic acid*: Low levels cause scurvy, and some research indicates low vitamin C levels may increase the risk for developing asthma

What are the bioflavonoids, often called "vitamin P"?

Bioflavonoids, or flavonoids, are often called "vitamin P," but in reality, they do not follow the true definition of a vitamin; they actually act more like an antioxidant. They are water soluble, and are companions to vitamin C (they were discovered about the same time). There are at least 500 naturally occurring varieties of bioflavonoids, which give color to fruits, flowers, leaves, and stems of plants. (For more details about bioflavonoids [flavonoids], see the chapter "The Basics of Nutrition: Macronutrients and Non-nutrients.")

Are some vitamins toxic to humans?

As with many things, moderation is the key when it comes to vitamins—whether you are taking supplements, eating fortified foods, or even ingesting certain foods with more of a specific vitamin (for example, beta carotene in carrots)—because too much of a certain vitamin may be toxic to humans. For example, there is a condition called hypervitaminosis, in which too much of certain vitamin supplements are ingested—and thus harms a person's health. This occurred in the late twentieth century, when some studies indicated an epidemic of hypervitaminosis D in children following the excessive fortification of vitamin D in milk (such is not the case now).

In another study, it was shown that hypervitaminosis D in adults was most often caused by megadoses of vitamin D supplements—in which many people took 50,000 international units (IUs) per day of vitamin D for several months, most often based on erroneous information from certain advertisements. (The recommended daily allowance [RDA] for most adults is 400 to 600 IU of vitamin D a day, with higher amounts to treat certain medical conditions under a doctor's care). The main consequence of hypervitaminosis D is a buildup of calcium in the blood (called hypercalcemia) that causes such symptoms as a poor appetite, nausea, and even vomiting, along with possible kidney or liver problems.

MINERALS

What are minerals?

In general, mineral content in organisms is determined by all the elements that remain as ash when animal or plant tissues are burned. For humans, minerals make up about three to five percent of a person's (male and female) average body weight.

How are minerals divided?

Minerals for human health are divided based on their daily dietary requirement—generally classified as macrominerals, trace (or micro) minerals, and electrolytes. The macrominerals include calcium, phosphorus, and magnesium; they are called macrominerals because you not only need these minerals, but you can also store larger amounts of them in your body. Trace minerals include iron, fluoride, manganese, iodine, selenium, zinc, molybdenum, chromium, and copper; they are called trace because your body needs only a small amount of these minerals—and they are stored in extremely small quantities in your system. Finally, the electrolytes are involved in generating electric impulses to transport nerve messages, and to maintain the proper balance of fluids and body chemicals in your body; they in-

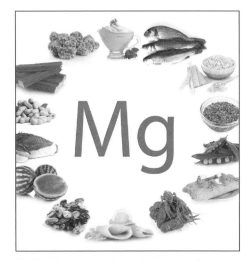

Foods high in magnesium include nuts and seeds, dark leafy greens, fish, beans and lentils, avocados, whole grains, dried fruit, low-fat dairy products, bananas, and dark chocolate.

clude sodium, potassium, chloride, and in some texts, bicarbonate is included. Overall, all of these minerals are necessary for a body to stay healthy—and because our bodies can't generate them, we must obtain these minerals from our food.

What are the most necessary minerals for our health?

The body needs a good amount of minerals—a combination of macrominerals, trace minerals, and electrolytes. The following chart lists these major minerals (not all are listed) and their role in human health:

Essential Minerals

Mineral	Essential for Health
MACROMINERALS	
Calcium	Best for building bones and teeth, and vital to muscle and nerve function; helps in blood clotting, and helps to maintain stable blood pressure
Magnesium	Helps to stimulate bone growth; helps with metabolism and the functioning of muscles
Phosphorus	Found in some body enzymes; helps bones and teeth to be strong; necessary for metabolism
TRACE MINERALS (OR MICROMINERALS)	
Chromium	Helps insulin to metabolize glucose in the body
Copper	Needed for iron absorption in the body; helps with connective tissues, nerve fibers, and red blood cells, along with being a component of several of the body's enzymes
Fluoride	Helps the body maintain strong bones and teeth
Iodine	Helps the body make thyroid hormones
Iron	Necessary to produce hemoglobin, the way the body transports oxygen
Manganese	Necessary for metabolism since it is a component of many body enzymes; helps in the formation of bones and tendons
Molybdenum	Necessary for the storage of iron in the body; necessary for metabolism because it is a component of many body enzymes
Selenium	Works with vitamin E to protect cell membranes from oxidation
Zinc	Helps certain enzymes in metabolism; necessary for growth and reproduction, along with supporting the body's immune system
ELECTROLYTES	
Chloride	Helps to keep our body's chemistry stable; used to make our digestive juices; seawater has almost the same concentration of chloride ion as human body fluids
Potassium	Necessary to maintain our body's fluid balance; helps our metabolism and muscle function
Sodium	Along with potassium, it helps to maintain the body's fluid balance; it also helps with muscle function
Bicarbonate	Listed in some research as an electrolyte; acts as a buffer to maintain the body's normal levels of acidity in the blood and other fluids

How do macrominerals affect humans?

Of the 3 to 5 percent of minerals in the average human body, macrominerals make up the majority—calcium, magnesium, and phosphorus. Most of the macrominerals are stored in the bones, but they also circulate in the blood. And similar to vitamins, the best sources of macrominerals for the human body are natural—in other words, ingest foods and not supplements if possible.

What are the best food sources for the major minerals?

There are many good food sources of minerals. The following chart lists the best foods to eat—the natural way to give our body the major minerals it needs (not all are listed):

Food Sources for Essential Minerals

Mineral	Best Food Sources
MACROMINERALS	
Calcium	Milk and milk products; fortified drinks, such as soy; canned sardines and salmon, with bones; some dark green vegetables; tofu and some tofu products
Magnesium	Many leafy green vegetables; whole grain products, such as bread and cereals; poultry, fish, eggs, nuts, and milk
Phosphorus	Found in most meats, fish, egg yolks, legumes, and dairy products; also found in soft drinks
TRACE MINERALS (OR MICROMINERALS)	
Chromium	Whole grain products and brewer's yeast; liver and chicken; cheese; mushrooms; molasses
Copper	Mainly from liver and shellfish; legumes and nuts; prunes
Fluoride	Mostly from fluorinated water; found in some teas
Iodine	Mostly from iodized salt, seafood, and foods grown in iodine-rich soils
Iron	From many sources, such as liver, meat, and seafoods; eggs; legumes, leafy greens, and dried fruits; whole grains, nuts, and seeds; some fortified cereals or other products
Manganese	Some teas; nuts, legumes, whole grains, and bran; leafy greens; egg yolks
Molybdenum	Liver and other organ meats; whole grain products, nuts, legumes; dark green leafy vegetables
Selenium	Brazil and other nuts; poultry, seafood, and organ meats; whole grain products, nuts, and brown rice; onions, garlic, and mushrooms
Zinc	Oysters and certain meats; yogurt and milk; eggs; wheat germ and nuts
ELECTROLYTES	
Chloride	Table salt; seafood and some meats; milk; eggs
Potassium	Avocados, bananas, citrus and dried fruits; whole grain products; legumes and many vegetables
Sodium	Table salt; seafood; some seasonings and dairy products; almost all processed foods
Bicarbonate	Can help balance electrolytes in the body

Why is calcium important for human health?

Calcium is one of the most important macrominerals for human health. Not only is it the most abundant mineral in the body, but it is the fifth most abundant substance in the Earth's crust. To break it down, about 99 percent of your body's calcium is deposited in the bones and teeth (the calcium in the bones is in constant flux depending on your diet or body's needs); the remaining 1 percent is found in the soft tissues, intracellular fluids, and blood. In the average adult male, overall calcium weighs about 2.16 to 2.78 pounds (980 to 1,260 grams); for the average adult female, it weighs about 1.68 to 1.98 pounds (760 to 900 grams).

What are some of the tasks calcium has in the human body?

Calcium has many tasks in the human body. For example, calcium is necessary for the development and maintenance of bone structure (and its rigidity), it helps in the blood's clotting process, it aids nerve transmission (and the connected muscle stimulation), it helps the parathyroid hormone to function, and it helps to metabolize vitamin D, to name a few of its functions.

What are the best natural sources of calcium?

Some of the best calcium sources are milk, cheese, yogurt, and other dairy products, and are good choices for those who can tolerate lactose. Calcium can also be found in fortified

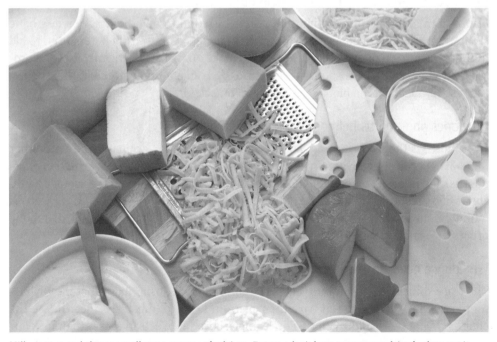

Milk, yogurt, and cheese are all great sources of calcium. But you don't have to consume dairy foods to get it; many vegetables and fruits also contain calcium.

soy, rice, and almond drinks; tofu and other soybean products; canned sardines and salmon (if you eat the bones); and a variety of vegetables and fruits, such as broccoli. As with all nutrients, there are exceptions: for example, for postmenopausal women who are at risk for developing osteoporosis, and certain others who cannot ingest milk or soy products, supplements may be the best way to obtain calcium. Check with your doctor to identify sources of calcium—ones that your body can best absorb for your special circumstance.

What can interfere with the absorption of calcium?

Researchers know that vitamins A, C, and D—along with phosphorus, if it does not exceed the amount of calcium—help to aid in calcium absorption in the human body. But there are numerous ways in which the absorption of calcium in the body is affected. For example, certain oxalates found in vegetables such as spinach and beets can interfere with calcium absorption in the body. In addition, if you eat excessive amounts of foods containing fat, protein, or sugar, all three can combine with calcium—creating an insoluble compound that the body can't absorb. And if you ingest too much phosphorus or manganese can hinder the absorption of calcium. In fact, too little calcium and too much phosphorus in the American diet is well documented—especially when many typical diets include soda, diet soda, and processed foods (like luncheon meats and cheese)—which may be why many people in the United States are calcium deficient. (For more about calcium and disease, see the chapter "Nutrition and Allergies, Illnesses, and Diseases.")

How does the mineral magnesium help our health?

Magnesium, like calcium and phosphorus, is essential to help build the body's bone strength; it is also needed for muscle function, metabolism (mostly for energy), to aid in the transmission of nerve impulses, and to make our cells' genetic material and proteins. Average adults have about 60 percent of their magnesium stored in their bones; the rest circulates in the blood or is stored in muscle tissue.

How does phosphorus help our bodies remain healthy?

Phosphorus is the second most plentiful mineral in the body—and it works with other minerals, specifically calcium (in fact, many foods high in calcium are also high in phosphorus) and fluoride, to maintain healthy, strong bones and teeth. In the average adult, about 85 percent of the mineral is found in the bones, while the other 15 percent is found in the body's soft tissues. It is also necessary for many of our metabolic processes—and especially helps in the storage and release of energy.

Why do we need trace minerals for our health?

The trace minerals—chromium, copper, fluoride, iodine, iron, manganese, molybdenum, selenium, and zinc—all have their place in terms of our body's health (see the chart above for more information). For example, chromium acts like a key to unlock our insulin—and without it, insulin would have a difficult time controlling our blood sugar; it is also helps to build proteins. Copper is needed to make red blood cells, skin pigment, connective tissues, and even nerve fibers—not to mention, it helps the body to absorb iron. And iron is necessary for the pigment (color) in our blood—specifically the red blood cells that carry oxygen throughout our entire body.

Why is chromium deficiency often found in the United States?

Chromium is an important trace mineral because it helps regulate blood sugar levels—in other words, it is important in carbohydrate metabolism that helps fuel the body. It is thought that chromium deficiencies are found more often in the United States than in other regions because of the soil—it does not contain an adequate supply of the mineral, and therefore cannot be absorbed by the foods we grow. Americans also eat a great deal of processed foods, sugar, and other refined carbohydrates—all of which lead to chromium loss. In addition, the most vulnerable groups for chromium deficiency include the elderly, people who are engaged in regular strenuous activities (such as runners), and women who are pregnant (mainly because the fetus uses so much chromium).

What trace mineral was once thought to help build muscle and burn fat?

As with many food and nutrition ideas over the years, some nutrition "trends" are simply inaccurate. For example, in the late twentieth century, it was thought that the trace mineral chromium would help people with their diets and to build muscle tissue at the same time. Thus many people turned to a chromium supplement sold as "chromium picolinate," which claimed to bulk up muscles while reducing body fat. Researchers have yet to find such a connection when it comes to weight loss; but that being said, the jury is still out when it comes to chromium's effect on our muscles.

Does the body really need copper?

Copper is considered an essential trace mineral for many reasons, especially its involvement in the synthesis of hemoglobin—the part of our blood that carries oxygen throughout the body. It is also considered one of the most important blood antioxidants and helps cell membranes remain healthy. It is also present in many enzymes that break down or build up body tissue; aids in the conversion of the amino acid tyrosine into a dark pigment (called melanin) that helps to color our hair and skin; and helps in the synthesis of phospholipids—substances needed to form the protective covers around our nerve fibers.

Why do we need fluoride?

Fluoride is the active form of fluorine, but it is not as "needed" in our diet as many of the other trace minerals. Most of us know about fluoride as the substance that helps prevent cavities, but it is also thought to be helpful in maintaining strong bones (by increasing the deposition of calcium). There are two types of fluorides: sodium fluoride, which is added to drinking water, and calcium fluoride, which is found in nature. (For more about the controversy concerning fluoride and drinking water, see the chapter "Controversies with Food, Beverages, and Nutrition.")

What trace mineral has only one known function in humans?

There is one trace mineral that has only one known function in humans: iodine is essential to make thyroid hormones. A deficiency can result in overgrown thyroid glands, or goiter, and sometimes can lead to hypothyroidism, or a low output of the thyroid hormone, that can cause weight gain, being cold most of the time, and a sluggish metabolism.

What is iron-deficiency anemia?

Iron-deficiency anemia is also called hypochromic anemia. It occurs when the amount of hemoglobin in the red blood cells is reduced—and as a result, the cells become smaller. Because of this, the oxygen-carrying capacity of the blood is reduced. Those at risk are usually women of child-bearing years (especially pregnant or lactating), older infants, children, and people with certain dietary restrictions, such as diabetics, the elderly, low-income people, and minorities; it is also estimated that one in four college women is deficient in iron—from both menstruation and an inadequate diet while in school. (For more about iron-deficiency anemia, see "Nutrition in Allergies, Illnesses, and Diseases.")

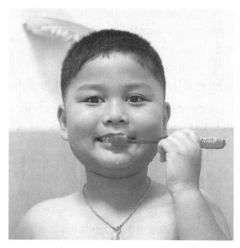

Since fluoride was added to our toothpaste and water supply, cavity rates have dropped in the United States.

Do we recycle iron in our systems?

It may sound funny, but yes: When the body breaks down old red blood cells, it actually recycles the iron. Thus, a healthy adult male will lose about 0.00003 ounce (1 milligram) of iron a day; for a healthy adult female who is still menstruating, the loss is about 0.000045 ounces (1.5 milligrams) per day. This is not enough to cause concern to a healthy adult who eats a balanced diet—especially foods that contain sufficient iron for that person's size, height, and age. But there are exceptions: menstruating and pregnant women, infants and preschool children, some athletes, people with certain dietary restrictions, or people with certain illnesses (or even taking medications) that may restrict the absorption of the mineral often have iron deficiencies.

Why do we need to eat foods with manganese and molybdenum?

There is a reason for needing the trace minerals manganese and molybdenum in our diet—especially because they are components of many enzymes in our body. In addition, manganese (also thought of as an antioxidant) is important to our metabolism and is needed to build strong bones and tendons. Molybdenum helps to regulate our iron storage, and aids in the production of our urine. Traces of molybdenum are found in almost all plant and animal tissues, but it is rare on Earth itself—and it is often lost in foods that are refined and processed.

Why is selenium so necessary to our bodies?

Selenium is an essential mineral; it is also thought of as an antioxidant, as it interacts with vitamin E to prevent free radicals. (For more about antioxidants, see this chapter and the chapter "The Basics of Nutrition: Macronutrients and Non-nutrients.") Research also indicates that selenium can help prevent many diseases, such as cancer, stroke, cirrhosis, arthritis, and emphysema by boosting the immune system. Overall, our liver, heart, spleen, and kidneys contain around five times as much selenium as in our muscles and other tissues. Other research also indicates that selenium may help relieve arthritis, help prevent cataracts, and even protect against alcoholic liver disease.

Do we need electrolytes for our health?

Yes, the body does need electrolytes—as they are essential to our nerve and muscle function, and also help to maintain the proper balance of our body's fluids. Chemically, they are substances that become ions in a (usually) liquid solution—and have the ability to conduct electricity. Most of us have heard of our body's "electrolyte balance," especially in terms of exercise. Some strenuous activities can cause the body to have an imbalance of electrolytes; for example, excessive sweating from extreme exercise can cause a deficiency in chloride. This is why many of the so-called "sport drinks" contain elements to help regain your electrolyte balance after strenuous exercise.

What is chloride?

Chloride (it is sometimes listed as chlorine) may be familiar to many of us as one part of the molecule that makes up table salt (sodium chloride), but it is also an important mineral to our bodies. In particular, it is necessary in the production of hydrochloric acid—the acid the stomach uses to digest what we eat (especially proteins and rough fibrous foods). It is also necessary for nerve conduction and helps regulate the acidic and basic (alkaline) balance (pH) of our blood (For more about pH, see this chapter.)

What is potassium?

Potassium, along with sodium, is a very necessary mineral that helps to regulate the body's balance of fluids. It is also necessary for our metabolism, helps in the

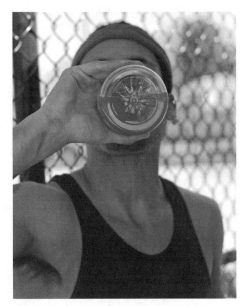

Sport drinks include minerals that are lost through perspiration from vigorous exercise. It isn't enough to just drink water.

transmission of nerve impulses, and is needed for muscle function. It also regulates the transfer of nutrients to the cells, and functions in the chemical reactions within the cells. It is important to our body's sugar levels—helping to convert glucose into glycogen so it can be stored in the liver. Potassium also helps stimulate the kidneys to eliminate our toxic body wastes—and even acts with sodium to help normalize our heartbeats.

What is the difference between salt and sodium?

Although sodium and salt are used interchangeably, they are two different terms. Table salt is sodium chloride, and there are other salts, such as sodium bicarbonate, whereas sodium is a chemical element. Sodium occurs naturally in our foods, and salt is the most common source of the sodium we consume.

What are the various types of salt?

There are many types of edible salt and all are nearly the same: sodium chloride, sometimes with natural minerals or added chemicals. Table salt is either extracted from rocks or produced from seawater in evaporation ponds; it comes in the form of iodized table salt, including a small amount of potassium iodide and dextrose (to stabilize the iodide; the iodine aids thyroid function), or plain table salt (including an anticaking agent like calcium silicate). Kosher salt is flaky and coarse; contrary to what most people think, it is not "saltier" than table salt, but dissolves faster on the tongue, which enhances its taste. Canning and pickling salts are fine grained and may contain anticaking agents (usually yellow prussiate of soda, or sodium ferrocyanide). Gourmet sea salts are course or fine, usually produced in evaporation ponds, and contain mostly sodium chloride, with about

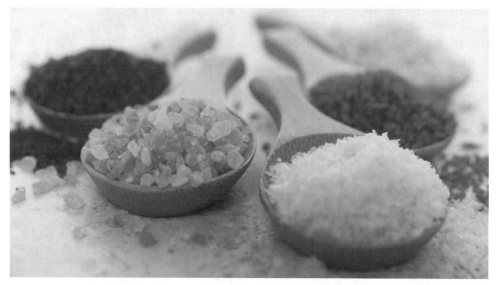

Some health food advocates suggest that sea salts (a variety are shown here) are better for you than regular iodized salts, but no research has thus far supported this position.

1 or 2 percent calcium and magnesium chlorides; they also come as grey salts, in which the unrefined salts still retain some of the natural clays and trace elements; and *fleur de sel* (French for "flower of salt") is from the smaller, more delicate crystals that are skimmed from the top of the evaporation ponds. There are also light salts (half-and-half blends of table salt and potassium chloride), seasoned salts (salts with various herbs and spices added), and salt substitutes (usually 100 percent potassium chloride).

Why is salt (sodium) good and bad for us?

Salt (and sodium, the element that joins with chlorine to form table salt) is good for us because it is needed for several critical functions: It helps us to maintain our blood pressure; keep our acidic and basic (alkaline) balance in our body's fluids; it can help our nerve cells transmit signals throughout the body (especially to the brain); it helps our muscles to move and function; and helps us to maintain the fluid balance in the body. But it can also be bad for us—causing fluid retention or even helping to raise blood pressure (although this is somewhat debated) if too much is ingested, especially if a person has a predisposition toward retaining fluids or has blood pressure problems.

Is sea salt better than table salt?

If you believe the media, you would think that table salts and sea salts were different, but in reality both contain sodium (as sodium chloride). Most sea salts come from dehydrating salts in areas near oceans or seas or from salt mines. Although sea salts may have more mineral content than regular table salt (which may include fillers to avoid clumping), the sodium content is similar. And to date, although many salt sellers want to convince you otherwise, there are no documented health advantages to sea salt.

What can cause sodium levels to fluctuate in the body?

Low sodium levels can be caused by many things, including starvation, vomiting, diarrhea, extreme sweating, or any condition that involves a great amount of water being lost

What is pH?

The term *pH* is a chemical term taken from the French phrase *l'puissance d'hydrogen*, meaning "the power of hydrogen." The pH is based on a scale that ranges from zero to fourteen, with a pH of 1 being very acidic, pH of 7 being neutral, and pH of 14 being very basic (alkaline). For example, battery acid has a pH of about 0; human stomach acid has a pH from 1 to 3; lemon juice has a pH of about 2.3; tomatoes, grapes, and bananas have a pH of 4.6; black coffee has a pH of about 5; urine is about a pH of 5 to 7; saliva has a pH between 6.2 to 7.4; our blood has a pH of around 7.3–7.5 (a bit alkaline); seawater has a pH of 7.8 to 8.3; and oven cleaner has a pH of about 13.

from the body. If there is a good deal of water loss and sodium remains, it can lead to what is called water intoxication, which can often lead to anorexia, apathy, and muscle twitches. In this case, the fluids need to be replaced before replacing sodium—because without liquids, the body cannot absorb the sodium. (For more about salt, see the chapter "Nutrition and You.")

Why is bicarbonate important to the body?

Overall, bicarbonates in our system help to maintain the pH of our blood and other fluids—or the balance between acidic and basic (for more about pH, see Sidebar). The kidneys and lungs usually help the body to maintain the pH—for instance, the kidneys remove bicarbonate from the blood if the pH is too high. But sometimes the levels can be affected by certain foods or medications. Thus, a doctor will often measure bicarbonate levels to determine if a patient has problems with acidity in the body.

What are symptoms of deficiencies of certain minerals?

There are several symptoms of macromineral, trace mineral, and electrolyte deficiencies. The following chart lists minerals (not all are listed) and their major deficiency symptom(s):

Symptoms Due to Mineral Deficiencies

Mineral	Result of Deficiency
MACROMINERALS	
Calcium	In children, rickets; in at-risk people, osteoporosis (brittle, porous bones); it may also indicate a lack of vitamin D, which helps the body to absorb calcium
Magnesium	Deficiency is rare, but can be depleted by alcoholism, long-term diarrhea, liver or kidney disease, and severe diabetes
Phosphorus	Lack of appetite, weight loss, or even obesity; it may cause irregular breathing, mental and physical fatigue, and nervous disorders
TRACE MINERALS (OR MICROMINERALS)	
Chromium	Even slight deficiencies can lead to problems with metabolizing glucose, and upset the function of the body's insulin levels
Copper	Although rare, deficiencies include low blood levels in children with edema or iron-deficiency anemia; in adults it may lead to general weakness, impaired respiration, and skin sores
Fluoride	Poor tooth development and dental caries
Iodine	Enlarged thyroid (goiter) and hypothyroidism (low secretion of thyroid hormones); can lead to hardening of the arteries, obesity, sluggish metabolism, dry hair, slow mental reactions, rapid pulse, heart palpitations, tremors, nervousness, and irritability
Iron	Most common is iron-deficiency anemia; can lead to constipation, brittle nails or ridges in nails, lethargy, apathy, pale pallor, reduced brain function, headaches, and heart enlargement; can cause some unusual food cravings (such as for ice, clay, and other nonfood items)

Symptoms Due to Mineral Deficiencies

Mineral	Result of Deficiency
Manganese	Mostly affects glucose tolerance, resulting in the inability to remove excess sugar from the blood by oxidation and/or storage, causing diabetes; can cause atherosclerosis; severe deficiencies can cause paralysis, convulsions, blindness, and deafness in infants; in adults, can cause dizziness, ear noises, and hearing loss
Molybdenum	Excessive deficiencies may cause fast heartbeat, increased rate of breathing, and visual problems
Selenium	May cause premature aging; major deficiencies may cause cataracts, liver necrosis, and growth retardation; low levels have been associated with several types of cancer, including bladder and colon cancers
Zinc	May show up in a diet high in grains and cereals and low in animal protein; it can cause retarded growth, delayed sexual maturity, and cause wounds to take longer to heal; it can cause brittle nails, and white spots on the nail may be a sign; it can also cause irregular menstrual cycles in teenaged girls and painful knee and hip joints in teens of both sexes
ELECTROLYTES	
Chloride	A deficiency can cause hair and tooth loss, poor muscular contractions, and impaired digestion; it also usually means there is a deficiency of sodium in the body
Potassium	An abnormal decrease (hypokalemia) or increase (hyperkalemia) affects the nervous system, and both can increase the chance for arrhythmias (irregular heartbeats); both can also affect the kidneys
Sodium	A major deficiency can cause intestinal gas, weight loss, poor memory, short attention span, difficulty in concentrating, muscles weakness, low blood sugar, and heart palpitations
Bicarbonate	Listed in most research as an electrolyte; difficult to determine in some cases, and deficiencies are often connected to other diseases, such as kidney disease, respiratory function, and metabolic conditions

What is pica?

Pica—from the Latin word for magpie, a kind of bird known to eat almost anything—is an eating disorder in which a person has an addictive craving for nonfood substances. (Other animals have been reported to have pica, too, including dogs and cats). A person with pica may eat nonfood substances, including dirt, clay, paint, fabrics, stones, and chalk. The term *geophagy*—or eating dirt or clay—is one of the most common forms of pica. To date, there is no test for pica, and a person is diagnosed with pica if he or she eats nonnormal items for one month or longer.

Many researchers believe pica is caused by a mineral-deficient diet, especially iron-deficiency anemia or a zinc deficiency. It also seems to occur in people with lower than normal nutrient levels and poor nutrition, even bordering on malnutrition; and there has even been thought to be a relationship between the ingestion of too much lead and pica. (This was a great concern in the late twentieth century, as many old houses con-

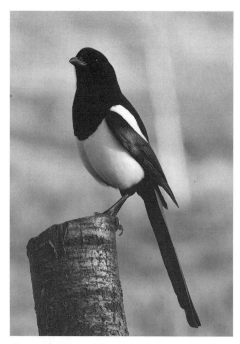
The word pica comes from the Latin word for magpie. Magpies are famous for eating just about anything, and pica is a disorder in which a sufferer can't help eating non-food items.

tained lead paint—and young children ingested lead via dirt, paper, and paint, often resulting in lead intoxication; for more about lead, see below.) But eating clay and chalk may not be because a person has a mineral deficiency—Native Americans make an acorn bread using clay, and certain stores in the southern United States used to sell particular types of chalky dirt for consumption.

Can some minor trace minerals be bad for our bodies?

Yes, there are minor trace minerals that can harm our overall health, either through ingestion or exposure to environmental pollutants. For example, aluminum is a trace mineral, but it can be dangerous (even fatal) if ingested in excessive amounts. It is known to weaken the living tissues of our alimentary canal (the "tube" that carries and digests our food from our mouths to our anuses); in particular, it binds to other substances that our body needs—and can even destroy certain needed vitamins in our systems. Cadmium is a trace mineral, but is very toxic—and has no biological function in humans, although it is found primarily in refined foods such as flour, rice, and white sugar; it is also present in the air, via cigarette smoke (in fact, a smoker going through one pack of cigarettes a day deposits 2 to 4 micrograms of cadmium into his or her lungs, which some research shows may help cause pulmonary emphysema) and some factory pollution; but because cadmium is poorly absorbed, it is not a major problem. Another potentially detrimental mineral is beryllium. If exposed to this mineral in excess, the body's storage of magnesium can be depleted; beryllium can also, if absorbed into the bloodstream, settle in vital organs and cause them to not function correctly.

Can some minerals be helpful *and* toxic to humans?

Yes, like certain vitamins, there are many minerals that can be helpful, and yet toxic, to humans—especially in large doses or through environmental pollution. For example, the mineral nickel is an essential trace mineral found in the body—and can be a factor in the maintaining the integrity of our hormones, lipids, and cell membranes, and also acts to stabilize our DNA and RNA (nucleic acids).

But nickel can also be toxic to humans if the levels are too high. One simple, well-known, and localized example is allergic reactions to piercings of the ear (and other body parts) because … as some earring posts contain nickel alloys. With a more severe exposure, such as when nickel combines with carbon monoxide to form nickel carbonyl in many industrial processes, the results can include headaches, vertigo, nausea, respiratory problems, skin rashes, chest pain, and coughing.

Is the mineral lead toxic to humans?

Yes, lead is a highly toxic trace mineral. The human body can tolerate only 1 to 2 milligrams (about 0.00003 ounce) of lead without suffering toxic effects. Overall, lead can enter our body via our skin and the gastrointestinal tract; because lead is poorly absorbed it is usually excreted in the feces. But when lead is absorbed, it is stored in our bones and soft tissues (including our liver). For most people, if lead is consumed, the body keeps pace by excreting the mineral; thus, the body does not retain as much lead. If the body can't keep up, lead toxicity can result, causing such symptoms as abnormal brain function (including learning disorders, reading problems, and slower reflexes), problems with the central nervous system, and anemia.

Why was lead such a problem in the past?

There have been many problems with lead toxicity in the past. For example, when foods or drinks are stored in lead-glazed earthenware pottery (fired at too low a temperature), lead may leach from the container into the food or drink. One classic example comes from ancient Roman times, when pottery, pipes, and other objects contained lead, and the mineral was ingested by many (for more about lead in ancient times, see the chapter "Nutrition throughout the Centuries"). Before 1930, American homes had lead piping, and if the region had soft and/or acidic water, lead would often leach into the drinking water, causing lead poisoning in many people. (It was 1986 before building regulations prohibited the use of lead solder to connect copper piping in homes.)

By the mid-1900s, it was determined that many older homes and structures contained lead paint. Young children—who naturally chew on things, including windowsills, walls, and floors—would become contaminated and experience learning disabilities. In addition, food was canned in lead-soldered containers (a process stopped in the late 1980s); and there were lead-based paints, cosmetics, and plaster, and even cigarettes had lead (from lead-containing insecticides applied to the tobacco). Probably the most insidious exposure came from motor vehicles

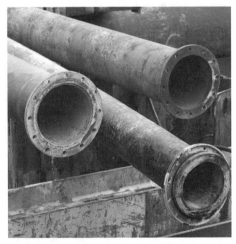

Old lead pipes like these once leached the metal into water supplies, making people sick. Interestingly, the same thing happened during the days of the Roman Empire because they used lead pipes, too.

(again, this especially affected young children playing in and eating dirt and grass in their front yards near roadways), which is why lead-free gasoline was developed.

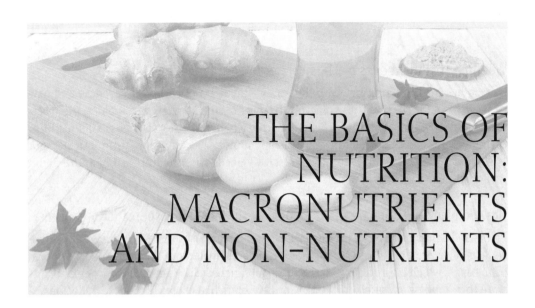

THE BASICS OF NUTRITION: MACRONUTRIENTS AND NON-NUTRIENTS

MACRONUTRIENTS

What are macronutrients?

As the term *macro* implies (*macro* is Greek for "big" or "far"), macronutrients are the larger (molecule-wise) nutrients needed for the body to exist—and we need them in large amounts. They are vital to every function in our bodies, mainly because they are the elements that give us fuel (energy) to keep our systems working. This fuel is familiar to all of us—in the form of carbohydrates, fats, and protein, and the foods that contain them.

Why are the three main macronutrients important to our health?

The three main macronutrients in our diet—proteins, fats (lipids), and carbohydrates—are the most important ways we have to obtain fuel (or energy) for our bodies. And although many cells prefer carbohydrates as a major energy source, fats and proteins are also broken down to provide energy. Lipids are broken down into simpler and more stable substances—scientists say that the fats are catabolized—into polymers our body needs, glycerol, and fatty acids, which are then used for cell respiration. Proteins are also catabolized into their certain amino acids, which are then fed into the process of glycolysis, also known as the Krebs cycle, and give us energy.

What is the Krebs cycle?

The Krebs cycle (also referred to as the citric acid cycle) is central to the body's aerobic, or oxygen-consuming, metabolism. In general, the cycle allows our cells to gain energy from glucose (what we commonly call sugar); the carbon dioxide we exhale is a result of the breakdown of the glucose, which occurs during the energy-obtaining phase of our aerobic cells' respiration. This process was discovered in 1937 by the German chemist Hans Adolf Krebs (1900–1981), who received the 1953 Nobel Prize for his discovery.

What macronutrient does our body prefer to burn for energy?

Our bodies most often prefer carbohydrates—made up of carbon, hydrogen, and oxygen—to burn for energy. These macronutrients are smaller than fats, making them easier to burn, while proteins provide energy when nothing else is available. Plus, carbohydrates can be stored for later use, and almost every system—from our nervous and renal systems to our brain and muscles—needs carbohydrates. (For more about carbohydrates, see this chapter.)

How do plant and animal cells store glucose, or the energy source for organisms?

Plants and animals use glucose (sugar) as their main energy source, but the way this molecule is stored differs between them. For example, animals store their glucose in the form of glycogen, which is formed by a series of long, branched chains of glucose, whereas plants store their glucose as starch, formed by long, unbranched chains of glucose molecules.

How do our muscles obtain energy?

The muscle cells that make up our muscles use various sources to power their contractions. For example, if they need quick energy, they can use stored molecules in the cells (adenosine triphosphate [ATP] and creatine phosphate), which are usually depleted after about 20 seconds of activity. Then the muscles switch to other sources—especially glycogen, a carbohydrate made up of a string of glucose molecules. It is this glycogen that helps you make it through your workouts—from lifting weights to running—and it all originates with the foods you ingest. The following chart lists the major sources of energy for our systems and where they are stored in the body.

Sources of Energy in Our Bodies

Source	Storage Site
Carbohydrates	Glycogen; there is an average of 500 grams stored most of the time in the average human, mainly in the liver and skeletal muscles.
Fats (lipids)	Adipose tissue (although it has several other tasks) stores energy in our system as fats (in the form of triglycerides); it is estimated that a healthy adult male has 12 to 18 percent body fat, while healthy adult females carry about 12 to 25 percent body fat.
Protein	This source is found throughout the body, and is usually the body's last choice as an energy source.

What is the difference between the terms *aerobic* and *anaerobic*?

The term *aerobic* refers to organisms that require oxygen to exist; for example, most living organisms need oxygen to stay alive. As humans, our cells get energy by using oxygen to help fuel our metabolism; as we breath, the molecule oxygen is taken in, converted by our cells, and used to keep us alive. *Anaerobic* refers to organisms that need little or no oxygen to exist. It often refers to bacteria, such as those found in the dark, nonoxygenated recesses of the human small intestines where foods are broken down so that we can more easily absorb nutrients.

What is a calorie in terms of nutrition?

In terms of nutrition, calories are a measure of the energy produced after we digest and metabolize our foods. The resulting energy not only keeps us alive, but it replaces the

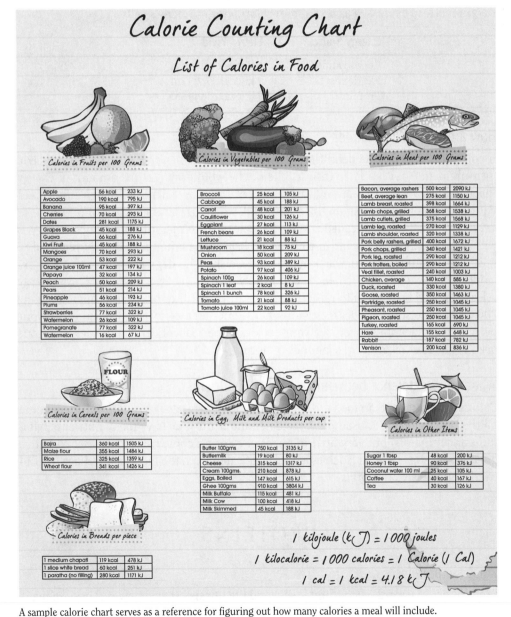

Calorie Counting Chart

List of Calories in Food

Calories in Fruits per 100 Grams

Apple	56 kcal	233 kJ
Avocado	190 kcal	795 kJ
Banana	95 kcal	397 kJ
Cherries	70 kcal	293 kJ
Dates	281 kcal	1175 kJ
Grapes Black	45 kcal	188 kJ
Guava	66 kcal	276 kJ
Kiwi Fruit	45 kcal	188 kJ
Mangoes	70 kcal	293 kJ
Orange	53 kcal	222 kJ
Orange juice 100ml	47 kcal	197 kJ
Papaya	32 kcal	134 kJ
Peach	50 kcal	209 kJ
Pears	51 kcal	214 kJ
Pineapple	46 kcal	193 kJ
Plums	56 kcal	234 kJ
Strawberries	77 kcal	322 kJ
Watermelon	26 kcal	109 kJ
Pomegranate	77 kcal	322 kJ
Watermelon	16 kcal	67 kJ

Calories in Vegetables per 100 Grams

Broccoli	25 kcal	105 kJ
Cabbage	45 kcal	188 kJ
Carrot	48 kcal	201 kJ
Cauliflower	30 kcal	126 kJ
Eggplant	27 kcal	113 kJ
French beans	26 kcal	109 kJ
Lettuce	21 kcal	88 kJ
Mushroom	18 kcal	75 kJ
Onion	50 kcal	209 kJ
Peas	93 kcal	389 kJ
Potato	97 kcal	406 kJ
Spinach 100g	26 kcal	109 kJ
Spinach 1 leaf	2 kcal	8 kJ
Spinach 1 bunch	78 kcal	326 kJ
Tomato	21 kcal	88 kJ
Tomato juice 100ml	22 kcal	92 kJ

Calories in Meat per 100 Grams

Bacon, average rashers	500 kcal	2090 kJ
Beef, average lean	275 kcal	1150 kJ
Lamb breast, roasted	398 kcal	1664 kJ
Lamb chops, grilled	368 kcal	1538 kJ
Lamb cutlets, grilled	375 kcal	1568 kJ
Lamb leg, roasted	270 kcal	1129 kJ
Lamb shoulder, roasted	320 kcal	1338 kJ
Pork belly rashers, grilled	400 kcal	1672 kJ
Pork chops, grilled	340 kcal	1421 kJ
Pork leg, roasted	290 kcal	1212 kJ
Pork trotters, boiled	290 kcal	1212 kJ
Veal fillet, roasted	240 kcal	1003 kJ
Chicken, average	140 kcal	585 kJ
Duck, roasted	330 kcal	1380 kJ
Goose, roasted	350 kcal	1463 kJ
Partridge, roasted	250 kcal	1045 kJ
Pheasant, roasted	250 kcal	1045 kJ
Pigeon, roasted	250 kcal	1045 kJ
Turkey, roasted	165 kcal	690 kJ
Hare	155 kcal	648 kJ
Rabbit	187 kcal	782 kJ
Venison	200 kcal	836 kJ

Calories in Cereals per 100 Grams

Bajra	360 kcal	1505 kJ
Maize flour	355 kcal	1484 kJ
Rice	325 kcal	1359 kJ
Wheat flour	341 kcal	1426 kJ

Calories in Egg, Milk and Milk Products per cup

Butter 100gms	750 kcal	3135 kJ
Buttermilk	19 kcal	80 kJ
Cheese	315 kcal	1317 kJ
Cream 100gms.	210 kcal	878 kJ
Eggs, Boiled	147 kcal	615 kJ
Ghee 100gms	910 kcal	3804 kJ
Milk Buffalo	115 kcal	481 kJ
Milk Cow	100 kcal	418 kJ
Milk Skimmed	45 kcal	188 kJ

Calories in Other Items

Sugar 1 tbsp	48 kcal	200 kJ
Honey 1 tbsp	90 kcal	376 kJ
Coconut water 100 ml	25 kcal	105 kJ
Coffee	40 kcal	167 kJ
Tea	30 kcal	126 kJ

Calories in Breads per piece

1 medium chapati	119 kcal	478 kJ
1 slice white bread	60 kcal	251 kJ
1 paratha (no filling)	280 kcal	1171 kJ

1 kilojoule (kJ) = 1000 joules

1 kilocalorie = 1000 calories = 1 Calorie (1 Cal)

1 cal = 1 kcal = 4.18 kJ

A sample calorie chart serves as a reference for figuring out how many calories a meal will include.

molecules we lose and helps us to run, jump, sit, and do everything in between. But in order to have calories, a food must be able to release energy of some sort for the body to use. If not, it is usually not considered a "food" in the true sense of the word.

How much average energy comes from the three major macronutrients?

Various molecules have a certain energy that is used by our body's cells. The following chart lists the energy source and the energy yield in kilocalorie per gram (the kilocalorie/gram is also expressed as a kilogram calorie) for our body's cells:

Energy Source	Energy Yield
Carbohydrate	4 kilocalorie/gram
Fat (lipids)	9 kilocalorie/gram
Protein	4 kilocalorie/gram

How are calories measured?

If you ask a chemist the definition of a calorie (and remember, scientists use metric measurements), with a lowercase "c," he or she would say it is the amount of energy (heat) required to raise 1 gram (1 milliliter) of water by 1 degree Celsius (1.8 degrees Fahrenheit). A nutritionist, on the other hand, would use an uppercase "C" or the term *kilocalorie* (or kcal; also called a kilogram calorie)—to measure how much energy is within each type of nutrient. In this case, a kcal is the amount of energy required to raise 1 kilogram (1 liter) of water by 1 degree Celsius (1.8 degrees Fahrenheit). For example, if a chocolate chip cookie is completely incinerated, the amount of heat energy released would be enough to raise the temperature of 1 liter of water by approximately 300 degrees Celsius (572 degrees Fahrenheit). But don't worry about burning out your oven if you accidentally overbake your cookies—the real conversion to energy in your oven is not as efficient as in a laboratory setting.

What is the difference between calories and nutrients?

Calories and nutrients in food are really two different things—and both vary depending on the type of food. For example, vegetables and fruits may have many nutrients (vitamins and minerals) but very little in terms of calories; conversely, foods that contain a great deal of sugar and fat, such as a doughnut eaten from the local bakery, have few nutrients but plenty of calories.

PROTEINS

What are proteins?

Proteins do, in a word, everything—allowing life to exist as we know it. They are made up of amino acids (about 20)—or a carbon atom attached to a hydrogen atom, an amino group, an acid group, and a side chain (the nitrogen in amino acids makes proteins different from carbohydrates and fats). Each type of protein contains a different number, combination, and order of the amino acids.

Why are proteins necessary for human health?

Proteins' tasks are many: They are required for all metabolic reactions, are important to the body's structures like muscles, regulate fluid balance and acidity, aid in tissue repair and immune function, and act as both transporters and signal receptors in cells. Every phase of a person's life needs proteins—and they are especially helpful to growing children, teens, and pregnant women (and fetuses).

What happens to the proteins in an egg when it is cooked?

The "white" of an egg is rich in the protein called albumin. When subjected to high heat, the bonds that form the structure of albumin are irreversibly changed. This causes the clear, jellylike consistency of the egg to become firm and white in a process known as protein denaturation.

How does your body use proteins?

Our bodies use the various types of proteins in certain ways. The following chart lists the generic types of proteins and the examples of their functions (this is not a complete list—just some examples):

Proteins and Their Functions

Type of Protein	Examples of Functions
Defensive	Antibodies that respond to invasion
Enzymatic	Increase the rate of reactions; build and break down molecules
Hormonal	Insulin and glucagon, which control blood sugar
Receptor	Cell surface molecules that cause cells to respond to signals
Storage	Store amino acids for use in metabolic processes
Structural	Major components of muscles, skin, hair, and nails
Transport	Hemoglobin carries oxygen from lungs to cells

What are some problems associated with an insufficient intake of protein?

For most people—adults and children—an inadequate intake of protein can lead to several body-oriented problems. For example, because hair is made up primarily of protein molecules, a lack of protein in the diet will essentially cut off the supply, causing hairs to fall out or even slow down growth in order to conserve protein. Another problem with low protein intake is a decrease in lean body mass, which will compromise muscles and muscular strength. For example, with less protein consumed, it will take much longer for a person's muscles to recover after strength-training exercises.

How do you obtain essential amino acids—the building blocks of proteins?

Of the twenty amino acids used by humans as building blocks for proteins, eight (some research says nine) are essential. In other words, our bodies cannot synthesize them, nor can we survive without them. Luckily, all of the essential amino acids can be acquired by eating animal meat (complete proteins) and/or certain plant sources (complementary proteins).

In general, our bodies make proteins by combining the 20 amino acids—but adults have to obtain eight of these amino acids through their intake of food, while children usually need nine. And from these amino acids, the body can make the rest we need to survive. When a person eats animal protein foods, such as eggs and milk, he or she can obtain the eight or nine needed.

Why do vegetarians need to know about complementary proteins?

Many people who eat a vegetarian diet are often asked where they get their protein—that is, their essential amino acids—if not from animal meat. The answer is simple: There are plenty of proteins that can be obtained from plants—especially grains, seeds, nuts, some vegetables, and beans and their byproducts (such as tofu from soybeans)—that can help "replace" animal protein.

But vegetarians cannot obtain these amino acids from a single vegetable protein source, and thus must mix certain foods together to obtain an ample supply of necessary proteins. Called complementary proteins, the amino acids in legumes, such as peas, lentils, and beans, complement those in other foods, such as potatoes and some nuts. Thus, eating pasta and chickpeas in a soup or combining grains such as rice and beans is usually sufficient for a person's daily requirement of essential proteins.

What happens to proteins in our skin as we age?

There are a variety of molecular changes in our skin that show up as we age. For example, there is a slowdown in production of the proteins in the skin—collectively known as collagen. As the amount of collagen decreases with age, the skin loses elasticity and begins to sag, bag, and wrinkle. The loss of elasticity can be demonstrated by gently pinching a fold of skin on the back of your hand: The skin of young children will immediately return to its smooth form when released, while that of an elderly person will take longer.

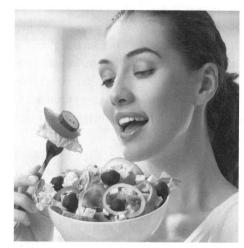

If one is not careful on a vegetarian diet, there is a chance he or she won't get enough proteins. Non-meat alternatives include nuts, seeds, grains, and beans.

What is a "Popeye" protein?

A family of proteins nicknamed "Popeye" was discovered only a decade ago. They are officially called "Popeye domain-containing proteins" (Popdc for short)—named after the cartoon character "Popeye the Sailor Man" because the protein is found in abundance in the muscles (the cartoon character was always flexing his muscles).

Usually, when under stress, the release of the hormone adrenaline—our heart's natural pacemaker—makes the heart beat faster, and thus deliver more oxygen around the body. But research in the lab has shown that when mice lack Popdc proteins, the heart rate actually slows down when they are stressed; and it is known now that many elderly people's hearts slow in a similar way when under stress. The research also shows that these proteins—located in the outer membrane of the heart's specialized pacemaker cells—play an essential role in allowing our hearts to respond to the stresses we encounter. Thus, scientists hope that a better understanding of Popdc will lead to new treatments for abnormal heart rhythms.

How does too much protein affect a person?

The typical Western diet usually contains more than enough protein—and because excess protein is used as energy or stored, excess protein can lead to an imbalance in your body. (In developing countries, where certain protein-rich food supplies are limited, the lack of protein intake is more of a problem.) For example, too much protein in your diet can cause calcium loss; high protein diets, especially those based on animal products, can increase your cholesterol levels, causing blockages in the arteries that lead to strokes or heart attacks; problems with your liver, brain, and nervous system; and even nausea and diarrhea.

How much protein does an adult—male or female—need?

The Institute of Medicine (IOM) recommends that daily protein be 10 to 35 percent of your daily caloric intake—in other words, the calories you take in from all the foods you eat during the day. The reason for the wide range is based on several factors. For example, an average healthy male should get about 56 grams of protein daily, an average healthy female should take in about 46 grams of protein a day, and people who are moderately or extremely active should take in more protein than people who are mostly sedentary. But if you're in doubt as to how much protein to eat, talk with your doctor or nutritionist about your specific circumstances to find out the best amount of protein to consume daily.

FATS AND FATTY ACIDS

What are fats?

Fat is considered a necessary nutrient for all humans, as it is essential for all our normal bodily functions; for example, polyunsaturated fats are often linked to a healthy cardiovascular system. Most foods contain some fat, which is good for us—mainly because humans also need fats to absorb certain vitamins (A, D, E, and K, in particular) and help other nutrients do their respective tasks. And fats also help us fuel-wise, often supplying us with energy we need to survive.

What are lipids?

In general, fats, oils, waxes, and certain sterols and esters fall into the lipid category; they dissolve in alcohol, but not in water. Along with proteins and carbohydrates, lipids are the main constituents of plant and animal (meaning humans, too) cells—and serve as an important source of food for the cells.

Why is the macronutrient "fat" healthy—and not so healthy—for humans?

Fats help to maintain normal growth and development, especially for children and teens, and they are a good source of energy. But fats have other tasks, including helping to cushion our organs (although an excessive amount of fat can cause organs to be moved, pushed, and even compressed). And as most of us know, fats provide better taste to many things we eat.

But there are down sides to fat: in particular, many people eat too many unhealthy fats, such as those found in fatty meats, hydrogenated oils, fried foods, and bakery goods. These unhealthy fats carry more calories than do carbohydrates and protein—in fact, each gram of fat is nine calories, versus four calories for carbohydrates and protein.

How does a person interpret how much fat to eat based on the daily calories he or she wants to consume?

Determining how much fat to eat—and remain healthy—each day is sometimes confusing. According to the American Heart Association (AHA), the average healthy adult should get about 30 percent or less of his or her total daily calories from dietary fats. For example, if you consume 2,000 calories per day, that means 65 grams or less of fat in your diet; if you consume 1,800 calories a day, it means about 60 grams or less of fat; and for 1,500 calories a day, about 50 grams or less of fat. Keep in mind, a teaspoon of fat (as oil, butter, animal fat, margarine, or shortening) has 5 grams of fat (and 45 calories), so 65 grams (if you consume 2,000 calories a day) of fat would equal about 13 teaspoons of those fats per day.

What are fatty acids?

The fats and oils in foods contain many types of fatty acids—what we call saturated and unsaturated (monounsaturated and polyunsaturated) fats—and all affect our bodies in different ways. In general, they are based on their chemical composition: there are about twenty-six common fatty acids, all with short or long chains of carbon atoms, and each with a space for a hydrogen atom. If every space is occupied, the fatty acid is called saturated; if two hydrogen positions are unfilled, a double bond will occur between two carbon atoms, thus the unsaturated fatty acid is called monounsaturated; and if four or more of the hydrogen spaces are unfilled, more of the double bonds will occur, and the unsaturated fatty acid is called polyunsaturated.

What's the connection between fatty acids and triglycerides?

When people mention the word "fat," they most often are referring to a type of lipid called a triglyceride. Natural fats from plants or animals are composed of three fatty acid molecules, all bound to a glycerol molecule (a type of alcohol)—which is where the "tri" in triglyceride originates. Triglycerides are found in fats and oils; the biggest difference between the oils and fats is their melting points—at room temperature, fats, such as lard, are solid, whereas oils, such as canola, are liquid. (For more about how triglycerides affect your health, see the chapter "Nutrition and Allergies, Illnesses, and Diseases.")

Why do "fats" have such a bad reputation—especially nutrition-wise?

The term *fat* often has an evil connotation when it comes to nutrition. In particular, it is often because we use the term *fat* to mean something we consume—*and* we use the term to refer to ourselves if we think we are too heavy in weight. Because the word "fat" has bad implications, the food industry has used the terms *fat-free* and *low-fat* to induce people to buy more products—many of which are no better than eating "fattening" foods! (For example, the food may be fat-free, but contain an abundance of sugar.)

Yes, too much of certain fats have been shown to cause obesity, which is caused by too much white adipose tissue (another name for body fat) in our systems. This excess can, and often does, lead to diabetes, heart disease, and other ailments when allowed to go unchecked. But there are also "good fats" (such as those in fish and olive oil) that have been shown to lower the risk for heart disease and keep our weight in check. As with everything, moderation is the key—as is eating the best types of oils and fats that are good for our bodies.

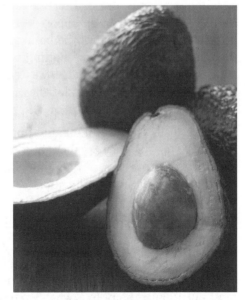

What is the difference between saturated and unsaturated fatty acids?

In general, saturated fats are solid at room temperatures (except palm, palm kernel, and some coconut oils); most animal fats, (meat, poultry, eggs, and dairy, such as butter and cheeses) are also saturated. The main problem with saturated fats involves how it raises blood cholesterol; this happens because these fats interfere with the removal of cholesterol from the blood.

Fat is not always bad. People need fats in their diets to help them absorb vitamins. Unsaturated fats, like those found in avocados, are good for us.

Unsaturated fats—or the polyunsaturated and monounsaturated fats—have been known to either lower, or to have no effect on the blood cholesterol. (But one caveat: When polyunsaturated fats are hydrogenated—which makes them firmer—they become more like saturated fats, and so can affect the body's blood cholesterol in the same way.) Monounsaturated fats are liquid at room temperature and are found in olive, canola, and peanut oils, along with some nuts, seeds, and avocados. These fats are also considered helpful to human health, as they also lower the "bad" low-density lipoprotein (LDL) cholesterol levels in the blood.

Is there such a thing as "an essential fatty acid"?

Yes, many nutritionists claim (but not all) that there are over 13 essential fatty acids. For example, alpha-linolenic acid (ALA, a type of omega-3 polyunsaturated fat) is thought to be an essential fatty acid found in soybean and canola oils and in flaxseed. Some research has shown that this fatty acid has many health benefits, especially to help the heart keep a strong and regular beat. In addition, another study showed that women who consumed the most alpha-linolenic acid had a significantly lower chance of dying from heart disease. But as with many studies in nutrition, there are researchers who question the various health benefit claims of these fatty acids.

What two types of polyunsaturated fats seem to help our health?

There are two types of polyunsaturated fats—or polyunsaturated fatty acids, or PUFAs—the two essential fatty acids called omega-3 and omega-6. They are considered essential fats; in other words, our body can't make them, so we must get them from our diet. Both are thought to play an important role in brain function, as well as aiding normal growth and development of the brain and eyes in infants. The omega-3 fats are also thought to help prevent blood clotting, which is known to often trigger strokes or heart attacks; they are also thought to lower triglycerides, thus decreasing the risk for a heart attack (thus, they are often called "heart-healthy" fats).

In general, along with the attributes listed above, omega-6s are thought to lower LDL (the "bad" cholesterol), and to improve insulin sensitivity. But they also have a "bad" side, too—as they are thought to increase inflammation in the body. (For more about the controversies surrounding omega-6 intake, see the chapter "Controversies with Food, Beverages, and Nutrition.")

Why do some researchers question the benefits of omega-3 and omega-6?

Many researchers say that a healthy diet consists of a balance of omega-3 and omega-6 fatty acids—but there are doubts among researchers. In particular, no one can decide the correct ratio of these fats to maintain our overall health. The closest balanced diet most nutritionists point to is what is referred to as the "Mediterranean diet," in which oils, whole grains, fish, fruits and vegetables, olive oil, and garlic, along with moderate wine consumption, seem to create a good balance between omega-3s and omega-6s.

(For more about the Mediterranean diet, see "Appendix 3: Comparing Diets.")

Are there different omega-3s?

Yes, there are different types of omega-3s. For example, the omega-3 fat found in walnuts and walnut oils is not the same as the omega-3 found in fish. The heart-healthy omega-3s from fish are omega-3 DHA (docosahexaenoic acid) and EPA (eicosapentaenoic acid); walnuts, and other foods, such as flaxseeds, contain an omega-3 called ALA (alpha-linolenic acid). Because our bodies do not make the ALA, it must be supplied by our diets; it is found in certain plant foods, such as flaxseeds and various nuts (see below). And although research shows that our bodies can make EPA and DHA from ALA, it doesn't always work (the body usually converts only about 20 percent of the ALA to EPA and DHA), which is why nutritionists often recommend eating fish to get the best EPA and DHA benefits.

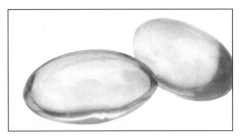

Fish oil caplets like these are one way to ingest omega-3s, but some have a fishy aftertaste. Krill oil pills with less aftertaste are also available.

How do omega-3 DHA and EPA help us health-wise?

Certain omega-3 fats have been shown to improve heart health and even help our moods. Of these fats, DHA (docosahexaenoic acid) and EPA (eicosapentaenoic acid) appear to be the healthiest. One reason is that they both make our cell membranes more fluid, which in turn, helps our brain, eyes, and nerve cells work more efficiently. They also appear to help reduce risk factors for heart disease, such as high blood pressure and high cholesterol, and inhibit the development of plaque and blood clots, lower triglycerides, and reduce cardiac arrhythmia (irregular heartbeats). In addition, omega-3 DHA is a major component of our cells' lipid (fat) content; and because each cell membrane's content of DHA is controlled by our genes, cells are not as easily affected by our DHA intake. (In fact, most of the fats in our brain's cell membranes, and 70 percent of the fats in our eyes' retinal cell membranes, are made of omega-3 DHA.)

What are some common foods that have omega-3 ALA?

There are many common foods that contain the several types of omega-3 fats. In particular, good sources of ALA (alpha-linolenic acid) are walnuts, flax and flaxseed oil, and canola, olive, and soybean oils. But note: if you eat these oils for their omega-3s, don't cook with the oil, as the heat can destroy most of the omega-3 fats.

What are the best sources of omega-3 DHA and EPA?

There are many natural and fortified sources of omega-3 DHA and EPA. Some of the most popular natural sources are fatty fish, such as salmon, anchovies, lake trout, tuna, mackerel, herring, and sardines (wild fish make DHA and EPA from the algae they eat), and seaweed (nori) and kelp (wakame, kombu, or dulse; all are algae that produce some

DHA and EPA). Fortified choices include eggs (hens naturally turn some of the omega-3s from flaxseed in their feed into DHA and EPA) and peanut butter (DHA and EPA usually come from added fish oil in this food).

Are there different types of omega-6s?

Yes, there are several different types of omega-6s; for example, many vegetable oils contain omega-6 fatty acids. One type is linoleic acid (LA; not to be confused with the omega-3 fatty acid, ALA, or alpha-linolenic acid). In this case, the LA is converted to another acid, GLA (gamma-linolenic acid) in the body (it is eventually broken down into AA, arachidonic acid)—an acid thought to reduce inflammation.

What are some sources of omega-6?

Omega-6 fats are found in plant sources; they are also liquid at room temperature, and include safflower, corn, and sunflower oils. Some nuts also contain omega-6s, including pecans, Brazil nuts, and almonds, and sunflower and sesame seeds.

Which is better to consume: the omega-3s or omega-6s?

There are many studies concerning the health benefits—or not—of omega-3s and omega-6s. Although most literature points to a healthy balance of the two fatty acids, there are some experts who disagree, saying that the ratio of both fatty acids is truly not significant, and that both are necessary for good health. The research continues, and for now, most experts recommend

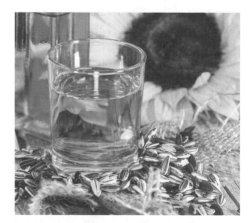

You can get omega-6 fats from sunflower oil, as well as from sunflower seeds.

moderate consumption of foods containing both of these fatty acids. (For more about the controversies behind the ingestion of omega-3 and omega-6 fatty acids, see the chapter "Controversies with Food, Beverages, and Nutrition.")

What are the various types of fats and their fat content?

There are numerous types of fat that we ingest. The following table shows some of the more common types of fat and their fat content, including fats classified as monounsaturated (a "good" fat that helps your health, for example, olive oil), saturated (a "bad" fat that can be detrimental to your health; especially when eaten in large quantities; for example, coconut oil is high in saturated fat), linoleic (or linoleic acid, a polyunsaturated omega-6 fatty acid; for example, sunflower oil is high in linoleic acid), and alpha-linoleic (or alpha-linoleic acid, an essential omega-3 fatty acid; for example, flaxseed oil is high in alpha-linoleic acid):

Types of Fat and Their Fat Content (in grams per tablespoon)

Oil Source	Total Fat	Saturated	Unsaturated	Alpha-Linoleic Acid	Other
Beef Tallow	6.4	5.4	0.4	0.1	0.5
Butter	7.2	3.3	0.3	0.2	0.5
Canola Oil	1.0	8.2	2.8	1.3	0.7
Chicken Fat	3.8	5.7	2.5	0.1	0.7
Cocoa Butter	8.1	4.5	0.4	0.6	–
Coconut Oil	11.8	0.8	0.2	0.8	–
Corn Oil	1.7	3.3	7.9	0.1	0.6
Cottonseed Oil	3.5	2.4	7.0	0.7	–
Flaxseed Oil	1.3	2.5	2.2	8.0	–
Olive Oil	1.8	10.0	1.1	0.1	0.5
Palm Oil	6.7	5.0	1.2	0.7	–
Palm Kernel Oil	11.1	1.6	0.2	0.7	–
Peanut Oil	2.3	6.2	4.3	0.7	–
Pork Fat (Lard)	5.0	5.8	1.3	0.1	0.6
Safflower Oil	0.8	10.2	2.0	0.6	–
Sesame Oil	1.9	5.4	5.6	0.7	–
Soybean Oil	2.0	3.2	6.9	0.9	0.6
Sunflower Oil	1.4	2.7	8.9	0.6	–

Source: U.S.D.A. Nutrient Database.

What are trans fats?

Trans fats (or trans fatty acids) are created through an industrial process, although a small amount is found naturally in some meat and dairy products, including beef, pork, lamb, and butterfat. The mechanical process adds hydrogen to liquid vegetable oils to make them solid—usually listed as "partially hydrogenated oils"—which makes the oil less likely to spoil and gives the foods that contain trans fats a much longer shelf life. Before the 1990s, few researchers realized the damage to human health caused by trans fats; studies soon showed that trans fats could raise a person's "bad" LDL cholesterol and lower a person's "good" HDL cholesterol, contributing to coronary heart disease. In fact, researchers now know that trans fats may even raise your LDL more than saturated fats. (For more about how trans fats affect humans, see the chapter "Nutrition and Allergies, Illnesses, and Diseases.")

How can you stay away from trans fats in your diet?

Overall, the American Heart Association recommends that only about 1 percent of your total daily calories should be from trans fats—or none at all—because they do not appear to provide any health benefits. If you buy packaged foods, such as snacks, crackers, and some bakery goods (such as cookies and cakes), and fried foods (such as doughnuts and french fries), make sure a product is trans-fat-free (but also be aware that a product label can claim to be trans-fat-free if there is less than 0.5 grams of trans fats).

The best way to determine if a product really does have trans fats is to check the ingredient list, and stay away from the ones that read "hydrogenated oil" or "partially hydrogenated oil" if you want to cut down on trans fats. And remember, even if you make your cookies and cakes from scratch, some of the highest amounts of trans fats are found in shortenings and some margarines used for baked goods. In fact, you probably eat enough naturally occurring trans fats daily from animal products, such as milk and meat, which are definitely less harmful than processed trans fats.

How have trans fats in foods changed in the past, and how may they change in the future?

The amount of trans fatty acids in foods has changed in the past decade, and there have been even greater changes in the amount consumed. In particular, according to a 2012 study of American adults, from the Centers for Disease Control and Prevention (CDC), blood levels of trans fats dropped around 58 percent between 2000 and 2009. The main reasons for this drop were not only greater awareness of how trans fats affect us, but also that manufacturers have significantly reduced the amount of trans fats in packaged food. In fact, according to the Grocery Manufacturers Association, since 2005, food makers have lowered the amount of trans fats in food products by more than 70 percent.

In 2013, the U.S. Food and Drug Administration (FDA) ruled for the first time that trans fats are not truly safe in foods (in fact, they never ruled officially that trans fats *were* safe in foods). The ruling was not a surprise—after all, trans fats have been blamed for contributing to strokes, heart attacks, and other cardiovascular ailments. In the future, if the ruling leads to an overall ban of trans fats, it means that certain fast food restaurants, bakeries, and sundry other food manufacturers will have to eliminate trans fats completely from their products—something many researchers (along with patients and their doctors) hope will slow down cardiovascular diseases. This doesn't mean everyone is (or will be) complying with less trans fats in foods. For example, some restaurants still use oils that contain trans fats for cooking fried foods—thus a large serving of french fries at such places can contain 5 grams or more of trans fats. In addition, some manufacturers have been replacing trans fats with other ingredients, including tropical oils such as coconut, palm kernel, and palm oils. But all these oils contain saturated fats that, like trans fats, raise your LDL cholesterol and contribute to heart disease.

CARBOHYDRATES

What are carbohydrates?

Carbohydrates are one of the three major macronutrients needed by the body for energy. They are classified by their chemical structure and digestibility—and further divided into two groups, simple and complex. The simple carbohydrates are the sugars; they most often form crystals that dissolve in water. Found in a variety of fruits and some vegetables—along with processed sugars such as table and brown sugars, and honey—simple carbohydrates are easily digested.

Complex carbohydrates cover a wide range and have various textures, colors, molecular structures, and flavors. They are all formed by complex chains of sugars, and are classified as starches or fibers. The starches—found in many grains, vegetables, and some fruits—can be broken down and metabolized by our body's digestive system. However, fibers cannot be broken down by our systems (we lack the enzymes to break down the fiber's cellulose and other woody parts), but they are still an important part of our digestive system, promoting some colon functions, and may even help prevent some types of cancer and other diseases.

How else are carbohydrates classified?

Carbohydrates are classified several other ways, as well. One way is by their overall length, by which they are divided into monosaccharides, disaccharides, and polysaccharides. They are even broken down further. For example, the monosaccharides (single sugars) are identified by the number of carbon molecules they contain: triose, with three carbon molecules; pentose, with five; and hexose, with six. Another classification is based on the carbohydrate's function. For example, glycogen and starch are called storage polysaccharides, because both store energy for the body.

Why are carbohydrates so important to our health?

Carbohydrates are considered one of our body's main sources of energy, and they are the most easily converted compounds that fuel our body's needs. Depending on the type of carbohydrate, they are also important for the central nervous system, kidneys, and brain, and also help with our gastrointestinal tract, especially in eliminating waste. Found in many foods, they are also easily stored in our bodies for later use, when we need the energy.

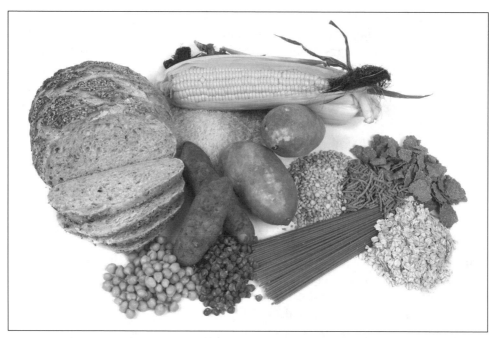

Foods rich in complex carbohydrates include corn, potatoes, and whole-grain breads. These foods give you energy and are important for the health of your brain, kidneys, and nervous system.

What are the best carbohydrates for our health?

The best carbohydrates are those from grains, fruits, vegetables, and low-fat milk products. The majority of these foods contain more vitamins and minerals and fewer calories—unlike such foods as bakery products and sweets. These latter carbohydrates may give us energy, but also plenty of calories that only contribute to excess weight and the risk for some diseases, such as diabetes.

Can dense carbohydrates that are high in fat and calories affect our sleep?

Yes, it is possible for high-fat and -calorie carbohydrate foods to affect our sleep. One good example is the holiday season, when high-calorie, fat-laden, sugary foods seem to abound at parties and get-togethers—all of which affect certain hormones in our body. In particular, the hormone leptin is influenced by eating a surplus of these foods. Usually associated with metabolism and appetite, the leptin levels change as we eat more carbohydrates, disrupting our sleep patterns—which, in turn, changes the leptin levels even more. This causes us to want more and more of these types of foods, which leads to more sleep disruption in a sort of endless loop of eating—and as a side "dish," we often gain weight.

What is refined sugar?

The refined sugar most of us find in our cupboards is actually a relatively new food in the human diet—developed only since the 1500s. Scientists divide sugar into intrinsic sugar (or sugar that we taste in fruits and some vegetables) and extrinsic sugar (or sugar added to food during preparation, processing, or while being consumed). The main sources of all our sugars are sugar cane and sugar beets (although beet sugar is not exclusively used in cooking—it is usually added to the sugar cane sugar to add bulk; however, you can find it in some health food stores as beet sugar). In general, the refined, white sugar most of us ingest is 99.9 percent sucrose, a disaccharide (double sugar) made up of two monosaccharides (single sugars) that has virtually no nutritional elements (which is why white sugar is often referred to as "empty calories" or even "junk food").

How do calories differ between the various types of sugar most used for cooking?

Although all forms of sugar have about the same energy value—4 calories per gram—not all sugars are alike in calories because of their texture and structure. The following chart lists the approximate calories of several familiar types of sugar used for cooking:

Type of Sugar	Calories in a Cup
Confectionery sugar*	385
Brown sugar, packed	820
Brown sugar, unpacked	551
White, refined sugar	770

*Confectionery sugar is merely pulverized refined sugar, but because of its consistency when measured, it has fewer calories.

What are the various names for sugar listed on a food label?

Sugars are listed on a food label in various ways—but as most nutritionists will tell you, sugar is sugar. Besides looking for the word "sugar," you can also look for the words "sucrose" (the refined crystallized white sugar in our sugar bowls); "dextrose" (pure glucose, or a sugar made of only one molecule); "maltose" (a sugar from starch, most often grains); "lactose" (milk sugar); "corn syrup" (manufactured from corn and containing various amounts of glucose, maltose, and dextrose); "brown sugar" (refined sugar coated with molasses [the molasses is taken out, then added back in] or even an artificial caramel coloring); "maltodextrin" (made from maltose and dextrose); "fructose" (sugar from fruit and maple sap); "raw sugar" (less refined white sugar with a minute amount of molasses); "high-fructose corn syrup" (concentrated corn syrup made of mostly fructose); "white grape juice" (a purified version of fructose); and "glucose" (known as blood sugar, dextrose, or grape sugar). (For more about controversies with sugar, especially high-fructose corn syrup, see the chapter "Controversies with Food, Beverages, and Nutrition.")

What amount of sugar can we eat every day?

The American Heart Association recommends that women get no more than 100 calories a day from added sugar from any source; this equals about 6 teaspoons of sugar a day. Most men should get no more than 150 calories a day from added sugar, or about 9 teaspoons a day. This applies to the average healthy individual, not a person who may have restrictions on his or her sugar intake, such as people with type 1 or type 2 diabetes.

Why does the American Heart Association suggest cutting back on sugar consumption?

According to the American Heart Association, the average healthy adult should have a certain daily maximum amount of sugar. The reason has to do with (of course) our health, especially because of what sugar does to our bodies. For example, too much sugar can damage the fine filtration system of the kidneys, leading to renal disease (and another connection: diabetes is one of the main causes of kidney failure); sugar can cause inflammation, especially to the linings of arteries leading to the heart, and

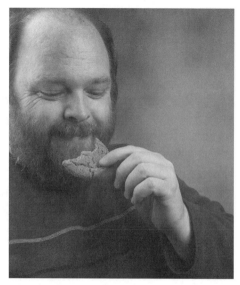

Americans eat a lot of sugar, and not just in sweets. Sugar in the form of high fructose corn syrup is commonly added to many processed boxed and canned foods.

also impairs the arteries' ability to respond to the heart's need for more blood; sugar also makes the platelets in our blood "stickier"; and the inflammatory factors in sugar can even exacerbate arthritis in some people.

What are some "healthier" natural sweeteners?

Sugar isn't just the type you find on the grocery shelf when it's time to make holiday cookies. It also comes in many other natural forms—some that are thought to be a bit healthier than the ubiquitous white, refined, processed sugars. The most familiar—from good to better, mainly according to the extent of their processing and/how they are assimilated into our bodies—are listed below:

Good and Bad Sweeteners

Type of Sweetener	Comments
Good Sweeteners	
Evaporated cane juice	This is the sweet liquid from sugar cane before refining and bleaching; the liquid is evaporated to form crystals—thus, it is truly just sugar
Agave	Extracted from a plant that looks similar to an aloe; dissolves easily and is used as a sweetener; contrary to some advertising, not everyone agrees that agave is healthier than most other sweeteners
Turbinado sugar	Although this is a true sugar, it is not as processed as white sugar; also called demerara, it is made from boiling down the sugar cane, resulting in a brownish crystal that still contains some molasses

Better Sweeteners

Maple sugar and syrup	Made by boiling down the sap of sugar maple trees; use pure 100 percent maple sugar (artificial maple syrup is maple-flavored high-fructose corn syrup with food coloring)
Honey	From flower nectar gathered by bees; best when eaten pure and raw, not processed, because it contains more healthy enzymes and minerals that support immune function
Brown rice syrup	Made from rice (not corn, as in corn syrup); often used in energy bars; good for people who are gluten-intolerant
Stevia	This sweetener is from the South American stevia plant (*Stevia rebaudiana*); the leaves are dried and powdered for baking, or used fresh in teas

How is maple syrup produced?

Maple sap is harvested from sugar maple trees (*Acer saccharum*) as temperatures fluctuate between freezing at night and thawing during the day, mainly in the cooler temperate regions. The maple trees are "tapped": tubes called spiles are driven into the sapwood and the dripping sap is collected in pails hanging beneath the spiles, an image most of us have seen in pictures or in person in the New England area in late February and early March. The tree makes starch during the previous summer, and it is stored in

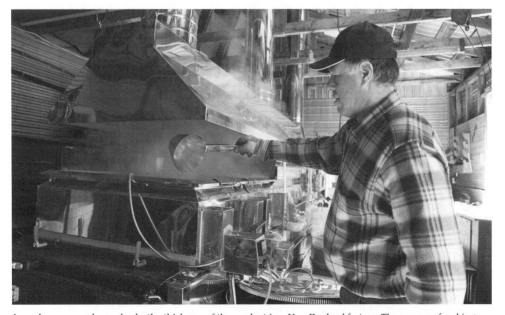

A maple syrup producer checks the thickness of the product in a New England factory. The process of making syryp from tree sap dates back to pre-colonial Vermont when Native Americans discovered they could boil the sap into a sweet, viscous liquid.

Why is "pancake syrup" (not true maple syrup) a concern?

Because maple syrup is expensive, most people turn to "pancake syrup," which is made mostly of sugar, water, and coloring. But there is also one ingredient that is a concern to health researchers: the caramel coloring often used in syrups to give the liquid its amber hue. This additive, found in most pancake syrups, and also other foods, such as baked goods, soy sauce, and some drinks (mostly dark-colored cola-type drinks), is called 4-Mel. Not only does it have no nutritional benefits, it is also considered a potential carcinogen. (Although it can be created when maple sap is converted to syrup, the amounts are negligible.) According to the World Health Organization, more studies need to be done, as the chemical has caused cancer in laboratory mice and it may also cause cancer in people as well. Thus, the main concerns are children and adults who eat pancake syrup on a regular, daily basis—and who also consume other products that contain 4-Mel.

the tree just under the bark (called the xylem sapwood); during the day, warmer temperatures create a positive pressure in the xylem sapwood, causing the sugary sap to push its way out the tapped tube, usually at a rate of 100 to 400 drops per minute. After collection, the sap is heated to get rid of most of the water content and leave the thick syrup. There is a reason for the high price of maple syrup: it takes 40 parts maple sap to make 1 part maple syrup (or 10 gallons of sap to make 1 quart of syrup).

But not every year is good for collecting maple syrup, because the flow stops (or never truly starts) when temperatures drop below freezing; and if the buds start to come out before the sap is collected, the tree's energy is sent to the buds, not to making sap. For example, in 2014, after record low temperatures were recorded in the northeastern United States well into March, maple syrup producers were unable to harvest their usual amount of sap—thus, supplies of syrup were lower and prices were higher.

What are artificial sweeteners?

Artificial sweeteners are added to many foods—or come in packets or containers for you to add to food—and (artificially) provide a sweet taste without the calories. Unlike regular sugars, artificial sweeteners do not cause tooth decay, and for diabetics they also offer a way of eating "sweets" (no glucose) without increasing blood sugar levels. Of course, not everyone agrees that artificial sweeteners are good for you, and there are many people who are allergic to several brands. (For more about the controversies surrounding artificial sweeteners, see the chapter "Controversies with Food, Beverages, and Nutrition.")

How do artificial sweeteners compare to refined sugar?

Many artificial sweeteners are much "sweeter" tasting than the same amount of refined sugar. For example, aspartame (marketed under the brand NutraSweet or Equal) is made from the amino acids phenylalanine and aspartic acid, and is a sweetener that's about 200 times sweeter than regular sugar. Saccharin is another artificial sweetener (marketed under the brands Sweet'N Low or Hermesetas)—the oldest on the market—and is about 300 times sweeter than sugar. There is also sucralose (sold under the brand name Splenda), which has 600 times the sweetening power of sugar.

What protein helps us taste any type of sugar?

One reason why sugars—no matter if they are artificial or natural—taste so sweet to us has to do with sweet receptors on our tongue. When a molecule of any sugar hits the tongue, it binds to a protein called T1r3, thought to be the primary receptor for sweet substances. Similar to most protein receptors, T1r3 has what looks like a pocket in which small molecules can enter and then bind. When we eat refined sugar

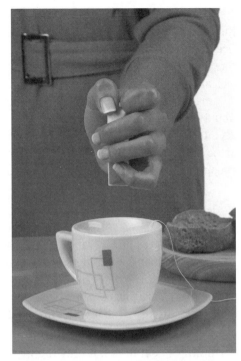

Today there are many types of artificial sweeteners, such as saccharine, sucralose, and aspartame, but people are starting to fear they might have bad side effects when used over time.

(sucrose), it binds to the T1r3, and a signal is transferred to the brain that you have just munched on something sweet. (The enzymes in your body help to metabolize the sugar, releasing energy; if we take in too many calories, the metabolized sucrose will cause fat to be deposited in our bodies, which is why excess sugar can make us gain weight.) Even if you eat something with the artificial sweetener saccharin, it will bind to the T1r3, but even more strongly than sucrose—which is why this artificial sweetener tastes around 300 times sweeter than the same amount of sucrose. (In this case, the saccharin has no calories after it is metabolized; thus, eating such sugars will not cause a weight gain.)

Are there any guidelines concerning the consumption of artificial sweeteners?

Yes, there are some guidelines put out by several groups, including the World Health Organization, that suggest the quantity of artificial sweeteners you can safely consume (although for many people, it is best not to consume any artificial sweeteners, especially people who have allergic reactions to sweeteners such as aspartame). Called the Acceptable Daily Intake, or ADI, it is based on the average daily amount a person can consume over a lifetime—in terms of any additive in foods, including artificial sweeteners—without causing any harm. This, of course, applies only to average healthy adults. (For more about ADI, see the chapter "Nutrition throughout Life.")

The basic formula is based on a certain ADI number and your weight: For example, if you weigh 100 pounds, multiply the ADI number for a certain sweetener times your weight—the number is how much of the sweetener in milligrams, per day, you can safely consume. For example, the American Cancer Society lists the safe amount of aspartame: A typical adult weighing 165 pounds (75 kilograms) can safely consume about 3,750 milligrams per day. Most sodas can contain about 180 milligrams of aspartame—meaning you would have to drink about 21 cans of such sodas a day in order to reach your daily limit. It's interesting to note, too, that in other countries, the amounts are different; for example, in the United Kingdom, the ADI for aspartame is 40 milligrams per kilogram of body weight, as opposed to the limit in the United States of 50 milligrams per kilogram of body weight.

What are sugar-alcohols?

Sugar-alcohols, or polyols, are reduced calorie sweeteners (also called sugar substitutes) used in sugar-free gums, candy, some chocolates, ice cream, and many baked goods. They include many sweeteners, such as sorbitol, xylitol, maltitol, and lactitol. For example, xylitol can be naturally occurring in many fruits and vegetables (it's mostly produced from birch trees), but also can be synthetically made. It is used in some toothpastes to make the product taste better, and in many candies and gums.

But some nutritionists warn consumers about foods containing these sweeteners. For example, xylitol is not only highly processed, but is also hydrogenated. And like many of the sugar-alcohols, it is known to cause bloating or diarrhea in people who are sensitive to it, especially those who consume large amounts of foods that contain the sweetener (children are especially affected, because of their smaller size).

What is the sugar that comes from milk?

Most of the sugars that humans use for energy come from plants. But there is one sugar that does not—called lactose, or milk sugar. Many people are lactose intolerant, meaning they lack (or have little) of the enzyme lactase in their digestive system that breaks down

What recent study showed a possible connection between fiber and slowing prostate cancer?

One recent study from the University of Colorado's Cancer Center showed that fiber may help slow the progression of prostate cancer in men. Researchers know that fiber is good for the heart and digestion, but they also found that phytic acid, a nondigestible carbohydrate found in fiber-rich foods, may actually slow the growth of prostate tumors. According to the study's lead scientist, the phytic acid didn't stop the tumor from developing, but it seemed to cut off the energy supply to the tumor in several ways, including reducing the amount of energy-giving glucose pumped into the cells.

the lactose in milk into the sugars glucose and galactose. Don't confuse this sugar with other sweeteners—most people who are lactose intolerant have no problem with sugars from other sources. (For more about lactose intolerance, see the chapter, "Nutrition and Allergies, Illnesses, and Diseases.")

What are fibrous carbohydrates?

Fibrous carbohydrates are not like sugar or starch carbohydrates, because the body cannot use them for energy, but they are still important for the body's overall health. In fact, "fibrous carbohydrate" is merely another name for "fiber"!

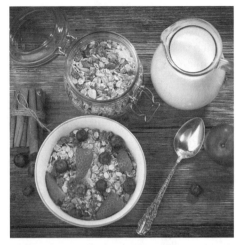

One way to get some dietary fiber is from breakfast cereals. A high-fiber diet may lower cholesterol and reduce the chance of contracting some forms of cancer.

What is soluble and insoluble dietary fiber?

Dietary fiber is the indigestible part of plant foods—and is known now to be an important aspect of the human daily diet, especially to prevent illness and to maintain health. Fiber comes in two categories—soluble (or viscous) and insoluble, with most plants having both types of fibers (although some have more of one than the other). The soluble fibers dissolve in water and stick together; they include such foods as oatmeal, oat bran, lentils, barley, and even pectin-rich fruits such as apples and strawberries. Insoluble fiber does not dissolve in water, and passes through the digestive system chewed, but otherwise the same. Foods with insoluble fiber include the edible skins of many fruits (such as apples, pears, and peaches), wheat bran, brown rice, and whole wheat products.

Can a high-fiber diet lower your cholesterol?

Some research indicates that just adding 10 grams of soluble fiber to your diet (the Institute of Medicine recommends women consume 21 to 25 grams and men 30 to 38 grams of dietary fiber daily) may help decrease your blood cholesterol levels (except for people with gastrointestinal problems who have to watch their fiber intake; contact your health-care provider for individual fiber guidelines). In fact, some research indicates that a high-fiber diet is even more effective in lowering cholesterol levels than a diet that is low in saturated fat.

What is the difference between fiber, grains, and seeds?

One of the more confusing topics is defining fiber versus grains versus seeds. Besides the fact that all of them have nutritional value, the following list gives the most common definition of each:

Fiber—As seen above, dietary fiber is defined as the part of a plant that your body's digestive system cannot readily digest. Fiber can come from vegetables, such as peas; fruits, such as strawberries; and grains, such as oatmeal and barley. Thus "grain" and "fiber" are sometimes used in the same sentence, such as "The grain barley has plenty of fiber."

Grains—Grains are made from wheat, rice, oats, corn, or other cereal products (no vegetables or fruits). They are usually eaten whole ("whole grains," such as whole oats and cornmeal, and bulgur) or milled (such as rice and wheat flours).

Seeds—Many grains are actually the seeds of plants; for example, teff, sesame, and wheat are actually the seeds of the plant. The seeds are collected, separated from the stalks, and from there, processed or eaten whole, depending on the type of seed. In addition, seeds can come from vegetables (for example, pumpkin seeds) and flowers (such as sunflower seeds).

What are the more nutritious grains and seeds?

Not every grain is alike. The following list gives some more well-known grains and seeds, along with some interesting facts about their nutritional benefits (for more about these seeds and grains as flours, see below):

Alfalfa seeds—These seeds are rich in minerals (phosphorus, calcium, iron, and potassium) and vitamins A, C, D, E, and K. Most people sprout these seeds or use them whole in baking.

Barley—Barley is thought to have originated in Syria or Northern Egypt. It is actually a member of the grass family, and may have been one of humans' earliest foods. It is rich in many of the B vitamins and phosphorus, and can be hulled (husk removed, bran not) or pearled (husk and bran removed).

Buckwheat—This is actually not a true grain, but a member of the buckwheat family that includes rhubarb, knotweed, dock, and sorrel. It is also called buckwheat groats or kasha, and is rich in protein and several B vitamins, bioflavonoids, phosphorus, and molybdenum.

Bulgur—Bulgur is found as cracked and roasted (precooked) whole-wheat kernels; it has a nutty flavor and cooks relatively fast. Like most wheat products, it is high in B vitamins, vitamin E, and many phytochemicals.

Cornmeal—Cornmeal is from dried corn, which is a giant grass; it comes in several forms, such as polenta (coarse cornmeal) or regular cornmeal. It has been used in many countries for centuries, and is rich in several of the B vitamins.

Cracked wheat—This looks like bulgur, but it is not precooked. As a wheat product, when not processed or milled, it is high in B vitamins, vitamin E, and many phytochemicals.

Kamut—This grain comes from the wheat family; it has an abundance of fiber and protein—more than many other grains. It is available as rice-looking grains or flattened as flakes, and has a buttery taste.

Millet—Millet is a member of the grass family, and is thought to be the staple grain for more than a third of the world's population. It is high in protein and rich in many of the B vitamins and the minerals calcium, phosphorus, and molybdenum. It is also a source of tryptophan, a precursor of serotonin (which helps regulate appetite, sleep patterns, and mood).

Oats—Oats are called a cereal grass, and may be the world's most important edible grain; it comes most often as rolled or steel-cut oats. It is rich in starch, protein, and many of the B vitamins.

Rye—Rye is a nonwheat grain and is found most often in the form of rye berries, flakes, or flour. It is high in fiber (as long as the bran and germ are still retained), and rich in potassium, iron, vitamin B_6, thiamin, niacin, and magnesium.

Teff—Teff has been eaten in Africa for centuries and is thought to be the world's smallest grain. It contains about 10 grams of protein per cup, and has a great deal of calcium, fiber, and B vitamins.

Triticale—Triticale is a rye-wheat hybrid, and usually come in the form of berries. It is very high in protein, and iron, calcium, thiamin, folate, and manganese.

What are chia seeds?

Chia seeds have been in the media lately, mainly referred to as a staple of the "Aztec Diet," an eating plan that highlights the seeds that were once important to the health of the ancient Aztec and Mayan empires. There is good reason for the interest in this seed (although not the diet): it is the highest plant source known to date of omega-3 fatty acids, in the form of ALA (apha-linolenic acid). It also is a complete protein, has more fiber than flaxseed, and has many nutrients, including niacin and magnesium, and antioxidants. Compared to flax, chia has 2 grams of omega-3 (versus flax with 2), 4 grams of fiber (flax has 3), 2 grams of protein (same as flax), and 53 calories (flax has 55) per tablespoon. Although some studies show that chia seeds may lower the risk for cardiovascular disease, this idea is still debated in the health literature. But one study shows promise for those with diabetes: Participants who ate bread containing chia seeds showed lower spikes in blood sugar after eating, along with the feeling of being full for longer.

The best idea is to eat chia seeds in various foods, such as baked goods or even sprinkled on a salad. But beware: People who are sensitive to mustard seeds, sesame

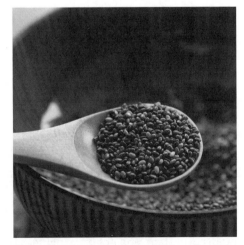

Chia seeds—yes, the same plant that is used in Chia Pets® that you see in commercials!—were eaten by the ancient Aztecs and Mayans.

seeds, oregano, or thyme may be allergic to chia. In addition, check with your doctor before eating chia seeds, especially if you are taking blood thinners or other heart medication.

Why are whole grains so important to nutrition?

Whole grains are important to human nutrition, as long as you're not allergic to gluten (for more about gluten intolerance, see the chapter "Nutrition and Allergies, Illnesses, and Diseases"). Although most are not a complete source of protein, whole grains are an excellent source of starchy carbohydrates and dietary fiber. In addition, whole grains in particular are a good way to take in niacin, vitamin E, riboflavin, phytochemicals (such as lignans and saponins), and other dietary nutrients necessary for good health. The reason nutritionists suggest eating whole grains has to do with the plant itself: the most valuable nutrients are found in the germ and the outer covering. When grains are refined and made into flour or meal, the germ and covering are removed. But whole grains keep both the germ and outer covering, thus retaining nutrients—which also includes much more fiber than refined flours.

Why are quinoa seeds considered to be a "complete" protein?

Quinoa is one of many nonanimal foods that are considered to be a complete protein (another is chia). It is often called a grain, but is actually a seed in the beet and spinach family (*Chenopodiaceae*). It is grown mostly in the Andes of South America, with Bolivia and Peru accounting for 90 percent of the world's production. Some research indicates it has been grown there for more than 5,000 years, as it is one of the few crops that grow well in the poor soil of the dry Andes Mountains. And although the leafy greens of the quinoa plant are edible, its seeds are more well known and eaten more frequently.

The seeds contain many nutrients; a one-cup serving (from ¼ cup dried quinoa) has more iron than any unfortified grain product—at about 4 milligrams. It also has magnesium, phosphorus, potassium, zinc, and numerous B vitamins, including B_6, folate, niacin, and thiamine. It has only 160 calories in the one cup of cooked grain, with 7 grams of protein, and not only includes the amino acid lysine, but is also a good source of saponins, a phytochemical said to help prevent cancer and lower the risk for heart disease.

Is brown rice more nutritious than white rice?

Yes, brown rice is considered to be more nutritious than white rice. All rice starts out "brown," but when some rice is milled, the outer bran layer and nutrient-rich rice germ are scraped away. This creates the white rice that is much faster to cook, and is fluffier and lighter in color. But white rice also loses its fiber and B vitamins when milled, and to compensate, most commercial white rice producers enrich the rice. Thus, many nutrition-conscience buyers pick brown rice for meals if they want the natural nutrients from the rice, not the added nutrients (and often less in amounts). The following chart shows the general nutritional differences between cups of white and brown rice:

White vs. Brown Rice

Nutrient	White Rice	Brown Rice
Fiber (grams)	4.1	4.9
Protein (grams)	0.38	1.25
Calories (or energy)	223.0	232.0
Thiamine (milligrams)	0.04	0.18
Riboflavin (milligrams)	0.02	0.04
Niacin (milligrams)	0.8	2.7
Iron (milligrams)	0.4	1.0
Potassium (milligrams)	57.0	137.0
Magnesium (milligrams)	15.28	60.3
Zinc (milligrams)	0.76	1.25

How did flour develop over time?

For centuries, people have been grinding many types of seeds to make various flours. At first, seeds were roasted and ground by a millstone to make them easier to eat; the ground seeds eventually were mixed with water, forming a crude bread. As more sophisticated methods became available, seeds were ground, sifted, and stored—with today's flours used for producing everything from breads and pastas to being used as thickening agents.

How healthy are flours?

Overall, flour has a high concentration of calories because the water has been removed; for example, one cup of cornmeal flour has about 400 calories, whereas one cup of cooked corn has only about 100 calories. The main nutritional problem with flour is that most of it is milled and processed, meaning many nutrients are lost.

That being said, and although many nutritionists emphasize getting most of your nutrients and fiber from vegetables and fruits, flours still have several health benefits. For example, they are a concentrated source of starch; some have a high-fiber content (especially if they are whole grain or lightly milled or refined); and enriched flours often are nutritional sources of iron and B vitamins.

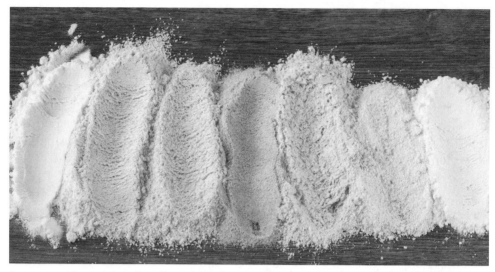

Seven types of flour are shown here (from left to right): all-purpose flour, rye flour, oatmeal, buckwheat flour, wholewheat flour, cornmeal, rice flour. Flour, because it is dense and has little water, provides a high concentration of calories.

What are some types of flour and their nutritional values?

There are numerous types of flour that many of us use or eat every day—from the toast or bagel we eat for breakfast and the bread we eat with our dinner to the cake we bake for a special occasion. The following chart lists some common flours and their general nutritional attributes (most information is from the Academy of Nutrition and Dietetics):

Common Flours and Their Nutritional Value

Flour Type	Nutritional Attributes
Almond	Also called almond meal, it is made by grinding blanched almonds; it has a short shelf-life, and is mostly used in pastries, baked goods, and dessert fillings, not breads; about one-quarter cup of almond flour has 6 grams of protein, 3.5 grams of fiber, and 60 milligrams of calcium; it is low in carbohydrates and has about 14 grams of fat in one-quarter cup, but it is nearly all unsaturated; gluten-free
Amaranth	High in complete protein; contains more of the amino acid lysine than most other flours; from ancient seed, it has a slightly sweet, nutty flavor; gluten-free
Arrowroot	A flour that is made from maranta roots; it is one of the most digestible flours
Barley	Flour from milled pearl or whole grain barley; has about 4 grams of fiber (soluble) in one-quarter cup; used as a thickener in soups, stews, and sauces
Buckwheat	Made by grinding buckwheat, which is not technically a grain, but is a cousin of the rhubarb plant; its seeds are considered the same seeds as kasha, and have a grassy flavor; it comes as white buckwheat and whole buckwheat, which has a stronger flavor and more nutrients than white; overall, it is high in lysine, magnesium, and manganese; gluten-free

Common Flours and Their Nutritional Value

Flour Type	Nutritional Attributes
Cornmeal	Not as nutritious as most flours but, when combined with beans and other legumes, provides a complete protein
Fish	A flour made by grinding up whole, dried, defatted fish; high in calcium and protein
Flaxseed	Also called flaxseed meal, it is made by grinding whole flaxseed; it is high in lignans, omega-3 fatty acids, and fiber (2 tablespoons has 4 grams of fiber); it is often used in baked goods as a substitute for eggs or fats; gluten-free
Oat	Made by grinding whole oat groats; it is high in soluble fiber and some B vitamins, calcium, and phosphorus; it is mostly used in breads and has a rich, nutty flavor and denser texture than other flours; gluten-free
Potato	Made by grinding whole, dried potatoes; one-quarter cup has 2.5 grams of fiber; like most potato foods, it is high in potassium (one-quarter cup has 400 milligrams of potassium); it is used to thicken liquids (in soups, stews, or sauces) and in breads (it makes them more moist and extends their freshness); gluten-free
Pumpernickel	(See Rye)
Rice, brown	Made by grinding unpolished brown rice; one-quarter cup has 2 grams of fiber (white rice flour, most often made from short grained rice, has about 1 gram of fiber); it is used for baked goods and as coating for lightly fried or sautéed foods (often as a substitute for all purpose flour); it has a nutty flavor; gluten-free
Rye	High in fiber as long as the bran and germ are retained; it is heavy and dark, with less gluten than all-purpose or whole-wheat flour and produces heavy breads (pumpernickel flour is dark rye flour made from whole grains); one-quarter cup has about 5 grams of fiber and 4 grams of protein; it is high in iron, and low in sugar and fats
Sorghum	Made by grinding sorghum; it is high in antioxidants and some fiber (one-quarter cup has about 2 grams of fiber); it has a mild flavor and is used in breads, baked goods, pastas, and cereals; gluten-free
Soy	Made by grinding soybeans; it is high in protein and low in carbohydrates and fats; it is a good source of calcium, iron, and magnesium; one-quarter cup has 10 grams of protein, 8 grams total carbohydrates, and 3 grams of fiber; used as a whole-wheat or all-purpose flour substitute, or as an ingredient in breads, baked goods, or even pancake mixes and cereals; gluten-free
Spelt	Made by grinding spelt, a cousin of the wheat plant; one-quarter cup contains 4 grams of protein, 4 grams of fiber, and 1.5 grams of iron; it has a light nutty flavor; often substituted for wheat flours in baking
Triticale	A hybrid of wheat and rye; rich in several of the B vitamins; high in protein, and often mixed with wheat flour to increase its nutritional value

What is gluten?

Gluten is a substance found mostly in wheat; the amount varies in such flours as rye and barley. The gluten in certain flours is responsible for the rising of the bread: when the flour and yeast are mixed with a liquid, the gluten proteins absorb the liquid and makes the dough elastic. This also allows the yeast's released gases to be trapped, which makes the baked good lighter, mainly because of the "holes" the gases produce. (For more about bread, see the chapter "Food Chemistry and Nutrition.")

Why are grains good—and bad—for some people?

Although grains have not been in the human diet for long, they do offer a relatively easy ways to obtain some nutrients—along with being more economical than other dietary foods, such as meat and fish—for a large number of people. Although a person's entire diet should not consist only of grains, most nutritionists believe that a balanced diet should include some grains. The best choices are whole grains, which are less processed than milled grains; these grains contain a good deal of vitamins and minerals, along with dietary fiber and starchy carbohydrates.

But not all grains are good for people. Those who suffer from what is called gluten intolerance have a slight to moderate—usually gastrointestinal—reaction to cereal grain products, especially wheat; celiac disease is a more severe intolerance to grain products, resulting in more extreme gastrointestinal and other health problems. (For more about gluten intolerance and celiac disease, see the chapter "Nutrition and Allergies, Illnesses, and Diseases.")

Are there gluten-free grains?

Yes, there are grains that are "gluten-free." For example, the grains millet and teff are gluten-free; plus, foods made with corn, rice, potato, or soy flour are usually gluten-free. But be aware: Check labels to see if there are any non-gluten-free ingredients if you can't

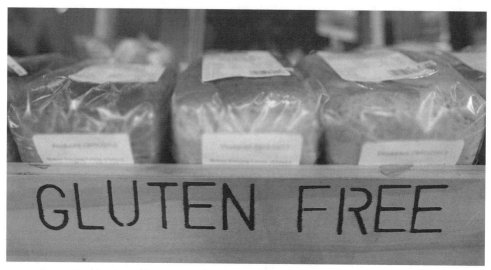

Some people who suffer from celiac disease or gluten intolerance may need to switch to breads made from gluten-free grains to avoid gastrointestinal distress.

have wheat products. This is particularly important if heavier grains, such as barley, are listed in the ingredients, because wheat flour is often added to a dough to make the prepared food lighter.

What are non-nutrients?

Contrary to popular belief, there is more to nutrition than just vitamins and minerals. Scientists classify these substances as non-nutrients (or nonnutrients)—all of which play an important role in keeping our bodies healthy. Included in this list are the non-nutrient antioxidants, bioflavonoids, and even water.

ANTIOXIDANTS

What are antioxidants?

In general, antioxidants are any substance—and there are many—that helps to eliminate free radicals in our bodies. For example, antioxidants include the micronutrients vitamins C and E, and the non-nutrients anthocyanidins and quercetin. Because your body is subjected to oxidation (similar to what happens when a cut apple is exposed to air)—our bodies "age" over time. This oxidation can eventually damage your cells and organs; in fact, it is known that oxidation (called oxidative stress) is a factor in almost all of the degenerative diseases, and is why our bodies (inside and out) age as we get older. The antioxidants in foods help to keep these free radicals at bay—and without such antioxidants, the oxidation can eventually lead to heart disease, cancer, and age-related declines in our body and minds. (For more about antioxidants, free radicals, and vitamins, see the chapter "The Basics of Nutrition: Micronutrients.")

Are there any non-nutrient antioxidants?

Yes, like the nutrient antioxidants—or vitamins and minerals that act like or are considered to be antioxidants—there are several major non-nutrient antioxidants and other substances that protect the human body from free radicals (the byproducts of oxidation). They include the antioxidants known as carotenoids, phytochemicals, and polyphenols; and the compounds called phytoestrogens. (For more about micronutrients as antioxidants, see the chapter "The Basics of Nutrition: Micronutrients.")

Are there health benefits when you eat foods that contain more than one type of antioxidant?

Yes, there are definite health benefits when you eat foods that contain more than one type of antioxidant (and most plant-based foods do contain more than one). This is because different types of antioxidants fight different oxidants, and the antioxidants will often work together to refresh one another, enhance the absorption in your system, and even increase the antioxidant activity. For example, some people put a pinch of cayenne (a spicy spice) in their green tea; both contain certain types of antioxidants and this boosts the green tea's antioxidants by almost 100 times. By using a small amount of black pepper with turmeric, it helps you better absorb the spice's antioxidants; and even a few leaves of the marjoram plant (an herb) in a salad can boost the antioxidant activity over 100 percent.

What are the non-nutrient antioxidants called carotenoids?

Carotenoids are non-nutrient antioxidants that help destroy free-radical-causing agents. There are many carotenoids, including beta carotene (which the body turns into vitamin A), lutein, and lycopene. They are found in colorful fruits and vegetables, such as carrots and dark leafy greens.

What are the non-nutrient antioxidants called phytochemicals?

Phytochemicals (sometimes called phytonutrients) act like non-nutrient antioxidants, and are found in fruits and vegetables. They are thought to have evolved naturally in plants, as a way that vegetables and fruits protect themselves from the sun's damaging rays. There are many types of phytochemicals—including polyphenols and bioflavonoids—found in such foods as soybeans and soy products, and hot chili peppers, tomatoes, broccoli, citrus fruits, berries, apricots, garlic, and onions.

How do phytochemicals affect our health?

Although there are many differences in opinion about phytochemicals, almost all scientists agree these chemical compounds seem to be good for our health. For example, some phytochemicals seem to stimulate enzymes; some seem to have antibacterial properties, physically binding to a cell wall and stopping a pathogen from adhering to the cell; and others appear to interfere with DNA replication, and thus are often thought to play a role in cancer prevention. But don't imagine that you can just take them as supplements and not eat your vegetables—eating natural phytochemicals is best for supporting health. In addition, scientists now realize that separating phytochemicals is not as effective for our health as eating foods in which many phytochemicals exist.

What are some examples of beneficial phytochemicals?

There are many phytochemicals that appear to be beneficial to human health. For example, curcumin is a compound that gives the spice turmeric its yellow color—and may be effective in the prevention of some inflammatory diseases. Another phytochemical is organosulfur, a compound associated with garlic—and often said to help prevent certain diseases. And there is even a phytochemical in celery called apigenin that works as an anti-inflammatory.

What are the non-nutrient antioxidants called polyphenols?

Polyphenols are specific types of phytochemicals that have antioxidant properties. They occur naturally in plants—and have several health perks, such as improved thinking, reducing the risk for heart disease, and reducing inflammation. Overall, it is thought that a high dietary intake of polyphenols is associated with longevity—one recent study showed that high polyphenol intake includes a 30 percent reduction in mortality in older adults. And with more than 8,000 phenolic compounds identified in plants, you have a great deal to choose from for longevity!

The many polyphenols seem to have some amount of antioxidant, anti-inflammatory, and/or anticarcinogenic effects. For example, the polyphenols called lignans—found in seeds such as flaxseeds, whole grains, legumes, and many fruits and vegetables—may play a role in preventing osteoporosis and cardiovascular diseases. In addition, there is evidence that foods containing polyphenols may help boost a person's insulin—and two of the best foods for such a task are raspberries and dark chocolate.

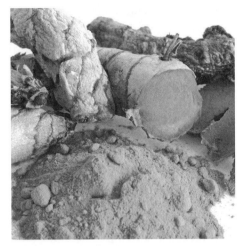

Curcumin is a compound that gives the spice turmeric (familiar in curry dishes, for example) its yellow color.

What are some foods containing healthy polyphenols?

Some of the best foods to eat that are rich in all types of healthy polyphenols are yams, onions, nuts, strawberries, raspberries, dark chocolate, legumes, apples, cereals, coffee, tea (green and black), and wine (see below for more about red wine and polyphenols).

What fruit is high in polyphenols, but only when it's raw?

One popular fruit is high in polyphenols: blueberries. But be aware: You have to eat them raw for the best benefits. If the berries are processed, by such methods as juicing and canning, it is thought that the polyphenol levels decrease by 22 to 81 percent. Further studies of baking, cooking, and proofing foods that contain blueberries showed that changes in several of the polyphenol levels had mixed results—some compounds dropped, some stayed the same, while others increased. For example, the anthocyanin levels dropped by 10 to 21 percent; quercetin remained constant; while the phenolic acid levels increased. In other words, the best way to eat blueberries for their high polyphenol content is to eat them raw—and be aware that your next piece of blueberry pie is giving you fewer antioxidants.

Is dark chocolate healthy to eat?

Dark chocolate is not only a favorite of chocoholics, but is also thought to be good for your health. In 2014, researchers discovered that dark chocolate helps restore flexibility to arteries, and also helps prevent white blood cells from sticking to the walls of the body's blood vessels—both factors that can cause arthrosclerosis (what is often called "hardening of the arteries," or blockage by plaque in the arteries). The dark chocolate ingredient thought to be responsible is flavanol, an antioxidant found in cocoa. Other studies have shown that the cocoa's flavanols (not all are created equal) may also help prevent obesity, as well as type 2 diabetes. Yet another study indicated that extra-dark chocolate (or "raw" non-Dutched cocoa) may benefit your memory and increase brain function. But health-care professionals warn that too much chocolate—whether it's dark or the more-fatty-milk chocolate—can cause weight gain and not help your health.

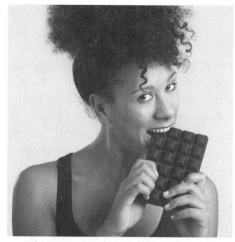

It was happy news for chocolate lovers when dietary experts declared that dark chocolate—at least, in small amounts—is actually good for your health! But the study has been highly debated since then.

Why is red wine sometimes healthy for people to drink?

When it comes to red wine, there are certain polyphenols that are abundant, and act as antioxidants by protecting the cells from damage as they go through oxidation. In particular, the skins and seeds of grapes, and red wine, contain resveratrol, one of many polyphenols. And because polyphenols may inhibit the oxidation of LDL—also known as "the bad cholesterol" in our system that can clog our blood vessels and often lead to heart disease and other health problems—a glass of red wine or two may help stave off such problems. But most doctors agree: Even though red wine may have helpful resveratrol, it is not wise to drink too much wine. As with everything in nutrition and health, moderation is the key.

Recent studies (highly debated) have also suggested that the polyphenols in red wine (and green tea) may inhibit prostate cancer growth—actually disrupting an important cell-signaling pathway necessary for the cancer to grow. It is hoped that this discovery may lead to the development of drugs that could stop or slow other cancer growth, such as colon, breast, and gastric cancers.

What is the mystery behind the polyphenols in red wine and grapes?

Researchers have had a difficult time pinpointing where the helpful polyphenols come from in red wine—are they truly from the grapes (skin, pulp, and seed), or do they develop after certain modifications take place in the wine's aging process? What scientists do know at this time is that grape and wine polyphenols are chemically distinct, and thus, their antioxidant activities are probably not the same. Either way, and no matter where they come from, these antioxidants are still considered by most researchers to be a good antiaging substance. But don't think you can only get these wonderful polyphenols by drinking wine or eating grapes—you can get the same antioxidants from other fruits and vegetables, such as cranberries, boiled peanuts, and blueberries—and even chocolate.

What recent study indicated that red wine and dark chocolate are not as healthy as we think?

A study in 2014 disappointed many lovers of red wine and dark chocolate: The antioxidant resveratrol found in red wine, chocolate, and grapes may not really be associated with longevity or a lower risk for cardiovascular disease, some cancers, and inflammation. The study looked at residents in two small Tuscany towns over several years; the researchers discovered that there was no real association between higher levels of resveratrol and a lower risk for heart disease or cancer—in fact, the lower rates of heart disease were in people with the lowest levels of resveratrol. The research doesn't surprise many scientists. Many believe it's not just a single substance in a certain food, such as resveratrol, that equates with a lower risk for any disease, but the combination of other ingredients in the foods. In other words, fruits and vegetables are loaded with a lot of phytochemicals (including resveratrol), which work together with the vitamins and minerals in the plant to help promote health and fight disease.

What are the non-nutrients called phytoestrogens?

The phytoestrogens are a group of natural compounds found in food that resemble the chemical estrogen; they are also considered to be phytochemicals. The most common products that contain phytoestrogens are soybeans and their related forms—such as soy milk, tofu, soy flour, tempeh, and miso.

Are foods that contain phytoestrogens controversial?

Yes, there have been several studies that list phytoestrogens, especially in soy products, as good, while other reports say the foods are harmful. Some research indicates that phytoestrogens affect male and female (especially postmenopausal) hormone levels to some extent; while other studies mention that the substances are too weak to cause the body to respond to the "pseudo-estrogen," and thus, problems with taking soy products for most people is not an issue. Either way, the connection between phytoestrogens and humans continues to be a highly debated subject. (For more about postmenopausal women and nutrition, see the chapter "Nutrition throughout Life"; for more about controversies and soy products, see the chapter "Controversies with Food, Beverages, and Nutrition.")

BIOFLAVONOIDS (FLAVONOIDS)

What are the bioflavonoids (or flavonoids)?

Bioflavonoids (or flavonoids; also often called vitamin P, although they are not true vitamins) are a group of phytochemicals thought to function as antioxidants; they are also considered to be a large family of polyphenolic compounds (for more about polyphenols, see above). They are a naturally occurring group—all with a common feature in their molecular structure—that acts primarily as plant pigments (giving plants their color) and flavorants. So far, scientists have identified more than 3,000 naturally occurring bioflavonoids. Overall, most bioflavonoids seem to play a role in cell-signaling pathways; they have also been suggested as the best substance to lower blood pressure, as found in such foods as raspberries and dark chocolate.

What are some common dietary bioflavonoids?

In most health literature, the dietary bioflavonoids (or flavonoids) are placed into many different classes; they include such classes as anthocyanidins (the most prevalent), flavanols, flavanones, flavonols, flavones, and isoflavones. The following lists these few classes and some foods rich in the specific bioflavonoid:

Foods Rich in Bioflavonoids

Bioflavonoid Class	Foods
Anthocyanidins	Red, purple, and blue berries; eggplant; red and purple grapes; red wine; purple cabbage
Flavanols	Divided into catechins (teas, especially green and white; dark chocolate; grapes; berries; and apples), theaflavins and thearubigins (teas such as black and oolong); and proanthocyanidins (chocolate, apples, berries, red grapes, and red wine)
Flavanones	Citrus fruits and juices (oranges and lemons, for examples)
Flavonols	Wide variety, such as yellow onions, scallions, kale, broccoli, apples, berries, and tea
Flavones	Parsley, thyme, celery, hot peppers
Isoflavones	Soybeans, soy products, legumes

What is the difference between anthocyanins and anthocyanidins?

Many times in the general media, the terms *anthocyanins* and *anthocyanidins* are used interchangeably—but there is a subtle difference. The anthocyanins are a class of bioflavonoid pigments; and after a certain type of reaction (hydrolysis), they produce what are called *anthocyanins*.

What are the connections between vitamin C and bioflavonoids?

Bioflavonoids are thought to apparently enhance the antioxidant effect of vitamin C (they were discovered at the same time, too). Still other research indicates that some bioflavonoids may help the body absorb and use vitamin C.

What are some foods high in a combination of different bioflavonoids?

There are many foods high in the various types of bioflavonoids—not just one. For example, foods rich in multiple bioflavonoids include black currants, broccoli, cherries, raspberries, green peppers, tomatoes, plums, cocoa (and dark chocolate), and even black tea and coffee.

In what ways do bioflavonoids protect the body?

The antioxidant-like benefits of bioflavonoids continue to be found—with the best sources being a wide variety of plant foods daily. In particular, studies have found that bioflavonoids improve capillary strength (smaller blood vessels in the body that allow oxygen, hormones, nutrients, and antibodies to travel from the bloodstream to individual cells) by helping the vessels' walls to remain strong. Bioflavonoids also seem to help prevent blood clot formation, especially important in treating phlebitis (the inflammation of a vein where clots may form), and to lower cholesterol. Some even destroy certain bacteria, retard food spoilage, and even protect humans from some foodborne infections.

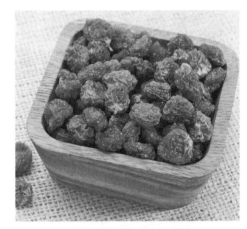

Dried goldenberry (*Physalis peruviana*) is a superfruit from Peru that is rich in antioxidants, vitamin A, bioflavonoids, and dietary fiber.

Can you be deficient in bioflavonoids?

Yes, like certain macronutrients and micronutrients, you can be deficient in bioflavonoids. In particular, the symptoms are similar to those of a vitamin C deficiency; they include an increased tendency to bleed or hemorrhage and bruise easily.

Why are bioflavonoids good for plants, in an indirect way?

Besides of the health benefits of bioflavonoids for most organisms, they contribute to the "continuation of species" effect when it comes to plants. In particular, bioflavonoids found in fruits attract animals by displaying colors such as yellow, red, blue, and purple; the animals eat the fruit and then disperse the plants' seeds, ensuring the plants' survival. Bioflavonoids are also the reason for the many colors of certain flowers—common in such plants as berries, eggplant, and citrus fruits, such as lemons and oranges—and thus attract insect pollinators, another way of continuing plant species.

What are some therapeutic uses of bioflavonoids?

Although several therapeutic uses of bioflavonoids are still being studied, the following list discusses a few of the more well-known connections:

Quercetin—This bioflavonoid is found in many fruits and vegetables, including apples, onions, tea, grapes, citrus fruits, cherries, and many other foods. It is thought that quercetin may improve lung function and help to lower the risk for asthma, emphysema, and other respiratory diseases. It has also been the subject of several prostate cancer studies, and is thought to help block male hormones that encourage the growth of cancer cells within the prostate.

Rutin—Rutin is a bioflavonoid found in such plants as buckwheat leaves. In particular, it has been studied for treating glaucoma, retinal bleeding in diabetics, and also to help reduce tissue damage from frostbite.

Hesperidin—This bioflavonoid is found in foods such as the peels of oranges, lemons, and other citrus fruits. It is thought to be helpful in treating bleeding abnormalities and for people who bruise easily.

What are citrus bioflavonoids?

Citrus bioflavonoids are just as they imply—citrus fruits containing bioflavonoids that improve our health. They include diosmin, hesperidin, rutin, naringin, tangeretin, diosmetin, narirutin, quercetin, and nobiletin. In Europe, the citrus bioflavonoids and related compounds are used to treat diseases specific to blood vessels (including hemorrhoids, easy bruising, and nosebleeds [especially diosmin and hesperidin]) and to treat problems in the lymphatic system (such as lymphedema, or arm swelling following breast cancer surgery). There is some debate as to how the citrus bioflavonoids respond in humans, and although it is thought that most bioflavonoids act like antioxidants, some researchers believe that the citrus bioflavonoids do not, but have a different "method" of helping our health.

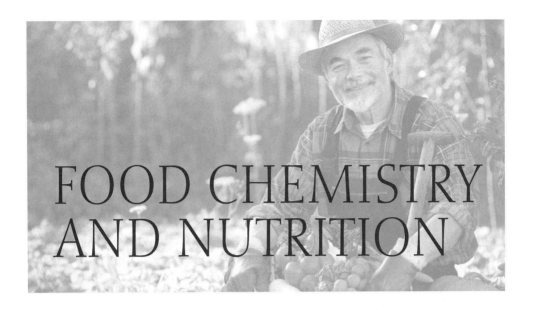

FOOD CHEMISTRY AND NUTRITION

FOODS DEFINED

What is the definition of food?

The definition of food is complex, mainly because that one word describes a number of things. In general, food covers anything we eat that has (and sometimes does not have) a nutritious value to maintain our health.

When it comes to nutrition and health, what matters is the way we approach our foods. For instance, we have to make a selection of foods that keep us healthy; we have to choose a cooking method (and recipe) that will not only match our cooking skills, but also be the most nutritious way to cook the foodstuff; and we have to make sure we eat enough—or not too much—of certain nutritious foods to maintain our health.

What are some chemical constituents of food?

Chemically speaking, almost all foods contain some type of carbon—from vegetables to meat. The biggest reasons for the different chemical compositions of foods are the source of the foods and the nutrients (or non-nutrients) they contain—for instance, from animals and plants to fungi, or from vitamin C and zinc to water.

How are certain nutrients destroyed—other than by cooking methods?

Various nutrients in foods are affected by cooking (see this chapter)—but also by other methods, such as the mechanical action of milling. For example, vitamin B_5 (pantothenic acid) decreases in foods, depending on the process: It decreases by about 33 percent during cooking; it is easily destroyed by heating in acids, such as vinegar, or basic sources (alkali), such as baking soda; about 50 percent is lost by the milling of flour that contains the vitamin; and a high, dry heat—such as that employed during dehydration of foods containing vitamin B$_5$—also destroys much of this vitamin.

INSIDE MEATS

How is meat defined?

In general, no matter what animal—from cows and lambs to pigs and buffalo—the "meat" many people eat is most often defined as the flesh of animals. Some people also define "meats" as only the flesh from mammals—or those raised for human consumption—but not from fish and sea creatures, poultry, and other organisms, even though these other animals also supply water, protein, fats, and carbohydrates. Another common way to define meats is as "red versus white" meats: The red meats "turn red" when proteins (myoglobin) in the animal's narrow muscle fibers are exposed to oxygen; most adult mammals (cows, cattle, sheep, etc.) are considered this type of meat. White meat refers to certain muscle fibers in an animal that are broader than those found in red meat—and usually includes the breast meat of chicken and turkey.

Are fish and seafood considered meat?

Yes, most fish and seafood are considered to be meat by most people, but they are often classified by themselves (something you often see in cookbook listings). But they really are meats, as—like meats from cattle, sheep, or any other "land" animal—fish and seafood have a combination of proteins, carbohydrates, fats, and calories that are readily available for human consumption. Most white-flesh fish are high in protein, low in fat (compared to most other sources of animal protein), loaded with vitamins and minerals, and with fewer calories. And most nutritionists who believe omega-3s are important to human health emphasize that certain fish—for instance, salmon, mackerel, herring, sardines, and sablefish—have some of the highest amounts of these healthy fatty acids. (For more about omega-3s and other fatty acids, see the chapter "The Basics of Nutrition: Macronutrients and Non-nutrients.")

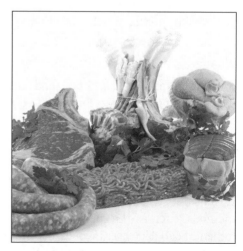

What is the overall content of most meats?

Overall, meat from mammal sources is mostly muscle, with surrounding fats, taken from various parts of an animal's

Meat is, simply, flesh from an animal. It contains protein, fats, water, and carbohydrates, primarily.

body; it is made up of roughly 70 to 75 percent water, 20 percent protein, 2 to 5 percent fat, 1 to 2 percent carbohydrates, and the rest is other assorted nonprotein substances. One reason why meat has some of the greatest nutritional values is because of the amino acids in the muscles (all needed for human health); the iron content; and with some meats, the abundance of essential fatty acids and B-complex vitamins (for more about nutrition and meats, see below).

What are the major parts of meat from most animals?

Most animal muscle (what we call meat) contains fiber, water, tissue, and fats. The following list describes several major parts of (most) animal muscle:

Muscle fiber—Each cut of meat has several thousand thin, several-inch-long, individual muscle fibers—all of which are finer than a human hair; each fiber is a single muscle cell made up of smaller, rod-shaped units called myofibrils. Wrapped in connective tissue, the individual fibers are seen as thin strands in the meat—what is often referred to as the grain of certain meats.

Connective tissues—The muscle fibers are held together by a thin, translucent sheath made up primarily of the protein called collagen, which also helps to attach the muscles to the bone.

Proteins—A meat's fibers are filled with filaments made up of two different proteins—actin and myosin. These protein filaments allow the animal's muscles to relax and contract.

Water—When you cook a piece of meat, it often appears to release "steam"—mainly because most meat (muscle) is made up of water. Most of the water in muscles is found in the myofibrils; the rest resides in the spaces between the muscle fibers.

Fat—In a piece of meat, fats are contained (and produced) in what are called adipose cells—a special form of connective tissue that also stores energy (for more about adipose cells, see the chapter "The Basics of Nutrition: Macronutrients and Non-nutrients"). Fat is most often found in two places on a piece of meat—the layer around the muscle and the fat as thin filaments running through the muscle (what is often referred to as marbling; see Sidebar).

What is marbling?

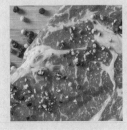 When discussing cuts of meat—especially beef—marbling refers to the fat (usually seen as small white flecks) throughout the red, uncooked muscle. Most chefs agree that more white flecks means a higher quality cut of meat. This is because fat contributes to—and is an indicator of—the tenderness, juiciness, and especially flavor of most pieces of meat.

Why is meat called a "prime food"?

Meat has had an important role in human evolution, and is often called a prime food, because it helps us produce energy, aids in the formation of tissue, and regulates some chemical reactions and physiologic processes in the body. And although most meat is about 70 to 75 percent water (usually higher in younger animals and lower in older animals), meat still provides enough nutrition to accomplish these tasks in the human body.

What are some differences in nutrients between some meats?

There are many meats, all with a certain nutritional content. The following table lists some of the more common ones, including the approximate number of calories, carbohydrates,* and fats based on a quarter pound of meat (4 ounces; 110 grams), which, in this list, also means fish. This data, and more about various meats and their nutritional values, can be found on the USDA site at http://ndb.nal.usda.gov/ndb/nutrients/index.

Meats and Their Nutrients

Meat Source	Calories	Carbohydrates	Fat
T-bone steak	450	0 grams	35 grams
Lamb	250	0 grams	14 grams
Pork (center loin)	205	0 grams	9 grams
Chicken (breast)	160	0 grams,	8 grams
Chicken (dark meat)	220	0 grams	15 grams
Fish (various)	110–140	0 grams	1–5 grams
Salmon (wild)	185	0 grams	8.5 grams

Note: The meats in this short list have no carbohydrates; this is because most carbohydrates are in breads, cereals, and other starchy foods, whereas certain meats have only a trace. For example, liver, bacon, and cured ham have a small amount of carbohydrates, whereas processed foods, such as some luncheon meats and sausages, have more carbohydrates.

Why is meat thought by many nutritionists to be important to human nutrition?

Many nutritionists believe that meat is an important component of a balanced diet. In general, meat is a valuable source of what is called "a high biological value protein," with the proteins containing all the essential amino acids beneficial to humans. Most meats also contain highly absorbable iron, along with the minerals zinc, selenium, and phosphorus; and meats can contain a good deal of water-soluble B-complex and some C vitamins, along with fat-soluble vitamins A, D, E, and K. And finally, when eaten in moderation—and depending on the animal species, what they were fed, or even if the cut of meat is from an internal or external part of the animal—the fat and fatty acid content of meat is often considered by some nutritionists to be important to human nutrition. (For more about meat and human evolution, see the chapter "Nutrition through the Centuries," for more about vitamins and minerals, see the chapter "The Basics of Nutrition: Micronutrients," and for more about fats, see the chapter "The Basics of Nutrition: Macronutrients and Non-nutrients.")

Why do some people disagree with eating meat?

Of course, the importance of meat in the human diet is often countered by those who eat a vegetarian or vegan diet. Vegetarians get most of their "missing" meat-based nutrients—or those not readily found in a plant-based diet—from various vegetables, fruits, certain vegetable oils,

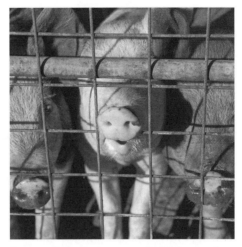

Some people don't eat meat on principle because they feel that farm animals are mistreated.

whole grains, and if needed (as is often the case with B_{12}), supplements. Many vegetarians and vegans stop eating meats for a variety of reasons, including wanting to stay away from the fats associated with meats; for personal reasons, such as religious beliefs; for environmental reasons, such as wanting to stop the elimination of forests for grazing animals; or they just don't believe in killing living organisms for food. For many vegans and vegetarians the idea of "cruelty-free" in terms of animals stretches into the clothes they choose to wear (none from animals, such as leather, feathers, wool, or fur) to the products they use (none tested on animals). (For more about vegetarian and vegan diets, see the chapter "Nutrition and You" and Appendix 3: "Comparing Diets.")

How do different meats—from cattle and pigs to poultry and fish—differ in protein content?

Many of the meats we eat have different amounts of protein. The following chart lists some of the more common meats, including fish, and their grams of protein content, per 100 grams of food (about 3.5 ounces), unless noted (written in grams to make the comparisons easier to see), as per the U.S. Department of Agriculture listing:

Meats and Their Protein Content

Meat	Protein in Grams
Beef, bottom sirloin, lean, cooked, roasted	22.39
Beef chuck for stew, cooked, braised	27.62
Beef, ground, 85% lean, patties, cooked, braised	22.04
Chicken broiler or fryer, drumstick, cooked or stewed	23.38
Chicken liver, cooked, pan-fried (for 1 liver)	11.34
Ground turkey, 85% lean, patties, broiled	22.00

Meats and Their Protein Content

Meat	Protein in Grams
Turkey thigh, from whole bird, roasted	23.55
Pork, cured, ham rump, bone in, roasted	22.12
Shrimp, cooked, breaded and fried	18.18
Halibut, Atlantic and Pacific, cooked with dry heat	19.16
Salmon, sockeye, cooked with dry heat	21.59
Tuna, light, canned in water, no salt, drained solids	21.68
Scallops (bay and sea), cooked, steamed	17.46

What are considered the best cuts of meat and why?

The best cuts of meat are usually considered to be those that are moist, not too fatty, and tender. For most meats (not including fish) that means the cuts from muscles that the animal did not use to move—such as those from the midsection. Those cuts that are from the hip or shoulder area are tougher meats and may need more marinating, tenderizing, and/or cooking to make them more edible.

How do certain meats become tough?

In many cases, the way meat is treated after an animal is slaughtered will often have a bearing on the tenderness or toughness of the piece. For example, since there is no blood flow anymore in the animal, there is a buildup of lactic acid that stays in the muscle. If the lactic acid amount is too high, the meat cannot bind to water, and it becomes pale and watery; if there is not enough lactic acid in the muscle, the meat becomes dry and tough. In addition, if a animal carcass is frozen too soon after the animal dies, the proteins actin and myosin bind together, causing the meat to be tough. This is often why meat is aged, allowing the enzymes in the muscle cells to break down the proteins and make the meat more tender. (For more about aging meats, see the chapter "Food Preservation and Nutrition.")

What is freezer burn, and how does it affect the meat?

Freezer burn occurs when a food is frozen and water vapor escapes from the food's surface. It is often associated with meat, al-

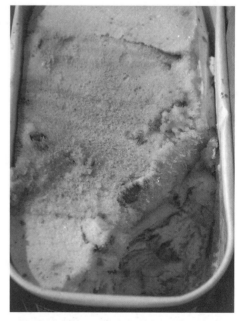

When foods are not sealed properly in a freezer, the result is freezer burn; water vapor escapes, leaving the food dry and tasteless.

though it can also happen to frozen vegetables and fruit. With frozen meat, the water vapor condenses on the interior of the package; this results in an off-colored piece of meat that is usually covered with ice crystals. Such meat should be avoided if seen in the meat department of your grocery store. It is usually safe to eat, but it means that moisture has escaped from the food—and that more often than not means a dry, tough piece of meat that often smells and tastes like the freezer!

The best way to stop freezer burn is to take the meat out of the package when you get back from the grocery (or local farm or farmer's market), wrap each chunk of meat individually (if applicable) in plastic or freezer paper—and put them in zipper-lock bags, pressing as much of the excess air from the bag as possible. According to the FDA, freezing foods at 0 degrees Fahrenheit (–18 degrees Celsius) can keep food safe indefinitely; but depending on the meat, if it is not eaten within a certain amount of time, the quality can be greatly affected. For example, raw hamburger, ground turkey, and stew meats can stay wrapped well in the freezer for three to four months without problems with quality; fresh whole chicken can last for about a year well-wrapped in the freezer; while bacon should be kept in the freezer for only about one month.

INSIDE VEGETABLES, FRUITS, AND LEGUMES

What part of a plant do humans benefit from the most?

The answer is simple: Humans benefit from all parts of a plant, from the roots to the stems and flowers (depending on the plant, of course). Plants are good for us because they combine water, carbon dioxide from the air, and nutrients from the soil—all necessary to humans' (and other organisms') health. Most plants are rich in vitamins A, C, and E, folate, and most of the B vitamins; in terms of minerals, they are rich in potassium and many others, depending on the vegetable. In addition, vegetables have high fiber, and are usually rich in bioflavonoids and antioxidants. Probably the only true drawback of vegetables is that some contain allergens that affect certain people. Otherwise, there's a reason why your mother always said, "Eat your vegetables!"

Why do humans (and other organisms) benefit from plant photosynthesis?

Photosynthesis is a process by which plants use energy from sunlight to manufacture food molecules from carbon dioxide (mostly from the air) and water (from the air and ground). The term is from the Greek word *photo*, meaning "light," and the Greek word *syntithenai*, meaning "to put together." First, sunlight is converted to chemical energy, with oxygen produced as a waste product (which is why greenhouses always make you feel so good—they are filled with oxygen released from the plants); second, a series of reactions convert carbon dioxide into organic compounds—mainly sugar molecules and other energy-containing products; and it is this sugar (or carbohydrates) that humans obtain when they eat vegetables. This is why many researchers state that photosynthesis is the process that provides food for the entire world. It is estimated that each year more than 250 billion metric tons of sugar are created through the photosynthesis process. It not only creates a source of food for the plants, but also provides nutrient-rich foods for all organisms that cannot internally produce their own food—including humans.

Why is plant chlorophyll important?

During photosynthesis, plant chlorophyll is the compound that turns carbon dioxide and water into carbohydrates (starches) while releasing oxygen into the atmosphere. It is also why plants are green in color—and many researchers believe it was color that helped ancient humans decide which vegetables were good to eat (see Sidebar). Chlorophyll is also found in other organisms, such as some algae, but in terms of eating, we associate the compound with plants.

If you have a garden, when is the best time to pick vegetables for eating?

If you have a garden (or know a local farmer who grows vegetables), there are times when certain vegetables should be picked for the best nutritional value. In particular, if a vegetable stays on the plant until it is ripe, it will contain more nutrients; if it is picked too early and ripens on your table or in a sunny window, it will have fewer nutrients. This is also why most growers who sell frozen vegetables will pick, blanch (cover with boiling water a very short time to kill off some of the enzymes that cause deterioration), and freeze ripe vegetables in the same day, which usually means the foods retain most of their nutrient value.

Is it good to refrigerate your vegetables?

The majority of research shows that the sooner you eat a vegetable—especially those picked from the garden or field—the more nutrients are available to your body. But depending on the vegetable, refrigeration can help preserve the food for a while, but not as long as most people think, or not as long as most people leave vegetables sitting in their refrigerator before they eat the food (or have to toss it out). Overall, there has been some research regarding the nutrient value of most vegetables over a wide range of conditions and for all nutrients, but not very much.

For example, a great deal of research has been done on the vitamin C content of

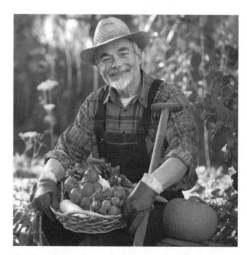

Good gardeners know that harvest time for fruits and veggies vary depending on where you live. Produce picked at its peak of ripeness has the most nutritional value.

How is the color of food thought to be tied to human evolution?

There are many colorful vegetables and fruits growing on the Earth—and one recent study explores a theory connecting foods' colors and human evolution. In particular, humans (and birds) are the only organisms thought to have color vision (or to see the full color spectrum). It's true that other species do see other "colors," but differently, such as bees seeing blue, violet, and purple as being the same hue. This human ability to see colors probably evolved as a way for us to not only see better, but to eat better. This is because most of the colorful fruits and vegetables are the most nutritious—from red peppers and purple potatoes to orange carrots—and are easily seen in a green background. For example, the deeper the red-purple of a vegetable, the higher the anthocyanin (a bioflavonoid that acts like an antioxidant) concentration, thought to be effective in reducing the risk for heart diseases, improving eyesight, and helping prevent certain cancers.

various vegetables, but little has been done on the losses of B-complex vitamins. There have also been some studies of specific vegetables; for example, there are studies that show that spinach loses much of its nutrient content after eight days in a refrigerator. In most studies, it also depends on the temperature of the refrigerator; in the spinach example, if the refrigerator was 39 degrees Fahrenheit (3.89 degrees Celsius), there was a 47 percent drop in folate after eight days; at 50 degrees Fahrenheit (10 degrees Celsius), the folate lost the same amount in six days.

Do frozen vegetables bought at the grocery store have nutritional value?

Most frozen vegetables you buy at the grocery store do not change nutritionally after they are in the deep freeze for a couple months. This is because more often than not, the vegetables come right out of the field and are blanched and frozen immediately. The exceptions include vegetables that are mishandled (frozen, thawed, and frozen again; you can usually tell by all the ice crystals in the bag of vegetables) or those vegetables frozen days after they were picked.

How do you store certain vegetables and fruits?

There are certain ways to store vegetables and fruits to help maintain their nutritional value. For example, don't expose vegetables to a hot environment, such as a car, truck, or RV, for a long time (unless they are snug in an efficient cooler or, in the case of a truck or RV, a refrigerator). The following list offers some other storage suggestions:

- There are some foods that can be stored on your counter, such as most fruits like oranges, pears, and even tomatoes (actually a fruit).

- Root vegetables, such as turnips, winter squash, and rutabaga, do best in a cool, dry spot with good circulation, such as an orchard rack.

If you live near a farmer's market around August and September in the Northern Hemisphere, there are usually plenty of people selling one of the more favorite flavorful vegetables—corn on the cob. But there's a reason why most of us ask if the corn was picked that day (or at least the day before): The corn is usually super sweet and packed with nutrients the day it's picked. But as it ages, nutrients disappear. Taste-wise, the sugar in the corn breaks down into starch—and if you've ever eaten week-old corn you know that it tastes almost like a starchy raw potato.

- Potatoes do better covered in a cool, somewhat dry place (the refrigerator is too humid); potatoes are also best stored in the dark because light turns the layer under the skin green—which is toxic to eat (just peel off the green parts of the potato skins to eat).

- Onions do well in a cool, dry place, and can be stored in a paper bag that has holes in it for circulation.

- Mushrooms can be stored in a paper bag (especially those that come from the grocery in plastic containers) in the refrigerator.

- Most greens (kale, swiss chard, spinach, etc.), summer squash, leeks, and almost all other vegetables not mentioned should be stored in the refrigerator. Many of these can also be blanched and frozen after picking for later use. (For more about freezing vegetables for nutrition, see the chapter "Food Preservation and Nutrition.")

Why is eating fruits good for your health?

Although some people are allergic to certain fruits, there are many that are good for your health. For example, fruits contain abundant antioxidants; studies show people who eat several servings of fruit a day cut their rates of cancer, heart attack, and stroke. Certain fruits, such as citrus, also contain abundant vitamin C; and brightly colored fruits are usually high in beta carotene (the precursor to vitamin A).

But of course, the amount of fruits you eat daily depends on your age, sex, and level of physical activity. For a look at general recommendations of how much fruit to eat, depending on age, you can go to the Internet site http://www.choosemyplate.gov/print pages/MyPlateFoodGroups/Fruits/food-groups.fruits-amount.pdf.

What are some of the best fruits for health?

There are a wide range of fruits—some familiar and some not so familiar—that are good for our health (as long as you're not allergic to them). For example, some of the best vitamin C-rich fruits are citrus fruits, strawberries, cantaloupe, kiwi, and mango. Some of the best fruits for beta carotene are cantaloupes, apricots, mango, and papaya. If you're looking for the best fiber-rich fruits, the best are apples, almost any type of berry, figs, and prunes. And for those of you who want to lose weight faster, some recent research indicates that eating pears and/or apples each day (10 ounces; or 300 grams) can help you (slowly) lose pounds.

What are the healthiest ways to get the most nutrition from fruits?

One way is to eat the freshest fruits you can find—but not everyone can live in a warm climate where fresh fruit is readily available. And because a fruit's nutrients and phytochemicals begin to deteriorate after they are picked, foods that travel a

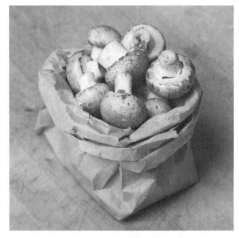

Mushrooms store well in a paper bag that is then placed in the refrigerator.

long way to get to the grocery can lose some of their nutritional value. Thus, one of the next best ways is to eat frozen fruits, which are significantly higher in vitamins and antioxidants than the fresh, "well-traveled" foods; this is because most of these fruits are picked and chilled at their peak ripeness, which means that many of the nutrients are locked in. Another way to get more of a fruit's nutrients is to eat dehydrated (usually said to be freeze-dried) foods—but beware that some of these fruits can be high in added sugar or sulfates (added as a preservative). Finally, if you decide to get some of your needed fruit nutrients from juices, be aware that many fruit juices are pasteurized, and heat destroys many of the nutrients; the best fruit drinks nutrient-wise are usually those that say 100 percent juice, with nothing else added.

Why are citrus fruits so nutritious?

There is a reason why nutritionists recommend several helpings of citrus fruits a day for a healthy diet (if you are not allergic to citrus): Most of these fruits are high in vitamin C, beta carotene (the precursor to vitamin A), potassium, and lesser amounts of other vitamins and minerals; they are high in fiber; depending on the fruit, they have various types of polyphenols; they are low in calories (when eaten fresh and by themselves); and they are a good source of energy because they contain natural sugars.

How do some fruits affect our intestines?

Fruits have a great deal of nutrition, but there are some fruits that respond "differently" in our bodies. For example, some fruits contain sugars that are easily absorbed into the bloodstream; others can cause gastrointestinal problems, as they ferment in the digestive tract and cause a buildup of gas. The reason for the difference has to do with a fruit's fructose to glucose ratio (the higher the ratio, the more "intestine-friendly" the fruit) and its fiber content. The intestine-friendly fruits include strawberries, raspberries, blackberries, pineapples, and oranges; the more intestine-unfriendly fruits include prunes, pears, peaches, and apples. This doesn't mean you should quit eating fruits that are less kind to your digestive tract—not everyone responds in the same way and for most people, eating fruit is a healthy choice for your overall diet. Plus, if you're ever constipated, sometimes the fruits with the lower fructose to glucose ratio can help!

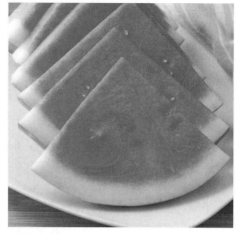

Seedless watermelons were first introduced to American markets in 1988.

What are seedless fruits?

There are many types of seedless plants found at the grocery stores and at farmers' markets—such as seedless grapes, watermelons, and naval oranges. These plants have to be grown in a certain way—created from plants that are either not fertilized by pollination or that don't develop mature seeds even though they are pollinated. For example, seedless grape growers take cuttings from the plants, root them, and then plant the plant cuttings. (The exact origin of seedless grapes is unknown, but many researchers believe the grapes were first cultivated thousands of years ago in present-day Iran or Afghanistan.) Another seedless plant is the watermelon—a relatively newcomer in the fruit world, first introduced in 1988. And navel oranges are oranges without seeds: a naturally occurring mutation created the first navel orange tree in an early nineteenth century Brazilian orchard; a bud from the mutant tree was grafted onto another orange tree to propagate the navel oranges we see in the stores today.

Do seedless fruits have nutritional value?

Yes, in most cases a seedless fruit will have almost the same nutritional value as a similar fruit with seeds. For example, seedless oranges, watermelons, and even bananas all have relatively the same nutrients as their "seeded" counterparts. Only one exception is often mentioned by nutritionists: Seeded grapes may offer a nutritional advantage over seedless grapes—mainly because grape seeds, although bitter tasting, have a good amount of protein, minerals, fiber, and fats.

Is there a difference between beans and legumes?

Yes, in a way, there is a difference between beans and legumes: legumes include all plants with seed-bearing pods that can be harvested and dried, a list that includes beans. In terms of eating and cooking, legumes are often called pulses, or the edible seeds of the annual plants. Not only are they good nutritionally for humans (and other animals), but they also fix nitrogen in the soil, a natural chemical that is taken up by many other plants when they grow.

What are the types of legumes?

There are around 13,000 different varieties of legumes—all of which vary greatly. They include vines (certain types of beans and peas); low-growing plants (such as lentils, soybeans, and bush beans); underground crops (such as peanuts—which are *not* nuts, despite their name); groundcover crops (such as alfalfa and clover); and even trees and shrubs (such as carob). Some nutritionists also consider some of the legumes to be vegetables, such as snap beans, mung beans, and fresh lima beans, mainly because they do not have as much fiber and other nutrients as the other "true" legumes.

Why do some people have flatulence when they eat beans, and is there a way to stop it?

Many people have flatulence, or gas—or bloating and burping—when they eat any type of bean. This is because of special types of bacteria that reside in our large intestines. If you consume beans, you may notice the gas later on in the day—this is because the gases from eating beans start to form when carbohydrates (called oligosaccharides) reach your large intestines. And if your digestive tract has a difficult time digesting the carbohydrates, these specialized bacteria within the large intestine take over for you. They can digest (and ferment) the oligosaccharides if you can't—and as they eat, they produce (mostly methane) gas in your lower intestine as a byproduct. (For more about flatulence, see the chapter "Nutrition in Eating and Drinking Choices.")

There have been many suggestions on how to cope with the flatulence caused by eating beans. After a while, most people will no longer have gas (or not that much gas) after they add beans to their diet. For the occasional bean eater, suggestions to stop the gas have included some "old wives' tales," including to add baking soda to the water. But most cooks agree that if you use the "quick-soak method" before you cook the beans, it can help reduce your gaseous feelings. (See this chapter for the "quick-soak" method.)

Do legumes have nutritional value?

All legumes are packed with nutritional value. They promote digestion and are excellent sources of antioxidants that scavenge free radicals from our bodies. Overall, legumes are rich in proteins (20 to 25 percent by weight), complex carbohydrates, and soluble fiber (which makes them good for our digestive tract). They also have a low glycemic index (important especially to diabetics for blood-sugar regulation), are considered heart healthy (the fiber content is said to lower cholesterol and

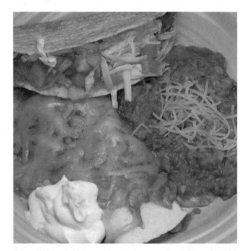

Legumes like these refried beans are a great source of protein, complex carbs, and antioxidants.

triglyceride, or blood fat, levels), and they are not expensive—thus, they are a main food staple in many places around the world.

And although all legumes have certain nutritional attributes, each type can also differ in the amount of nutrients they offer. For example, beans and lentils have a great deal of folic acid, magnesium, potassium, and B vitamins; lima beans are good sources of protein, iron, and vitamins A and C; and shelled beans are rich in thiamin, vitamin B_6, potassium, and magnesium.

What are certain types of beans and some of their nutritional attributes?

There are many beans in the world, some familiar and some not so familiar. The following chart lists some of the types of beans and their overall nutritional value—including fiber content:

Beans and Their Nutrients

Bean	Nutritional Value
Adzuki	These are smaller red beans than kidney beans; they have a lower amount of B vitamins, but are higher in mineral value than the kidney beans
Black bean	These sweet-tasting beans are also called turtle beans; the fiber content is about 7.5 grams per ½ cup; they are lower in folate than kidney beans
Black-eyed peas	These legumes have a fiber content of about 4.6 grams per ½ cup
Chickpeas	Also called garbanzo beans, they have a nutty flavor; they also have a fiber content of around 6.2 grams per ½ cup
Kidney beans	One of the most popular beans; they are vitamin- and mineral-rich, thus they are often said to be the most nutritious of the dried beans; have a fiber content of 6.1 grams per ½ cup
Lentils	One of a few beans that do not need to be soaked before using in a recipe; contain about 7.8 grams of fiber per ½ cup
Lima beans	contain about 6.6 grams of fiber per ½ cup; one of the most widely available beans and they are thought of as both a bean (dried and white) and a vegetable (when fresh and green)
Navy beans	A smaller version of the Great Northern beans; they have about 4.6 grams of fiber per ½ cup
Pinto beans	This mottled, multicolored bean has a fiber content of about 7.3 grams per ½ cup
Small red beans	These are smaller renditions of the red kidney beans, with about the same fiber and nutritional value
Soybeans	Used for a multitude of products, such as tofu, tempeh, soy milk, and so forth; they have about 5.2 grams of fiber per ½ cup
Split peas	Used in soups and stews mostly; like lentils, one of the few beans that does not have to be soaked before using in a recipe; they have about 8.1 grams of fiber per ½ cup
White beans	Also called Great Northern beans, they have a fiber content of about 5.7 grams per ½ cup

What are some beans that are often grown in home gardens?

There are different types of beans that can be grown in the home garden. For example, green beans—from yellow (often called waxed beans) and green to purple—are varieties of beans that are harvested at the immature stage while the pods and seeds are soft. The beans are either eaten right out of the shell (or cooked and eaten), or the entire bean pod and seeds can be eaten raw (or cooked and eaten).

In shelled varieties, only the seeds are eaten. For example, the dry shelling beans (*Phaseolus vulgaris*) are grown for drying, and include Tiger's Eye and Cannellini beans. Fava beans (*Vicia faba*) can be harvested and cooked as a green shelling bean and also allowed to dry. After drying, these beans can be stored in a cool, dry place; when needed for cooking, they are soaked in a liquid, cooked for a certain amount of time, and then used in a recipe. (For more about cooking beans, see below.)

How do you store dried beans?

Storing beans is not too difficult. As long as the beans have been dried correctly, they can be stored in a tightly covered container in a cool, dry place. Most beans will keep for about six months to a year after purchase, although many people have been able to keep beans for years under the right conditions. It is also recommended not to mix different types of beans together—various beans require different soaking and cooking times— or to mix older beans with new ones.

What are sprouts?

There are some legumes and seeds of certain vegetables that are not only nutritious as a cooked or raw food, but also as sprouts. The sprouts are actually young plants: The seeds of certain legumes, vegetables, or even flowers are allowed to grow in a moist environment—resulting in sprouts from the seeds several days later. For example, most beans and peas can be used, with sprouts from such legumes as mung beans, peas, and alfalfa; vegetable spouts include broccoli, kale, and radishes. Not all spouts have the same nutritional value. For example, broccoli sprouts are rich in sulforaphane, thought to be one of the most potent anticancer compounds from a natural source, and are rich in vitamin C, beta carotene, and folate, while radish spouts are high in vitamin C and fiber, but lower in such nutrients as iron and folate.

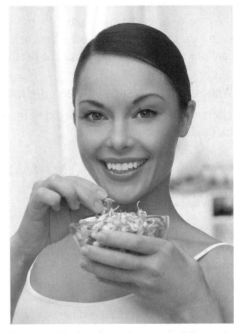

Bean sprouts are one type of young plant that people enjoy eating. They are tender and nutritious and add fiber to your diet.

What are micro-greens?

Micro-greens have just come into vogue in the past few years or so—and include most vegetables that can be grown and eaten when young. They include most of the green leafy vegetables, herbs, and some edible flowers, such as arugula, beets, basil, chard, onions, mustard, kale, and bok choy. Unlike sprouts that grow a certain length from their seed, micro-greens are planted in soil and allowed to grow only about two inches high; they are then clipped and used right away—to be eaten in salads, or cooked in various dishes. These immature, tiny, tender renditions of the larger plant are high in nutrients—although you have to eat more to get the most benefits.

COOKING FOODS

How do foods change when you cook them?

In general, and no matter what the cooking method, foods change when they are heated. This is because the molecules in the food—as they are heated by hot ovens or in skillets—speed up; the movement of the molecules from the heat bump into the "slower-moving" molecules in the colder food, causing the food's molecules to move and thus heat up. If the food changes color upon heating, it is usually because of gases driven from the food or chemical reactions that take place in the food as it is heated (see the Maillard reaction on page 100). For raw foods with thick cell walls, such as carrots and onions, the heat causes the cells to break down, making them tender. With more heating, the cells break down even further, resulting in mushy, but cooked vegetables; and for some foods, too much heat can make the foods taste bad, as the heating oxidizes some of the foods' natural oils.

What is the difference between the major ways of cooking foods?

There are many methods of cooking foods. The following chart lists the most popular methods and how they work:

Cooking Methods

Cooking Method	How It Works
Fry	Cooking using a thick layer of hot oil or fat (lard) in a skillet or pot; often used with food that is breaded or battered, with the food most often submerged in the oil for a specific time and the oil at a certain temperature
Sauté	Thin film of hot oil in a skillet that works best for thin foods (such as thin or small chunks of meat), and chopped vegetables
Grilling	Cooking on a grate over a fire (charcoal or gas; small or large fire); there is either a cover or not (with a cover this is similar to roasting)
Stew	Cooking by sautéing first, then further cooked at a simmer for a longer period
Boil	Cooking foods in boiling water for a certain time

Cooking Methods

Cooking Method	How It Works
Simmer	Cooking foods in a liquid just below the boiling point for a certain time
Poach	Cooking foods in a liquid—usually water—that is well below boiling point; the pot is usually covered to retain moisture and heat
Steam	Food that is allowed to cook over simmering water; it is a gentle way of cooking and usually does not cause the food to lose its flavor
Braise	Foods that are first sautéed, then water is added, the pan covered, and the food is simmered
Roast	Cooking foods in a hot oven, usually in a pan that catches the juices of the meats or with a bit of oil when cooking vegetables
Rotisserie	Slowly cooking food by surrounding it with heat like roasting, but most often the meat is rotated on a spit to make sure it is uniformly heated and cooked all over
Claypot cooking	Cooking in a pot made of clay, using the water-soaked pot to "steam" the food as it cooks (for more about claypots, see below)
Barbecue	Cook foods on a grate over a small, smoky fire; grills often have a hood to close for faster cooking
Sear	Cook on a hot, flat (usually metal, such as cast iron) surface for a short period of time (a few minutes); it is usually used to seal moisture in meat that will be cooked in other ways, such as baking or sautéing
Slow cooking	As the name implies, cooking foods in a somewhat low-temperature specialized pot for many hours that allows the flavors to meld together; it is usually used for stews and soups, and cooked in an electric slow cooker (for more about slow cookers, see below)
Sous vide	Cooking a sealed bag of food in a temperature-controlled (usually) hot water bath, usually for very long times (some foods up to 72 hours); it is from the French, translated as "under vacuum," and has often been sited as causing health problems as some foods remain raw or undercooked
Confit	Foods cooked slowly at low temperatures while submerged in liquid fat or oil; some also in sugar or liquid syrup (it is also used by some as a way to preserve certain foods)

Can some types of cooking affect your health?

Yes, some cooking techniques—and certain foods that are cooked—can affect your health. For example, some cooking practices encourage the formation of advanced glycation end products, or AGEs. These products have been linked to such negative effects as hardening and narrowing of the arteries; and it is thought that as you age, it becomes harder for your body to remove these AGEs. Some cooking methods form more AGEs than others, such as browning, grilling, broiling, and frying—especially of meats; the least are formed when you roast, boil, steam, or use a pressure or slow cooker. A "rule of thumb" is: high heat and lack of water usually cause more AGEs to form.

What is claypot cooking?

Claypot cooking, or cooking in a clay (terracotta) pot with top and bottom sections, is nothing new: the method has been used for cooking as far back as Roman times. The pots are soaked, absorbing the water; this generates moisture during cooking and prevents foods from drying out. It also means that a minimum of fat is used; and it creates a more flavorful dish, as the food's own juices mingle during cooking. In addition, the nutrients are better preserved because the foods cook in their own juices.

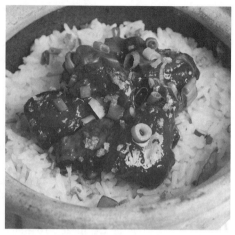

Claypot cooking is a method of heating up foods without using fat. Simply soak the pot in water before cooking and follow the recipe directions.

How does cooking affect a food's fat- and water-soluble vitamin content?

The effects of cooking on a food's vitamin content vary. In general, fat-soluble vitamins (for example, A, D, E, and especially K) will not be lost as much when the foods that contain them are cooked; whereas, water-soluble vitamins (the B-complex [with the exception of niacin] and vitamin C), especially when cooked with higher heat and/or more liquid, can lose much of their vitamin content. (For more about fat- and water-soluble vitamins, see the chapter "The Basics of Nutrition: Micronutrients.")

How do various cooking methods affect a food's mineral value?

Unlike with some vitamins, heating various foods does not affect the mineral content of most foods, with the exception of potassium, a mineral that escapes from food into the cooking liquid (although it's interesting to note it is not affected by heat). But all other minerals—from calcium and iodine to chromium and sodium in raw or cooked foods—are there for you when you ingest your foods.

What are slow cookers and pressure cookers?

A slow cooker is usually an electric appliance—sometimes called a crockpot—with an insert (ceramic or glass) near a heating element; it cooks for long periods of time, allowing tough meats to become tender and flavors to mingle. As for keeping the foods' vitamin and other nutrient values, there is some disagreement. Some people say slow cookers don't hurt the nutrient value of vitamins because the cooking temperatures are too low, and most "lost" vitamins would be in the liquids in the bottom of the cooker; in addition, many foods' nutrients are enhanced by cooking. Others say certain nutrients are lost by cooking the foods for so long; in particular, lycine, an amino acid, is mentioned, as it is often destroyed when cooking at lower temperatures.

A pressure cooker functions just as the words state: cooking using pressure. In pressure cooking, the air in the pan is withdrawn so a heat as high as 250 degrees Fahrenheit (121.1 degrees Celsius) can be maintained at 15 pounds of pressure (10 and 15 pounds of pressure are the most commonly used for home canning of foods). At that temperature and pressure, foods cook in only about one third of the usual total time it takes to cook conventionally at boiling temperatures. The nutrient values of the foods depend on what you put into the pressure cooker. For example, if you pressure cook carrots or spinach, the cooking makes more nutrients available; but water-soluble vitamins (C and B-complex, for example) are the hardest to retain when heating—and this includes the higher temperatures of the pressure cooker.

COOKING VEGETABLES AND LEGUMES

Are vegetables better for you cooked or raw?

According to research, this is not a "yes" or "no" question—that's because, depending on the vegetable, some active nutrients in vegetables are more available when cooked, while others are more prevalent when foods are eaten raw. For example, tomatoes are rich in the antioxidant lycopene when cooked, as opposed to eating them raw. But that does not mean raw tomatoes have no nutrient value—they are rich in other vitamins, minerals, and antioxidants, too.

How do you retain the nutrients in vegetables *before* cooking?

Although you will always lose some nutrients in your vegetables before (yes, raw vegetables contain nutrients, but if you let them sit around too long, they lose vitamins mostly) and during cooking, there are ways to minimize such losses. Here are just a few suggestions from the Food and Agriculture Organization of the United States:

- Do not soak your vegetables in water before you cook them—you can lose nutrients such as vitamin C (although cleaning and rinsing them is fine)
- One of the best ways to preserve water-soluble vitamins and minerals is to cut the vegetables into larger pieces or cook them whole
- Make sure the cooking time, temperature and amount of liquid is at a minimum when you cook vegetables
- Overall, nutritionists suggest that you gently and somewhat quickly cook your vegetables when necessary, with little water to protect the water-soluble vitamins. They also suggest covering the vegetables as the heat will cause the vegetables to release some of their water, helping to cook the food. And in most cases, consuming the broth means you get some of those nutrients

Are there foods in which cooking actually boosts nutrition?

Yes, not all cooking is bad for nutrients. For example, the amount of lycopene in tomatoes actually increases when they are cooked. One study in the early 2000s showed that one type of lycopene (cis-lycopene) in tomatoes rose by 35 percent after being cooked for 30 minutes at 190.4 degrees Fahrenheit (88 degrees Celsius). But it may not be only the lycopene that increases—some researchers believe that the heat breaks down the plant's cell walls, thus allowing our bodies to take in more lycopene.

But the results of cooking (or not cooking) are not as straightforward as it seems. For example, some research has shown that boiling carrots can help you absorb more beta carotene, the precursor to vitamin A, while other studies showed that boiling carrots leads to the loss of polyphenols. Still other vegetables make more antioxidants available to our bodies when they are either lightly steamed or boiled, such as cabbage, peppers, mushrooms, and spinach; although, on the other hand, researchers also note that boiling can destroy some of the vitamins in the vegetables—especially vitamin C.

What is caramelization?

Caramelization usually refers to vegetables. As they are roasted, the natural sugars become easier to taste. Caramelizing is actually a chemical reaction of sugar: as the sugar is heated to a certain point, the molecules begin to break apart. This creates new flavors, colors, and smells in the sugar—and since vegetables contain a great deal of natural sugars, caramelizing such foods as onions, carrots, and squash means they will have a more "sugary" taste. But don't confuse this with the term *browning*—that is usually only reserved for meats and breads, and involves the interaction of the heat, sugar molecules, and proteins in both foods (for more about browning, see this chapter and the Maillard reaction).

How do you stop some vitamins from "cooking away"?

Because many vitamins—except the more stable vitamin K and niacin (a B vitamin)—are often easily destroyed or depleted when steamed, cooked, boiled, or fried, there are some methods you can use to make sure you get the most vitamins from your vegetables. For example, if you cook in oil, use as little as possible so you don't lose the fat-soluble vitamins A and E.

What are the best ways to cook vegetables to save nutrients, especially antioxidants?

There are several ways to cook vegetables to retain their valuable nutrients. The following list describes some of those methods:

Baking or Roasting—Both these methods can preserve certain vegetable nutrients, but not all. For example, food researchers have found that baking ar-

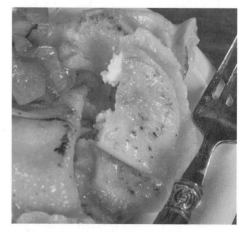

Caramelized onions with pierogies—mmmmm! Not to be confused with mere browning of vegetables, caramelization involves roasting to bring out the flavorful sugars.

How is vitamin C affected by cooking?

Water-soluble vitamin C is one of the most well-known nutrients, and it is probably the most relied upon for health. But cooking can take its toll on the vitamin. For example, not only is the vitamin sensitive to air (oxygen), it is definitely affected by high heat and cooking in a liquid. In fact, if you toss a vitamin C-rich vegetable in cold water, then heat it to boiling, for each minute it takes to go from cold to boiling, the vegetable will lose 20 percent of its vitamin C. This is because an enzyme that destroys vitamin C becomes more active as the temperature rises (but it stops destroying the vitamin at the boiling point). This is why many recipes say to add vegetables to already boiling water—or why steaming or cooking in a small amount of water retains more than twice as much vitamin C than boiling does. And if you put the food in the refrigerator after cooking, eat leftovers within two days—after about a day in the refrigerator (not freezer), the foods can lose up to 25 percent of their vitamin C, and after two days, about 50 percent. (For more about vitamin C, see the chapter "The Basics of Nutrition: Micronutrients.")

tichokes, asparagus, broccoli, and peppers retained their antioxidant levels, but baking carrots, Brussels sprouts, leeks, cauliflower, peas, zucchini, onions, beans, celery, beets, and garlic means a loss of antioxidants. The cases in which baking can really help *increase* antioxidants is with green beans, eggplant, corn, Swiss chard, and spinach.

Griddling—This method has only recently become popular, but has been in use for centuries. Many vegetables—especially beets, onions, Swiss chard, celery, and green beans—keep their antioxidants when cooked on griddles, or a flat metal surface. There is one caveat: Some researchers caution that the nonstick griddles may contain toxins; the alternative is to use a thick frying pan with no oil.

Microwaving—If you want to preserve antioxidants in food, researchers suggest microwaving; for example, microwaving broccoli can preserve up to 80 percent of its vitamin C. The exception is cauliflower, the only vegetable that loses 50 percent of its antioxidants when it is cooked in a microwave oven.

Sautéing and Stir-frying—Stir-frying or sautéing vegetables usually means using high heat and little oil, which often retains most of the nutrients; even some of the oils used in the sauté or stir-fry pan will help your body absorb the nutrients. The main reason is that both methods are quick, and the short amount of time the food is in the wok or skillet means less nutrient loss.

Steaming—This is probably the "worst" method on this list (although still better than frying or boiling; see below), but only if you let the foods stay too long in the steamer. If the food is *lightly* steamed, it is still a good way to preserve antioxidants in vegetables such as broccoli and zucchini.

How can you retain the most nutrients when you steam (or blanch) vegetables?

One reason steaming (or blanching, in which you put the vegetables into boiling water for a very short time, then immediately put into cold water to stop the cooking) isn't a good cooking method is that many vitamins and nutrients in vegetables are fat soluble; this means that, like sautéing, oils help your body absorb the nutrients much better. Thus, adding a bit of oil to the steamed vegetables can help—as long as the steaming keeps the food slightly crisp, not mushy. Another trick to make sure you keep as many nutrients as possible is to add a pinch of salt to the water. This will raise the boiling point and the steam created will be hotter, and thus will cook the vegetables faster.

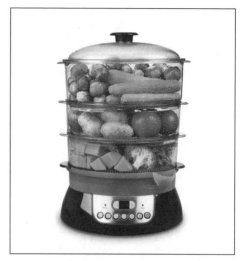

Steaming food is a cooking method that is not ideal for keeping vitamins and minerals in your food, especially if you only use water. Add some oil to help absorb these nutrients, instead.

How can you keep vegetables firm—and nutritious—if you roast them?

As in much of cooking, science steps in with answers. Most people know that browning makes meats taste better; and with vegetables, caramelizing brings out the natural sugars (for more about caramelization, see this chapter). But with vegetables, methods such as roasting make your carrots or sweet potatoes look wrinkled and withered as the food loses moisture—and nutrients. To make sure the vegetables don't wither, many cooks now use two methods: first steaming at a low temperature, then roasting. At low temperature, between 120 and 160 degrees Fahrenheit (48.9 to 71.1 degrees Celsius), an enzyme (called pectin methylesterase) allows the pectin in the vegetable's cell walls to bind better with the calcium already in the vegetable—and the food does not break down as fast; at higher heat, the enzyme is not active, and the cell walls break down faster. Thus, when it comes to vegetables such as potatoes, carrots, or cauliflower, sometimes steaming them first at a lower temperature, then roasting them at a higher temperature, works not only to make them taste better, but also to hold more nutrients.

What are some of the *worst* ways to cook vegetables and destroy nutrients?

Although there are exceptions, some of the worst ways to cook vegetables—especially those that destroy nutrients—include frying and boiling. Frying not only adds fats to your diet, but it can also cause a vegetable to lose 5 to 50 percent of its original nutrient values. Because boiling involves water, it also causes vegetables to lose antioxidants—especially peas, cauliflower, and zucchini (if you want to ingest the nutrient-rich water from boiling vegetables, you can add it to a soup or stew). There is one exception:

> ## Does a pinch of baking soda preserve the color of green foods when cooked?
>
> Yes, baking soda does keep green vegetables green after they are cooked, but there is a downside: the baking soda also breaks down the plants' tissues. This makes the vegetables mushy—and destroys most of the vitamins.

Researchers have found that boiling carrots causes their carotenoid content to rise even more than steaming them (for more about carotenoids, see the chapter "The Basics of Nutrition: Micronutrients").

Should you add baking soda when cooking legumes?

It is often recommended that you add baking soda when cooking legumes—especially beans—to help the food retain its color and freshness. Although the baking soda does help the beans look better, it also destroys their thiamine content.

How do you cook dried beans?

Dried beans should be cooked in a liquid to soften the cellulose fiber that "coats" the seeds. Cooking in a liquid also helps the bean to restore the moisture that was lost in the drying process, and brings out the flavor in the bean.

The cooking can be done in two ways—overnight soaking or what is called a quick soak. With the quick-soak method, the beans are rinsed and checked (mostly for stones that can accidentally be picked with the beans); the beans are placed in a saucepan with three times their volume of hot—for some beans, boiling—water, and allowed to boil for two minutes. The saucepan is then removed from the heat, and the beans are covered and soaked for an hour. After, the beans are drained and rinsed, and cooked with the correct amount of liquid and for the specific time for that bean type. In the traditional soaking method, again the beans are rinsed and checked; they are then put in a large bowl with three times their volume of hot water (some use boiling water). They are soaked between four hours to overnight (soybeans definitely have to be soaked for a full 12 hours); some people also change the soaking water a few times, but it's not necessary. After soaking, they are drained and rinsed, and cooked with the correct amount of liquid for the bean's specific cooking time.

How long should you cook certain legumes?

There are specific cooking times for certain beans, from adzuki beans to soybeans. The following chart lists the amount of time for each legume (*Note:* in general, 1 pound of dry beans equals two cups of soaked beans—and that yields 5 to 6 cups of cooked beans), from the U.S. Dry Bean Council:

99

Adzuki Beans—1 to 1½ hours
Baby Lima Beans—1 hour
Black Beans—1 to 1½ hours
Black Eyed Peas—30 minutes to 1 hour
Cranberry Beans—45 to 60 minutes
Garbanzo Beans (Chickpeas)—1 to 1½ hours
Great Northern Beans—45 to 60 minutes
Kidney Beans (light or dark)—1½ hours to 2 hours
Large Lima Beans (Butter Beans)—1 to 1½ hours
Navy Beans—1½ to 2 hours
Pinto Beans—1½ to 2 hours
Small Red Beans—1 to 1½ hours

COOKING MEAT

What is the Maillard reaction?

The Maillard reaction is why most people can enjoy the aroma of baked bread, roasted coffee, or even grilled hamburgers. It is also why breads turn brown on top, why soy sauce is brown, and why we can brown our meat on a grill. This chemical reaction was first identified by the French chemist Louis-Camille Maillard in a paper published in 1912, in which he observed how amino acids react with sugars by raising the temperatures of various foods. Thus, Maillard is often thought of as one of the founders of food science.

The reaction occurs when, for example, steak is cooked with high heat—most often when the surface temperature of the meat reaches more than 300 degrees Fahrenheit (148.9 degrees Celsius)—and not only is the food cooked, but the flavor also changes. This is due to several complex chemical interactions (in total, called the Maillard reaction) in which, simply put, the amino acids and reducing sugars (such as glucose and fructose in the meat) react to form new flavor compounds. As the cooking continues, these compounds form even more flavor compounds, until large molecules called melanoidin pigments form. This produces the brown color on the meat—and the flavors most of us associate with the taste and smell of "(something) on the grill" or roasted meats. There are also

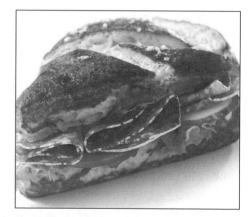

The Maillard reaction is what causes breads to brown on top and what gives that delicious aroma when they bake.

some variables that can affect the reaction, including if you are using frozen or fresh meats, if there is any moisture, or if the temperature is not high enough.

Is there a downside to the Maillard reaction?

Yes, according to research, there is a downside to the Maillard reaction: in particular, it can produce cancer-causing acrylamide and furans in some foods, especially highly processed or burnt meats. This is frequently noted in the media when it's "grilling season" (usually in the summer for both hemispheres), when viewers are advised to grill meat until it is cooked, but not until it is especially well-done. This is because the same heating processes that kill bacteria and produce such wonderful tastes and aromas can—if temperatures get too high—also create harmful chemicals in the meats. If such foods are eaten regularly, the chemicals can lead to problems in humans such as inflammation, diabetes, cancer, and even cardiovascular disease. (For more about cooked meats and health problems, see below.)

What are some definitions of cooked meat?

Meats usually have a number of definitions after they are cooked, including the following: well done (grey throughout); medium well (slightly pink center, thick grey around the edges); medium (pink center, with thinner grey edges); medium rare (pink throughout with a slightly red center, and the edges seared); rare (red center, with pink edges and a very thin grey or brown sear line around the outside); and black and blue (nearly raw). Which method results in the most nutritious meat is highly debatable, and often the type of cooking comes down to personal preference.

What ways of cooking meats are thought to be connected to cancer?

One of the most well-known foods that seems to be connected to cancer is meat, especially depending upon how the meat is cooked. For example, research has shown that cancer-causing substances called polycyclic aromatic hydrocarbons (PAHs) can form when meats are cooked at a high heat (PAHs are also present in cigarette smoke and car exhaust). When you cook meats at very high temperatures on the grill (either with charcoal, an electric element, or a gas flame), the meat drips a great deal of fat on the hot coals, causing smoke containing PAHs to fall back on the food, and you can even breathe the substances into your lungs. (Some people solve this problem by parboiling or slightly braising the meat before it's put on the grill to lessen the cooking time.) Although still being studied, some research indicates that there is an association between the consumption of these grilled meats and, in particular, the high incidence of colorectal cancer in the United States.

Another problem is substances called heterocyclic amines (HCAs), which occur when you cook meat, fish, and poultry at high temperatures. These can form when you grill, fry, or broil meat, especially red meats (some researchers believe this is why red meat is often connected to an increased incidence of certain cancers, such as colon cancer). And there are also problems with foods containing the preservative nitrate, which can create carcinogenic nitrosamines when cooked at high heat.

What recent study showed how beer can help grilled foods?

Because of the connection between the formation of polycyclic aromatic hydrocarbons (PAHs), grilled meats, and cancer, researchers have been attempting to find a way to reduce the formation of these harmful substances—and in 2014, researchers may have found one way to help. It is known that some beer, wine, or tea marinades can reduce some of the potential carcinogens in cooked meat, but the researchers concentrated on beer for this study. They marinated pork for four hours in nonalcoholic pilsner beer, regular pilsner beer, or black beer ale, along with a control piece of pork that had not been marinated, and grilled the meats on a charcoal grill until very well done. The black beer had the best effect, reducing the level of PAHs by more than half compared to the nonmarinated pork. Just why this occurs is not yet fully understood.

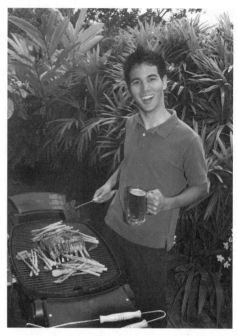

Don't just drink beer while you grill, cook with it! Cooking food in beer (or wine or tea marinade) can counter the carcinogens that might arise from charring meat.

NUTRITION IN EATING AND DRINKING CHOICES

THE BASICS OF EATING

What is a "superfood"?

"Superfood" is a somewhat trendy word to describe foods that have relatively high levels of certain vitamins, minerals, essential fatty acids, and/or phytochemicals. Because of this, they are usually said to have a positive effect on some aspect of our health. Some superfood definitions include meats (including fish), but mostly animals that are eaten without the skin or from lean cuts (low fat), and those raised in the most "natural" ways (*grass-fed* is the term often used for such meats as beef; *wild-caught* is used for most fish). They include beef, chicken, turkey, and salmon—all of which contain essential fats, minerals (such as zinc), and protein.

But most superfood definitions concentrate on plant-based foods, for example, vegetables, fruits, whole grains, beans, nuts, and seeds that contain enough nutritional value to enhance our health. One superfood may work to block the growth of cancer cells, while another one will boost the immune system to fight disease and infection. A good example is the allium family of plants: onions, garlic, shallots, and chives all help to boost the body's immune system, and in the case of garlic, it is said to also help prevent heart disease.

What is the difference between appetite and hunger?

There is a difference between the two terms *appetite* and *hunger*, although they are often used interchangeably. Appetite means a desire for food or drink (in which you have a physical craving or a strong liking to a food or drink), whereas hunger is the need for food. In fact, an appetizer is any food (or less often a drink) that excites your appetite—especially foods that are served before a meal to stimulate your appetite.

What is a "functional food"?

Functional foods are often highlighted in the media to describe certain foods that provide benefits beyond our basic nutritional needs. For example, one seed in particular seems to fit that definition: sunflower seeds, loved by humans and birds alike. These seeds are rich in several of the B vitamins; they also contain a good amount of calcium, phosphorus, and iron. As for antioxidants, they have both selenium and vitamin E, both of which are thought to fight cancer and lower the risk for heart disease.

SEEING, CHEWING, AND TASTING

How does digestion begin?

For most of us, digestion actually begins with sight and smell—we see the bakery, smell the aroma of bread and baked goods, and then see the food in the front window or behind the counter. This is when digestion begins: our appetite is stimulated, our mouth starts watering and even our stomachs begin to churn. The anticipation of eating kick-starts your digestive tract, brain, and even salivary glands into action; and if you're really hungry, there will also be a rumbling in your abdomen that accompanies the anticipation. (This is also why it's not wise to go grocery shopping on an empty stomach!)

How are teeth built to chew various foods?

Not all animals have the same teeth. It all depends on the animal's main diet—and whether they need to chew, cut, grind, slice, or crush their foods. For example, animals that eat only plants have sharp incisors to bite off grass, reeds, leaves, and other plant material; they also have flat molars for grinding and crushing plant material so it is better digested in their specific digestive tracts. Animals that eat meat usually have pointed incisors and very large canine teeth (dogs and cats come to mind), while their molars are rough and jagged to help them chew the flesh of other animals. Animals that eat plants and meat, such as bears, have modified versions of canines and molars so they can eat both types of food.

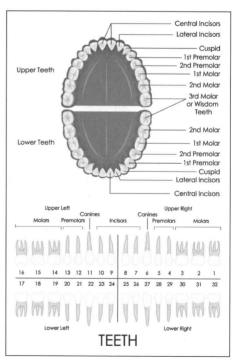

This diagram of human teeth reveals that we have a combination of teeth for cutting (incisors, cuspids), chewing, and grinding (molars and premolars) food.

When it comes to humans, researchers know (along with dentists, periodontists, and orthodontists) that not all teeth are created equal, which you can verify by just running your tongue around your teeth. Overall, however, most of us have certain teeth for specific reasons, similar to other animals that eat plants and meat. Our small mouth means we can eat only a small amount of food at a time; and by chewing our food well, we are helping our stomach (smaller chunks digest better) and small and large intestines to work better.

How does saliva help us when we eat?

The mouth's saliva—or as most of us call it, spit—is one of the body's best fluids to help with digestion. It has several functions:

Saliva helps us taste our foods—The liquid from the salivary glands helps us move the food around our tongue, bathing the food with the first digestive enzyme—called salivary amylase; fats are broken down to a certain point by another saliva enzyme called lingual lipase. These enzymes break down the chemical bonds between the carbohydrate molecules (or the starch in foods) and some fats—essentially preparing the food for the next part of the digestive tract.

Saliva helps us to swallow food without choking—This is why it's hard to swallow anything if your mouth is "dry" from a fever or lack of water. Saliva makes sure that when you eat anything from peanut butter to potatoes, the foods can slide down your 10-inch-long (25.4 centimeters) esophagus, the tube that connects the mouth to the stomach.

Saliva helps to fight germs—The enzymes in saliva help to keep your mouth clean and for some people, it also helps stop tooth decay and infection (this is also why many animals, such as cats, clean themselves with their specially adapted "cleansing" saliva). But not all saliva is helpful: some people also have certain bacteria in their saliva that actually promote tooth decay and infection.

Saliva goes "deeper"—Besides helping with digestion, tooth decay, and infection, saliva is also swallowed and goes through the digestive tract. It contains something called epidermal growth factor (EGF), which can help the growth and repair of injured or inflamed intestinal tissues.

How does human taste work?

Almost everyone has a different number of taste buds—and taste sensations—in their mouth, which is why there are so many cookbooks and recipes about how to fix a meal. Our ability to taste has to do with cells in our mouth (the taste buds); the distribution of the taste buds is believed to be genetically predetermined. It was once thought that certain tastes, such as saltiness or bitterness, were concentrated in certain sections of the tongue. But it is now known that the buds for various tastes are distributed all over the tongue, and throughout the mouth. The biggest difference between peoples' taste buds has to do with the number: some people can have ten times as many taste buds as another person.

Are taste and smell related?

Yes, the senses of taste and smell are intertwined, but they involve different types of receptor nerves that respond to various stimuli in specific ways—in the air (odorants, or odors in the air) and in foods (tastants, or chemicals in foods). The olfactory cells (smell nerves) become active by the odors around us; a small patch of these cells is found high up in the nose, and when a smell reaches the area, they send smell signals directly to the brain. The gustatory cells (taste nerves) are found as taste buds in the mouth and throat, most of which can be seen as tiny bumps; these cells react to tastants in foods and drinks (mixed with our saliva). The taste information is sent to surrounding nerve fibers—and on to the brain. In a short time after both types of cells are stimulated, they converge, allowing us to detect the flavors of the food.

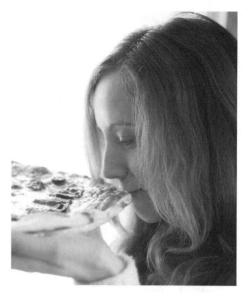

Your sense of smell adds to the sensation of food flavors by working in concert with taste receptors in the mouth.

Do humans have a good sense of smell?

No, humans are not able to smell as well as many other animals. In fact, humans have a mere five million scent receptors, while, for example, a bloodhound has about 300 million receptors. Or, in another comparison, a human's smell receptors are in a patch the size of a postage stamp, whereas a bloodhound's smell patch is the size of a handkerchief.

What is a supertaster versus a non-supertaster?

We all may know someone who eats very little or doesn't like any type of spice, herb, or harsh flavorings, and the reason may have to do with the person's number of taste buds. People called supertasters usually notice that certain foods seem to taste super-salty, sweeter, spicier, and/or more bitter than do people who are average (or below average) tasters. The main reason for this ability to "super-taste" is that supertasters have more taste buds than non-supertasters. This is also why non-supertasters tend to want more flavorings with their foods, and why they may prefer more flavorful ethnic foods: The non-supertasters have to eat more flavorful food so they can spread the taste over more parts of their mouth, whereas a small bit of super-flavored food usually overwhelms the supertaster's numerous taste buds. Some early research claimed that supertasters perceive foods to be ten times more intense than do non-supertasters, but later research showed that it is really about three times as much. The number changed because researchers found that there are other factors—such as

What basic "taste" was only recently confirmed?

Many of us remember the illustrations of the tongue from our grade school days—it was divided into salty, sweet, bitter, and sour areas of taste. Now researchers know that humans have taste buds all over their tongue and mouth, all representing these tastes in varying proportions.

But a "newer" taste was uncovered in the early 1900s, when Japanese physical chemist Kikunae Ikeda (1864–1936) extracted a white compound from giant sea kelp. He further used this to give broths a savory and meaty taste, even without meat in the pot. It was chemically a glutamate (a type of amino acid); he called it *umami*, after the taste it produced, the Japanese word for "savory." It took until around 2000 before molecular biologists discovered a receptor for the substance in the mouth—and umami became our fifth basic taste. In fact, in America, if someone says that a stew or soup has a "robust" or "full" flavor, they are usually describing umami without even knowing it.

aroma, how the food tastes in your mouth, if you wear dentures, and so on—that also affect taste.

DIGESTION

Why do we digest food?

The main reason humans digest foods is simple: By breaking down large food particles into smaller molecules, our digestive tracts can better absorb the nutrients from foods. In humans, from the mouth to the anus (called the alimentary canal), the length is about 30 feet (9.9 meters). It is lined with mostly smooth muscles that automatically push the digested foods along (an action called peristalsis; see below). Simply put, the digestion of various foods starts in the mouth, then on to the stomach and intestines; while there, food is further digested by enzyme secretions from the pancreas. The nutrients from the digested food are absorbed in the intestines, and after reaching the bloodstream are carried to the liver, where this organ prepares the nutrients for immediate use or stores the nutrients for later use.

What is the esophagus?

When you swallow, foods go into a long tube called the esophagus, directed by a flap of cartilage at the base of your throat (called the epiglottis). This flap is near the windpipe (trachea), the tube that leads into your lungs; the epiglottis closes when you swallow so the foods will not go into your windpipe. If you ever choke on food, it usually means the epiglottis didn't function properly, and you end up coughing to get the food away from your windpipe.

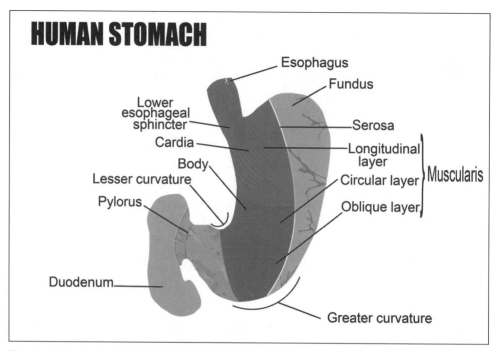

HUMAN STOMACH

Esophagus
Fundus
Lower esophageal sphincter
Serosa
Cardia
Longitudinal layer
Body
Circular layer } Muscularis
Lesser curvature
Oblique layer
Pylorus
Duodenum
Greater curvature

The stomach breaks down food and, at the same time, contains acids that kill potentially harmful bacteria, while helpful bacteria that live in the stomach also help your body extract nutrients.

What are some characteristics of the human stomach?

Unlike some animals, humans have only one stomach, which by volume represents about 17 to 21 percent of the total volume of the gastrointestinal tract. It is actually a mixing (combining and liquefying the foods we eat) and storage (regulating what enters the small intestines) chamber. The stomach helps us digest our foods, and gets the food ready for the small intestines, where the nutrients will be absorbed. And it's usually a one-way trip: Something called the cardiac sphincter stops foods in the stomach from backing up into the esophagus (if not, many people know this by the name "heartburn" or "acid reflux"). There is also another sphincter (pyloric) at the bottom of the stomach that keeps food in the stomach long enough to be digested before it goes into the small intestines.

The lining of the stomach secretes gastric juices, including hydrochloric acid—an acid that is strong enough to eat through meat and potent enough to kill off most of the harmful bacteria that may be in the food. In a way, it is also our body's way of disinfecting certain foods (although not all the bacteria get destroyed—some make it to the intestines to do other jobs for our body's absorption of foods and nutrients; for more about our gut's bacteria, see this chapter). Along with hydrochloric acid, enzymes are secreted, including the pepsins (the protein-splitting enzymes) and lipases (the fat-digesting enzymes); the acid and enzymes break down the solid foods into a liquid, creating what is called "chyme."

How does the human stomach survive its natural hydrochloric acid?

In general, the inner lining of the human stomach produces hydrochloric acid; in a chemistry lab, it is an acid with a pH of 2, or very acidic, but in the stomach, it is only mildly acidic, with a pH of around 4 to 5. Even though the acid is "mild," the stomach still has to have safeguards to protect its lining. This includes special epithelial (surface) cells that create a protective mucus layer. These cells release a basic (bicarbonate) solution; the higher pH (above a pH of 7) counteracts the acid, protecting the stomach from harsher digestive enzymes.

What is a stomach ulcer?

A stomach ulcer is often referred to as "the stomach lining eating itself." When a person contracts a gastric ulcer, it usually means that the stomach acids have reached the stomach tissues below the protective mucus layer. This often results in stomach pain, usually two to three hours after eating, or when the stomach is empty, which is why the pain sometimes calms down when a person eats or takes an antacid. A few decades ago, it was thought that ulcers occurred only from stress or worry—that people essentially ate holes in their stomachs from the acid buildup during times of stress. Today, several additional reasons have been found that lead to a gastric ulcer, including heavy drinking, smoking, hereditary predisposition, surgery, and even the heavy use of over-the-counter drugs, such as most nonsteroidal anti-inflammatory drugs (or NSAIDS), such as aspirin and ibuprofen).

But gastric ulcers differ from another type of stomach ulcer—one caused by bacteria that can disrupt the stomach's natural defenses. Now researchers know that over 90 percent of ulcers—called duodenal ulcers (because the stomach acid digests the lining of the duodenum)—are caused by bacteria called *Helicobacter pylori*. Most of these bacteria-based ulcers are treated with antibiotics and/or an acid reducer that often cures and prevents a reoccurrence of the ulcer. It is also suggested that people who have tendencies toward developing ulcers decrease their intake of caffeine, alcohol, and other stomach irritants, such as (if possible) aspirin and anti-inflammatory drugs.

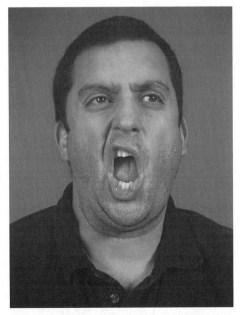

Why do we burp? Sometimes it's because bacteria in our intestines are producing excess gases that need to be released.

Why does my stomach rumble and why do I burp?

There are several reasons why your stomach rumbles—and why you do things like belch (burp). The most common reason for rumbling is that you're hungry or you're anticipating eating; it is caused by the stomach contracting and squeezing air in your digestive tract—making a noise as the air goes through. Belches usually occur when we are hungry or tense, from a mix of air and our saliva, or when the intestines produce gases from fermentation (mostly caused by our internal bacteria). This is why you sometimes burp without having eaten, as the upper digestive tract tries to eliminate the gas (air) you've swallowed during the day or from the gas from your intestines. Other times, belches occur as we eat and swallow air with our food. If you burp a great deal after a meal, one recommendation is to slow down your eating; swallowing fast means you also gulp down more air. Another suggestion is to, of course, relax before, during, and after you eat.

What are some natural juices in our digestive tracts that help break down foods?

There are many natural digestive juices that help break down food as it leaves the stomach, and which also help us to absorb nutrients in the food. For example, protease breaks down proteins; lipase breaks down fats; intestinal juices from the intestinal glands contain enzymes that break down carbohydrates and protein (and a few that break down fats); and amylase breaks down starches and glycogen.

How does our digestive tract "push" food along?

The major part of the body that pushes food along the digestive tract is the small intestine. This organ's surface has hundreds of folds, and is covered with constantly moving, fingerlike projections called villi that move the food through the intestines in a process called peristalsis. The villi are, in turn, made of several hundred cells, each covered with moving microscopic hairs called microvilli. The microvilli are responsible for trapping the nutrient molecules, drawing them into the body's cells underneath to be absorbed. When the food wastes reach the large intestines of the digestive tract, muscles move the foods from the top of the colon to the rectum, so you can eliminate the wastes.

Is there a time during the day when you absorb nutrients more efficiently?

According to most reliable studies, there is no time during the day that you absorb vitamins or minerals more efficiently—it is the same whether you ingest nutrients early or late. There are some caveats and exceptions, of course: For example, if you are under a doctor's care, and you have to take calcium—often true for pregnant or postmenopausal women, vegetarians, and vegans—calcium carbonate should be taken with meals, because your stomach acid will aid in the calcium absorption. (Of course, there are exceptions; for example, if you take thyroid medication, you should not consume foods with calcium before or right after taking your pill, as the calcium interferes with the absorption of the thyroid medication.) And if your doctor recommends the mineral iron—often true for women with heavy menstrual bleeding and for some vegetarians and vegans—it should be taken with water on an empty stomach, as a meal may reduce the absorption by 30 percent. It is also best taken with vitamin C, which helps your body better absorb the mineral.

How does the body absorb nutrients?

Within about three to four hours after eating, the body begins to absorb nutrients. The primary place in which absorption takes place is the small intestines; from there, the nutrients are passed into the bloodstream. The average human small intestine is about 20 feet (6.1 meters) in length; thus, the overall surface area for absorption is almost equal to the area of a quarter of a football field! It has three parts: the duodenum (about the first 12 inches [30 centimeters]), jejunum, and ileum. Nutrients that are either easily broken down or water-soluble are absorbed in this upper part of the small intestines. The duodenum is where calcium, vitamin A, and the B vitamins thiamin and riboflavin are absorbed; the jejunum absorbs fats; and vitamin B_{12} is absorbed by the ileum. After the nutrients are absorbed into the blood, they are carried to the liver; from there, the liver prepares the nutrients either for immediate use or for storage and future use.

What are the functions of the large intestine?

The large intestine, called the colon, has three functions: the removal undigested food (waste products left over after nutrients are absorbed), removal of excess water (around 90 percent of all the water we consume—even water in foods—is reabsorbed by both intestines), and the holding of certain bacteria that help us absorb nutrients. Foods that take longer to be digested can reach the large intestines; thus, the nutrients from these types of foods are absorbed in this intestine. In addition, most fiber that passes untouched through the digestive tract goes to the large intestine. Some of the fiber is digested by bacteria, which changes the fiber to glucose, while much of it is excreted. This dietary fiber is considered important as it actually "exercises" the large intestines—helping to maintain the health and tone of our intestinal muscles.

If fiber is good for digestion, how much do we need daily?

According to most nutritionists, we all need a certain average amount of fiber each day to keep our digestive systems in good working order—that is, if our bodies can easily digest fiber. But how much fiber do you need each day? The Institute of Medicine—a group that provides science-based advice on matters of medicine and health—as of 2012, has the following daily recommendations for adults (for more about fiber, see the chapter "The Basics of Nutrition: Macronutrients and Non-nutrients"):

Daily Recommended Fiber

	Age 50 or Younger	Age 51 or Older
Men	38 grams	30 grams
Women	25 grams	21 grams

Why do we have bacteria in our digestive tract?

All humans are born with no bacteria, but about two weeks after birth, our digestive tracts are colonized by a large population of "good" bacteria (unlike "bad" bacteria, such as bacteria that cause food poisoning). These tiny creatures stay with us most of our lives, with ups and downs in their numbers depending on what you eat, your health, or if you take antibiotics. Scientists estimate that at all times there are about 100 trillion bacteria in and on your body, with your intestinal tract (small and large intestines in particular) carrying most of those bacteria—for a healthy adult, about one or two pounds worth at a time.

These various types of bacteria should not make you squeamish—they are there for an important reason: to help you obtain nutrients you need from foods in order to survive. When your immune system is in top working order, the bacteria

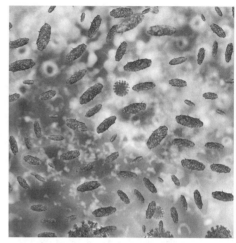

Not all bacteria are bad little microbes that need to be killed with disinfectant. Some, like those in your stomach that aid in digestion, are good for you.

also play a role in protecting our stomachs from "bad" bacteria that would otherwise rapidly grow. They also grow well in the sunlight- and oxygen-deprived environment of our guts, using our digested food as their source of nutrition; and they also help to synthesize some important nutrients our body needs, such as biotin and vitamin K, for good health. (For more about bacteria and our digestive tract health, see the chapter "Nutrition and Allergies, Illnesses, and Diseases.")

Does the stomach have a memory?

Yes, it appears that the stomach does have a memory—but not like the one we think of in association with our brains—and it is often referred to as the "gut brain." It is composed of about 500 million nerve cells that not only control the muscular contractions to move foods through your stomach to the small intestines, but may also communicate with the brain, letting us know when we're hungry or full. In the field of neurogastroenterology, researchers believe the gut brain evolved so digestion could happen somewhat autonomously and not include the "middleman," the spinal cord.

What causes flatulence?

Humans are not the only animals with flatulence—it is a process in almost all organisms, from your dog or cat to a snake. But for those humans who contribute methane gas to the atmosphere, it often has to do with the foods we eat and the bacteria that come in contact with that food. In fact, if you eat fruits, vegetables, whole grains, and other highly nutritious foods, it may be the price you pay for eating well!

In most cases, gas forms as intestinal bacteria ferment the remains of certain foods. For example, when you eat certain beans, some of the intestinal gases start when carbohydrates called oligosaccharides reach the large intestines. That is because, although your body has a hard time digesting these molecules efficiently, the bacteria are very efficient, and as they help you by digesting the oligosaccharides, they also produce gas as a byproduct. Other foods that cause flatulence are vegetables and fruits, such as broccoli, cabbage, corn, melons, and peppers. Flatulence can also be caused by certain conditions; for example, people who are lactose intolerant or have gluten intolerances will often experience bloating and accompanying flatulence if they eat an offending lactose- or gluten-rich food, respectively.

What ancient bacteria seem to be disappearing from people's digestive tracts?

According to recent studies, the *Helicobacter pylori*, ancient bacteria that have been in human digestive tracts for probably thousands of years, are now disappearing from our modern guts. In some ways it may be good, as these bacteria have been associated with the risk for gastric ulcers and cancer. But it's not really a good thing to most of us: The loss of *H pylori* means we are not as protected against several different types of cancer, asthma, and certain allergies. Most scientists don't understand why the bacteria are disappearing, but many associate the loss with our overuse of antibiotics. They reason that since the antibiotics cannot differentiate between "good" and "bad" bacteria in our guts, the *H pylori* are killed off when these drugs are ingested.

What are probiotics?

Probiotics are organisms that help our digestive tracts stay healthy and balanced, often referred to as our friendly or beneficial bacteria. (The term *probiotics* is the antithesis of antibiotics, compounds that suppress or destroy bacteria in our systems.) In terms of the human digestive system, probiotic types include the bacteria *Lactobacillus acidophilus* and *Lactobacillus rhamnosus* GG, and bifidobacteria.

There are various ways to make sure your gut contains these good bacteria. For example, many people consume fermented foods, such as yogurt, which can be helpful so long as the product contains "live cultures" of lactobacilli or bifidobacteria. And although

What bacteria seem to affect anxiety and depression?

Although the research was conducted on mice, researchers recently discovered that a certain bacterium may eventually help anxiety and depression in humans. They fed mice the bacterium *Lactobacillus rhamnosus*—a bacterium that is also found in a commercial (human) probiotic supplement—resulting in the mice showing fewer symptoms of anxiety and depression. The scientists believe the bacterium acts on what is called the central gamma-aminobutyric acid (GABA), which helps with the ups and downs of emotional behavior. The reason scientists are searching for the connection between this gut bacterium and the brain is obvious—especially if it is true in terms of humans.

there are many probiotics offered in pill or powder form as supplements, the consumer should be aware that the products vary in their effectiveness. This is mainly because of how the products were prepared, how they have been stored and handled (the bacteria don't like heat, so most products should be stored in the refrigerator), the types of bacteria the product contains, how much bacteria is said to be in the pill or powder, the expiration date on the product, and even how your system digests the pill or powder. (For more about probiotic diets, see the chapter "Nutrition and You.")

How can you naturally make your intestines "work well"?

There are several ways most of us can make our intestines naturally work well—or at least keep them healthy. And it has to do with foods. For example, some people

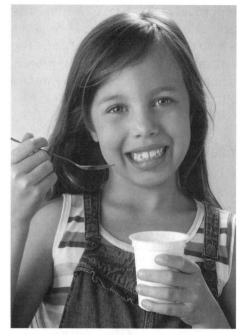

While you already have good bacteria in your digestive system, you can add to them by eating probiotic foods, such as yogurt.

help their digestive tract by eating prebiotic foods (foods that influence the microorganisms to grow) such as onions, garlic, and leeks; if possible, they eat yogurt or any fermented milk product (remember that pasteurized milk products, or those that have been sitting in the refrigerator for a long time, will have very few active bacteria). There are also studies that suggest opening your windows—the winds carry in soil particles that hold a great deal of bacteria (local bacteria are good for your system)—or taking walks in local parks or along hiking trails. And even our pets are mentioned in one study in which the researchers found that homes with dogs had more diverse microbes!

Can the microbes in your intestines make you fat?

Maybe. There is still a need for more research, but there is some indication that microbes in your gut may have an effect on your weight. One 2013 study showed that these intestinal organisms may be part of the weight gain puzzle—or why some people gain weight while others do not. It appears that there may be naturally occurring bacteria and other microbes (and some say perhaps viruses) in the body's intestinal tract that can influence our weight. The researchers think it may be the way the microbes respond to the foods we eat—and based on what types of microbes are in a person's gut, that person gains weight or not. If you have more efficient microbes (they break down foods better), the body will absorb more calories and gain weight; if you have more inefficient microbes, the body will be leaner, as there will be less absorption of calories.

Researchers stress that interfering with a person's natural microbes is not a quick fix to losing weight (and they still don't know which microbes do what), because there are other factors such as genetics, exercise, and daily dietary habits to consider. But this research may be a part of the overall puzzle of the obesity problem in the United States (and other countries): to date, the U.S. Centers for Disease Control and Prevention estimates that more than a third of adults and about 17 percent of children (triple the rates of a generation ago) are obese. (For more about obesity and nutrition, see the chapter "Nutrition and Allergies, Illnesses, and Diseases.")

What is an enzyme?

Enzymes are proteins that act as biological catalysts. They decrease the amount of energy needed (called activation energy) to start a metabolic reaction. Without enzymes, you would not be able to obtain energy and nutrients from your food. For example, a person with lactose intolerance cannot produce lactase, the enzyme that breaks down milk sugar (lactose) in most dairy products. Because of this, if any dairy is eaten, the milk sugar affects digestion, resulting in bloating, gas pains, and, if severe, vomiting and/or diarrhea. While this condition is not life threatening for most adults, it can have severe consequences for infants, children, and the elderly. (For more about lactose intolerance, see the chapter "Nutrition and Allergies, Illnesses, and Diseases.")

Do enzymes work only in specific environments?

Yes, enzymes do seem picky when it comes to their environment. This is because changes in temperature and pH can cause the structure of a protein to change. Thus, enzymes in our bodies have criteria that must be met in order for them to perform their functions. For example, the amylase that is active in the mouth cannot function in the acidic environment of the stomach; and pepsin, which breaks down proteins in the stomach, cannot function in the mouth. This is why it is important to take precautions when body temperature is higher than 104 degrees Fahrenheit (40 degrees Celsius) for any amount of time, as this changes the way proteins move through our system.

Who was the first to use the term *enzyme*?

Around 1876, German physiologist Wilhelm Kühne (1837–1900) proposed that the term *enzyme* be used to denote phenomena that occurred during fermentation. The word itself means "in yeast" and is derived from the Greek *en*, meaning "in," and *zyme*, meaning "yeast."

How many enzymes are found in the human body?

To date, scientists have identified about 75,000 enzymes in the human body. There are three major divisions: metabolic enzymes run our body's metabolic reactions, mainly for energy production; digestive enzymes break down and assimilate the foods we eat, and include the digestion of carbohydrates, fats, and proteins; and food enzymes are ob-

Why is eating slowly good for most people?

Nutritionists often emphasize the necessity of eating slowly, especially in our Western fast-paced society. There are several reasons, including the most obvious: Eating fast often gives you indigestion, never allows you to truly taste your food, and is often associated with stress. But the biggest advantage of slow eating is better digestion. Many nutritionists advocate chewing your food slower, not only so you can enjoy and savor the foods, but to break down foods so your digestive tract will work more efficiently at absorbing nutrients. This is particularly true for vegetables—the more you chew, the more the vegetables are broken down, and the easier it is for your gut to absorb the foods' nutrients. Even diet comes into play when it comes to slow eating—if you slow down your eating, you're more likely to eat less. This is because it takes about 15 minutes for your stomach to get the message to your brain that you're full. If you eat slower, it allows this time to pass—and you may not eat all those cheese and ground beef–covered nacho chips!

tained mostly from plants. (We can't make the last enzymes; we have to get them from foods such as raw fruits and vegetables.)

What are some foods that affect your metabolism?

As food goes through our bodies, there are chemical changes that occur in the foods' nutrients—from the time they are absorbed and become part of our system or are excreted. Metabolism is the conversion of these digested nutrients into components that give us energy—or that build and maintain our living tissues, from our cells to our organs The main components important to metabolism are glucose (from carbohydrates we eat), glycerol and fatty acids (from fats), and amino acids (from proteins). Each unit is important and is converted to either use for energy (such as carbohydrates converted to glucose, providing us with energy), or to release energy (such as some fats that are metabolized to produce heat or to be stored for later use).

IS IT GOOD FOR YOU?

Is tofu good for you?

Depending on your dietary needs, for some people, especially many vegetarians and vegans, the soybean product called tofu (made from puréed soybeans and often called soybean curd) is a nutritiously beneficial food. Not only is it low in calories and saturated fat, but it is high in protein, iron, B vitamins, potassium, zinc, and other minerals. It is also versatile: tofu cakes can vary in texture from soft to extra firm and can be stir-fried, grilled, baked, and mashed, or added to many other foods. Soy products such as tofu are often said to have a beneficial effect, fighting heart disease, some cancers, and osteoporosis, and, although this is debatable, are thought to help alleviate some menopausal symptoms.

But not everyone likes tofu—and there is a great deal of debate in the nutrition community concerning this particular soy product. Soy-contrary people mention that soy contains potent enzyme inhibitors that block enzymes that break down proteins (but research also shows that those inhibitors also can protect the body from certain cancers). The debate continues, but for most people, eating a moderate amount of tofu is fine, and may even be beneficial. (For more about tofu, see the chapters "Food Preservation and Nutrition" and "Controversies with Food, Beverages, and Nutrition.")

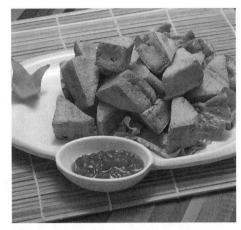

Tofu is a gelatinous curd made from puréed soybeans. It can be used as a meat substitute in many dishes because it can be cooked just like meat.

How nutritious are eggs?

Eggs are very nutritious and can be served in so many ways—and are found in so many food products and recipes! Overall, large whole eggs have an average of 70 calories, 4 to 5 grams of fat, 6 grams of protein, and about 185 milligrams of cholesterol.

Are eggs good for you?

Eggs, like some other foods, have been in and out of favor over the years. But overall, most nutritionists recommend eating eggs for the food's vitamins, proteins (containing all nine essential amino acids), and other nutrients that help a person's eyes, brain, and heart. In fact, many of the healthy nutrients in eggs, such as vitamins D, B_{12}, and E, along with omega-3 fatty acids and lutein, are known to increase in an egg when the laying hen is fed a good diet—in other words, when the chickens eat an organic, vegetarian diet that contains no animal fats or byproducts versus a more conventional diet.

Most of the negative press about eggs has come from the cholesterol content, especially for people who have high cholesterol. And while you should follow your doctor's or nutritionist's advice about what to eat, there has been a great deal of research on eggs, and most of it shows there is no evidence that people who eat more eggs have more heart attacks than those who eat few eggs. Of course, as with most things, moderation is the key.

What are dairy products?

Contrary to what you see in your grocery store's "dairy case," dairy products are considered to be only those foods that come from cow's milk—although this may include milk from other animals, such as sheep or goats. These products include milk (in most cases, whole, 1 or 2 percent, or skim), all types of cheeses, yogurts, ice cream, and such specialties as ricotta cheese. They *do not* include eggs, which come from poultry, but eggs often end up right next to the milk and cottage cheese in your grocery store, adding to the confusion.

If avocados have so much fat, why are they considered good for you?

Yes, the average avocado has 30 grams of fat, but two-thirds of those fats are the healthier monounsaturated fats (for more about fats, see the chapter "The Basics of Nutrition: Macronutrients and Non-nutrients"). They are available year-round, although the most famous avocado—the Hass—has a season from March to September. Avocados have been around a while, and were known by the Aztecs, who believed the food was an aphrodisiac. (The fruit was considered so potent that maidens were kept inside during the harvest!) Whether this is true or not, researchers do know that avocados are high in fiber, and have some potassium, magnesium, and protein—and are thought to lower "bad" LDL and boost "good" HDL cholesterols.

What are some of the lesser-known nutrient-rich greens?

Greens are usually found in the produce section of the grocery and are, as the name implies, in most cases green, and all are very nutritious. Most of us are familiar with the

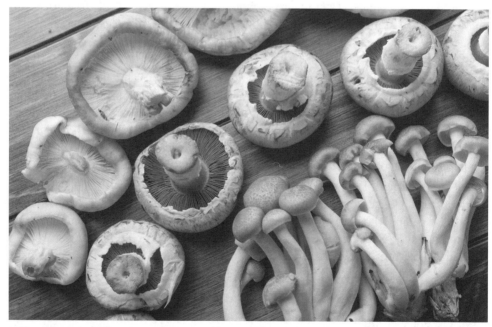

Different types of edible mushrooms (left to right): Brown beech mushrooms, Shimeji mushroom, and baby bella. Many people used to think mushrooms were mostly just cellulose and water, but they are now recognized for being rich in vitamin D, glutamic acid, selenium, riboflavin, zinc, potassium, and thiamin.

usual greens: different types of lettuce and spinach. Some of the lesser known, but still nutrient-rich, greens are as follows: escarole (mild in flavor, high in folate); kale (a bit bitter, but after a light freeze in the garden becomes sweeter; high in potassium and lutein); collards (taste between cabbage and kale; high in calcium, fiber, potassium, and vitamins C, A, and K); bok choy (a crunchy, almost cabbage-tasting green that is often used in a stir-fry; high in calcium); beet greens (the sweet tasting tops, either baby-sized or larger; high in calcium and potassium); and mustard greens (peppery taste; one of the highest in vitamin K of all vegetables).

Why are purple vegetables some of the best to eat?

Purple vegetables are high in anthocyanin, an antioxidant thought to protect against certain cancers, reduce the risk for heart disease and Parkinson disease, and improve your eyesight. In a recent study, when a group of obese people with high blood pressure ate two servings daily of steamed purple potatoes for a month, their blood pressure was lowered by 4 percent (around six points), suggesting purple potatoes are even more effective than oatmeal (a food often suggested to lower blood pressure). Other purple vegetables include the more commonly known eggplants, plums, and red cabbage. More recently, because of the interest in purple plants, growers have developed or discovered (in other countries) some more purple vegetables that are rich in antioxidants—such as sweet potatoes, asparagus, baby artichokes, carrots, cauliflower, peppers, tomatoes, and wax beans.

What are mushrooms and why are they considered to be beneficial to your health?

Mushrooms, as well as truffles (prized, more rare edible mushrooms), are classified as fungi. Edible mushrooms have several nutritional benefits: they are fat free and low in calories; they are rich in minerals, including potassium, selenium, riboflavin, thiamin, folate, and zinc; and when exposed to sunlight, mushrooms make vitamin D (similar to how we make vitamin D when sunlight hits our skin), which is why wild mushrooms in particular are high in the vitamin. (Most commercial mushrooms are grown in the dark, but lately, some producers have been exposing the fungi to light; these commercial mushrooms mention vitamin D on their labels.)

In addition, all mushrooms have a high concentration of glutamic acid—an amino acid that is thought to boost our immune systems. It is interesting to note, too, that glutamic acid is the naturally occurring form of monosodium glutamate (or what most of us know as MSG)—which is why mushrooms are used as a natural flavor enhancer in many recipes.

What are some edible mushrooms?

To date, there are approximately 200 varieties of edible mushrooms and about 70 species of poisonous ones (which is why it's important to know your mushrooms, especially if you gather them in the wild). The common white mushroom most of us recognize in the produce section of the grocery store was first cultivated by the French more than 300 years ago in abandoned gypsum quarries near Paris. Today they—and other types of

119

mushrooms—are cultivated all over the world. The following chart lists some of the more exotic cultivated and wild edible mushrooms:

Edible Mushrooms

Common Name	Scientific Name
American matsutake	*Tricholoma magnivelare*
Beech mushroom	*Hypsizygus tessulatus*
Blewit	*Lepista nuda*
Black truffle (*)	*Tuber melanosporum*
Chanterelle (*)	*Cantharellus cibarius*
Chicken mushroom	*Laetiporus sulphureus*
Golden mushroom	*Flammulina velutipes*
Honey mushroom	*Armillaria mellea*
Meadow mushroom	*Agaricus campestris* (and others)
Morels (*)	*Morchella esculenta* (and others)
Oyster mushroom	*Pleurotus ostreatus*
Porcini (*)	*Boletus edulis*
Portobello	*Agaricus bisporus*
Shiitake	*Lentinula edodes*
Straw mushroom	*Volvariella volvacea*
Trompette des morts (*)	*Craterellus cornucopioides*
White button	*Agaricus bisporus*
Wild Maitake (*)	*Grifola frondosa*

*Wild, edible mushrooms.

What is one of the oldest known plants grown for its seeds?

It is thought that one of the oldest known plants grown for its seeds—and its oil, too—is the sesame plant. It originated in the Mediterranean and African regions, and is especially important in Middle Eastern cooking, with such uses as sesame oil and tahini (ground sesame seeds). The famous phrase from *The Arabian Nights* that we are all familiar with—"Open sesame!"—actually is based on a part of the sesame plant's life cycle: When the seed pod reaches maturity, it literally bursts open.

What seed and its oils have been known for centuries to help our health?

One seed has been known for centuries to help our health: the flaxseed, either as a seed or as flaxseed oil. Greek physician Hippocrates (460–377 B.C.E.) thought of flaxseed as a medicine, and used it to relieve intestinal distress and even as a tea for sore throats. In the eighth century, King Charlemagne (c. 742–814) passed laws requiring the use of flaxseed by all his citizens. Today, flaxseed is thought of as one of the best natural sources of omega-3 fatty acids, lignans, and both soluble and insoluble fiber (for more about fatty acids and omega-3, see the chapter "The Basics of Nutrition: Macronutrients and Non-nutrients").

What somewhat controversial plant, as an oil, has potential health-promoting compounds?

Cannabis, often referred to as marijuana, is a hallucinogenic plant that is illegal according to U.S. federal law, although it has recently been legalized in some states, especially as medical marijuana. But there are also other forms of cannabis—including a close cousin called hemp (*Cannabis sativa L*; also called hempseed)—considered a low-hallucinogenic (often called nondrug) variety. Hempseed has a long history and has been eaten raw, cooked, or roasted; as hempseed oil, it has been used as a food and medicine in China for at least 3,000 years. Overall, hempseed has high

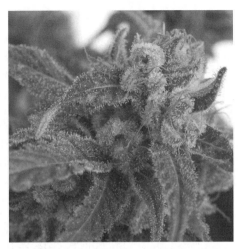

Marijuana can be classified as a depressant, stimulant, or hallucinogen because it can have any of these effects on those who smoke or ingest it.

levels of vitamins A, C, and E, along with beta carotene; it is also rich in proteins, oils, carbohydrates, many minerals (including phosphorus, potassium, and magnesium), and insoluble fibers.

Not much research had been conducted to check the oil's potential health benefits in the past decades, mainly because of the negativity and illegal use of high-hallucinogenic *Cannabis* (hempseed and all *Cannabis* varieties were banned in the late 1930s in the United States). But recently, in part because of the increased demand for healthy vegetable oils, research has shown that hempseed oil has health-promoting sterols, aliphatic alcohols, and linolenic acid—an omega-3 fatty acid. Thus, as more countries, including some states in the United States, legalize growing certain varieties of the plant—and as the stigma surrounding *Cannabis* changes—nutritionists may have another oil to suggest that promotes good health.

HERBS, SPICES, AND NUTRITION

What are herbs?

According to The Herb Society of America, the word "herb," like many plants (such as fungi and mosses), has more than one definition. Botanists, or scientists who study plants, describe herbs as "small, seed-bearing plants with fleshy, rather than woody, parts." But for most people who grow or study herbs, it also includes a wider range of plants—from perennial herbs to trees, shrubs, vines, and even more primitive plants. Overall, of the 250,000 species of flowering plants in the world, more than 20,000 (about 10 percent) are considered to be herbs.

How have herbs been used throughout history?

Humans have gathered and used many types and varieties of herbs for many reasons—from medicine to flavoring for other foods—and this "herbal lineage" would fill another book. Overall, it is thought that about 4,000 years ago, the Egyptians had the first herb gardens for religious reasons. Just a few centuries ago, herbs continued to be mostly associated with temples and the church, with the plants used for daily worship, ritual, or medicine (for example, the monasteries in Europe during the Middle Ages), and even for a show of power and money (for example, the formal herb gardens of the grand Châteaux de Villandry in France). But not every country (or continent) has the same types of plants; thus, the uses of many herbs have differed greatly over the centuries. In addition, many herbs from other parts of the world have been cultivated in other countries; for example, many European plants, such as certain types of oregano (for instance, *Origanum onities*, Greek/Turkish oregano native to the Mediterranean region) were brought to, and are now readily found in, the United States.

What is holy basil?

Holy or sacred basil (*Ocimum tenuiflorum*, or *Ocimum sanctum*), a member of the basil family, is a spicy, aromatic, shrubby perennial herb, and has become well known because it is revered in India. Medicinally, it is often recommended as a tea for sore throats; and because it also helps to cut off excessive cortisol production in the body, and thus cuts back inflammation, it is often suggested for arthritis. But more recent studies have shown that holy basil is also a mild nervine—or that it actually balances (and often uplifts) our moods—and for some people, that may also mean lower stress levels.

What are some common culinary herbs?

For herbs to be used in cooking, they usually have to offer some specific flavoring. Most culinary herbs are from the leaves of the plants—and sometimes they are represented by the herb's seeds (or fruits) or bulbs. The following table lists some of the more familiar culinary herbs—including the common and scientific names, the part used, and what the herb is often known for in terms of health (*Note*: some of the possible health benefits are debated or still being studied, so if you are ill, please consult your physician):

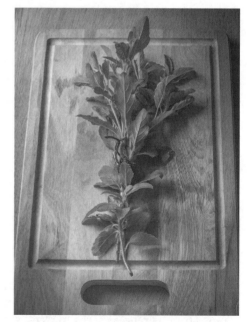

Revered in India, holy (sacred) basil can be brewed as a tea to help sore throats, and it also is a mood enhancer and anti-inflammatory.

Herbs and Their Uses

Common Name (Scientific Name)	Part(s) Used	Possible Health Benefit(s)
Sweet basil (*Ocimum basilicum*)	Leaves, flowers, oil	Good for digestion
Bay laurel (*Laurus nobilis*	Leaves	For indigestion (do not eat the leaves, but remove them after cooking)
Cumin (*Cuminum cyminum*)	Seeds, oil	Minor digestive problems
Dill (*Anethum graveolens*)	Seeds, leaves	For digestive disorders; some use as a mild diuretic
Garlic (*Allium sativum*)	Bulbs	Used to treat colds, and gastrointestinal problems; in onion family
Mustard (*Brassica nigra*) (black mustard seeds)	Seeds	Cabbage family; stimulate circulation and digestive tract
Onion (*Allium cepa*)	Bulb, some leaves	Protects against infection, reduces blood pressure and blood sugar levels
Oregano (*Origanum vulgare*)	Leaves	For colds and indigestion
Parsley (*Petroselinum crispum*)	Leaves	For many uses, including indigestion and menstrual complaints
Peppermint (*Mentha piperita*)	Leaves	Decongestant; improves digestion, mildly antiseptic
Common sage (*Salvia officinalis*)	Leaves, oil	Improves digestion; anti-inflammatory, relaxes spasms
Common thyme (*Thymus vulgaris*)	Leaves, oil	Improves digestion, controls coughing; antiseptic and antifungal

Why is garlic so good for your health?

Although many people steer clear of this member of the allium family, garlic has some major health benefits. With thousands of years of use, there must be some benefits to eating this herb: The ancient Egyptian healers and Alexander the Great (giving it to his troops) used it to build physical strength; the Chinese use it traditionally to lower blood pressure; and it was the nineteenth-century French chemist Louis Pasteur (1822–1895), who discovered the antiseptic properties of garlic (put to use during World Wars I and II). Scientists have now identified a compound in garlic called allicin (it varies in amount depending on the garlic variety). When chewed, cut, or cooked, the allicin undergoes a number of chemical reactions, forming sulfur compounds as the cells are disturbed, such as ajoene, allyl sulfides, and S-allyl cystein (SAC)—some of which are thought to have anticancer, anticlotting (thus reducing heart attacks), antifungal, antioxidant, and antihypertensive effects.

How do you get garlic's health benefits?

Don't think you'll get the same benefits from garlic supplements as with the real thing—it's been found that allicin is an unstable substance; in addition, putting it into

What discovery shows that spices were used as far back as 7,000 years ago?

A recent discovery by archaeologists in Denmark and Germany showed that flavorings were used in cuisine about the time the humans transitioned from hunting and gathering to agriculture. In particular, they found traces of the spice garlic mustard (*Alliaria petiolata*) in some charred pottery pieces that date from the Mesolithic-Neolithic times. (This plant is often thought of as a weed or an herb in some places, but in this study, it was called a spice.) This probably doesn't mean that these earlier humans ate the garlic mustard for nutrition—it has virtually no nutritional value—but ate it as a spice in other foods such as fish or other animal meats, since garlic mustard has a strong flavor.

pill form is difficult, as is getting the pill through our acidic stomachs (the acid destroys the allicin in the pill). Although there is no real consensus concerning how much garlic you should eat to benefit health, some people say a clove of raw garlic a day helps them to stay healthy. But overall, to make sure you get garlic's full nutritional power, start with raw garlic cloves. The cloves should be chopped or crushed, allowed to sit for about 10 minutes, and then cooked lightly. This allows the allicin and its potent derivatives to become active. (You can also use older garlic cloves that are sprouting—recent research indicates that such cloves may have even more antioxidant activity than fresh garlic!)

What are spices?

Spices are aromatic seasonings. They come from many different parts of specific plants; for example, they can come from bark (as in cinnamon), fruits and berries (as in black pepper), pods (as in vanilla), seeds (such as nutmeg), roots (also called rhizome, as in ginger), the styles (or spiny-filament center of a flower, as in saffron)—and even stems and outer coverings of the seeds (as in mace, from nutmeg).

What herbs and spices are thought to have antioxidants?

Several studies have shown that certain herbs and spices act as antioxidants—the molecules that help to rid our bodies of free radicals, or oxidants (also called oxidizing agents) that cause us to age, and can be triggers for cancers, heart disease, and even wrinkles (for more about antioxidants, see the chapter "The Basics of Nutrition: Macronutrients and Non-nutrients"). The most well-known antioxidant-rich herbs are rosehips (some claim rosehips have ten times the antioxidant value of wild blueberries, although the latter tastes better; it is also rich in vitamin C and bioflavonoids); rosemary, sage, thyme, and oregano (they contain aromatic phenols, and also have anti-inflammatory and immune-boosting benefits; most of the health benefits are stronger as

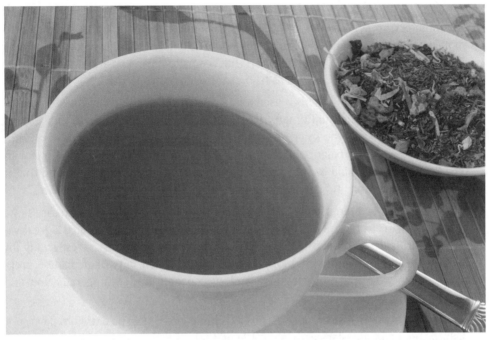

A cup of honey spice rooibos (red) tea can be sipped as a way to lower cholesterol and high blood pressure.

the herb is dried). The most well-known antioxidant-rich spices are turmeric, ginger, cloves, cumin, and cinnamon (for more about many of these spices, see below).

Many teas—considered herbs—contain antioxidants, too. For example, rooibos (or red) tea may help protect against high blood pressure and cholesterol levels; green tea (drinking this tea is the best way to obtain the antioxidants; it is also said to be beneficial for cardiovascular health, and helps your mood, mental alertness, and even skin health); white tea (it has three times the antioxidant power of green tea, and just a bit less caffeine); and oolong and black teas (fewer antioxidants than green or white, and with more caffeine—but still beneficial).

What spices are thought to be good for your health?

There are several spices thought to be good for a person's health. The following list offers a representative sampling of the more "healthy" spices:

Saffron—It is not only the taste that makes people want this spice (see above), it is also desirable for its medicinal properties. For example, saffron has been used in traditional Persian medicine as a mood booster, usually as a tea or in prepared rice, and even to relieve mild depression; other studies have found that saffron may also relieve symptoms of PMS (premenstrual syndrome).

Turmeric—Turmeric spice—the fragrant spice that gives most curries their yellow-orange color and is actually a member of the ginger family—has several health benefits.

125

For example, it is used in both Indian (ayurvedic) and Chinese medicine for its anti-inflammatory properties; also, in India it is used to relieve arthritis, and as a paste is applied to wounds to speed healing. Many research studies have been conducted on a compound in turmeric called curcumin that seems to have a positive effect on cholesterol levels and moods, as well as having antioxidant properties.

Cinnamon—Cinnamon has been used for centuries. It was prized by King Solomon, and the ancient Greeks and Romans used it to boost appetite and relieve indigestion. Today, people still use the spice for medicinal purposes, including some who claim that the spice can help balance cholesterol and control the blood sugar of people with type 2 diabetes (it is said to smooth out blood sugar spikes after meals), and that it helps relieve bloating and gas. The oil of cinnamon also acts as an antioxidant.

Ginger—Ginger is often used to relieve colds and stomach trouble; to help ease some types of arthritis (it has inflammatory-fighting compounds); and contains a great variety of antioxidant compounds. It is well-known for easing nausea—especially for people who have problems with motion sickness (such as on ships or airplanes), pregnant women with morning sickness, and even people undergoing radiation and chemotherapy treatment.

Cayenne—Cayenne (also erroneously called chili pepper) is a spice used to flavor hot dishes, and it contains capsaicin, a volatile oil that gives the spice its bite. It has been used as a topical painkiller (because of the capsaicin), and may help reduce the overall symptoms of a cold or flu. In an indirect way, it is also a mood booster—researchers believe the hot spice stimulates the body's production of endorphins, or our natural mood-boosting chemical. This is probably why many people feel good—albeit needing to "cool down" their mouths with milk or bread—after eating spicy food.

What is the most expensive spice in the world?

The world's most expensive spice is saffron, from the styles—spine-like filaments at the centers—of a flower called autumn crocus (*Crocus sativus*). The name comes from the Arabic word *za'faran*, meaning "yellow," and it is native to eastern Mediterranean countries and Asia Minor. The spice has a long history and was prized by many ancient civilizations, including Egypt, Assyria, Phoenicia, Persia, Crete, Greece, and Rome. It is easy to see why the spice is so coveted: around 70,000 flowers must be picked to yield 210,000 stigmas—which equal about one pound (0.45 kilogram) of the spice. In addition, these flowers bloom for only two weeks; the stigmas are picked during that time, and removed before the petals of the flower wilt. After being roasted, they are sold as powder or whole stigmas, and depending on where they come from, their prices range widely: to date, the prices can range from about $15 for 0.035 ounces (1 gram) and $2,700 per pound (454 grams) to up to $10,000 per pound.

What parts of plants are sources for spices?

There are many spices available, many of them grown in warmer climates, such as India and the Far East—too many to list here. But here are some of the more common spices, their scientific names, the parts used, and a few of the possible health benefits follows (*Note*: some of the possible health benefits are debated or still being studied, so if you are ill, please consult your physician). For more details about certain spices, see below:

Plant Sources of Spices

Spice (Scientific Name)	Part(s) Used	Possible Health Benefit
Allspice (*Pimenta dioica*)	Fruit/berries	For indigestion, gas, and nervous exhaustion
Black pepper (*Piper nigrum*)	Fruit	For indigestion and gas
Capsicum (*Capsicum annuum; Capsicum baccatum; Capsicum chinense; Capsicum frutescens*)	Fruit/seed	Stimulates circulation and the digestive tract; increases perspiration; capsaicin is the compound that causes the burn when you eat hot peppers
Cinnamon (*Cinnamomum zeylanicum*)	Inner bark	Ceylon cinnamon, although other cinnamons also work; stimulates circulation; good for gastrointestinal problems; antioxidant properties
Cloves (*Eugenia caryophyllata*; syn. *Syzygium aromaticum*)	Flower buds	For gastrointestinal problems; known to lessen toothaches; antioxidant properties

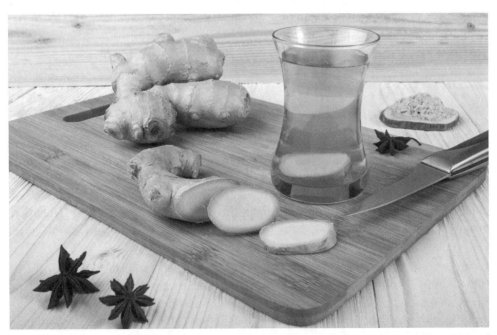

Ginger root can be ground up into food, sliced, or brewed in a tea. It is an antioxidant, anti-inflammatory, and stomach-soother that also helps relieve cold symptoms.

Plant Sources of Spices

Spice (Scientific Name)	Part(s) Used	Possible Health Benefit
Ginger (*Zingiber officinal*)	Root (rhizome)	Good for motion sickness, nausea, and indigestion; antioxidant properties
Mace (*Myristica fragrans*)	Seed (outer)	Outer covering of nutmeg seed, used for gastrointestinal problems
Nutmeg (*Myristica fragrans*)	Seed (inner)	Good for nervous and digestive system problems; often used for insomnia
Saffron (*Crocus sativus*)	Styles	Improves digestion and stimulates circulation, increases perspiration
Turmeric (*Curcuma longa*)	Root (rhizome)	For digestive and skin complaints; antioxidant properties
Vanilla (*Vanilla planifolia*)	Fruit (pods)	Improves digestion

What is curcumin—and can it affect your mood?

Yes, recent research has shown that the spice turmeric may contain an ingredient called curcumin (from *Curcuma*, a genus of eighty species in the family Zingiberaceae that includes the spice turmeric) that helps lift your mood. This compound apparently increases the brain's levels of serotonin, the neurotransmitter that makes people feel good. In fact, in another study, researchers found that taking 1,000 milligrams of curcumin was thought to be as effective as fluoxetine—the antidepressant better known as Prozac; in addition, curcumin appears to inhibit the production of monoamine oxidase, an enzyme that is associated with depression.

BEVERAGES AND NUTRITION

How nutritious are the various forms of milk?

If you live in the United States, you know that milk is often thought of as an important part of the diet. In fact, the government listing of foods we should eat each day includes dairy products—from milk and cheese to yogurt. This milk differs greatly from breast milk from a nursing mother (for more about breastfeeding, see the chapter "Nutrition throughout Life"); most milk we drink from the time we are weaned comes from cows, and secondarily, from goats, sheep, and even such animals as emus.

Cow's milk is the most consumed, and is widely available (most forms are fortified with vitamin D, too) as whole milk (not less than 3.25 percent fat), low fat (either 1 or 2 percent fat), and skim or fat-free milk (less than 0.5 percent. There is also cultured buttermilk, with less than 1 percent fat. Milk most often comes as a combination of pasteurized and homogenized (although raw milk is sometimes sold in specialty markets; some researchers [but not all] warn that raw milk often contains disease-causing or-

Has milk always had a dominant place in the American diet?

No, milk has not always been a staple food in the American diet as it is today. In the early twentieth century, milk was hard to keep, especially before refrigeration. It spoiled quickly, and often carried disease, and was mostly thought of as a spring drink, as the cows would have plenty of early grasses and be calving at that time; by winter, it was not as abundant. In order to make milk more available, milk had to be changed from its natural state to one that was pasteurized and homogenized—and thus began an industrial process to supply a great deal of milk to the general public, many of whom could now afford refrigerators. Interestingly enough, the milk was usually whole, and most people believed that skim milk was better to give to the hogs than to humans. This all changed after World War II, when the concern about heart disease intensified, and skim milk was proclaimed to be healthier than whole milk. (For more about controversies surrounding cow's milk, see the chapter "Controversies with Food, Beverages, and Nutrition.")

ganisms that are killed by pasteurization); milk is also often available as UHT (ultra-high temperature) or ultra-pasteurized, in which the milk is processed at high temperatures so it can be kept on grocery shelves for much longer.

Why are most soft drinks—or all—not nutritionally good for you?

Whether you call them soft drinks, sodas, or even pop, these drinks are actually filled with nothing more than water, flavoring, and sugar. Apart from an energy boost from the sugar (which is why soft drinks are often used when an ill patient can't take in other foods or liquids), and sometimes the caffeine, these drinks have little or no nutritional value. As with most sugary foods, when consumed in moderation, sodas are not harmful. But many people consume soda in large amounts, often to satisfy their hunger, and thus, soft drinks can easily take the place of essential nutrients in the diet.

In fact, most sodas contain such large amounts of sugar and acids that they can cause tooth decay, along with weight gain because of the empty calories they contain (for instance, there are about 100 calories in a 10-ounce bottle of cola). In particular, young children who drink soft drinks instead of 100 percent fruit juices and/or milk are losing necessary calcium and other nutrients for growth; and they may lose additional calcium because many of these drinks also contain a large amount of phosphates—chemicals that are known to weaken calcium absorption in the body.

Why are some health-care professionals concerned about people who drink too many sweetened drinks?

Because of the obesity problem in the United States, many health-care professionals—from nutritionists to doctors to health researchers—are scrutinizing the many foods and beverages that people seem to eat and drink in excess. One of these items is the loaded-with-sugar sweet drink—especially soda. Study after study has shown that these beverages are linked to obesity in adults and children.

It is thought that, on the average, Americans consume 200 to 300 more calories a day than they did 30 years ago. Some research indicates that nearly half of the extra calories come from sugary drinks that can pack on the fat. And although soft drink consumption is down since the late 1980s, recent studies don't point to just soft drinks—but even very sweet coffees that also contain plenty of calories that can lead to obesity. For children, the effects are even worse: a study in the late 2000s showed that a soft drink a day gives a child a 60 percent greater chance of becoming obese as a child and into adulthood.

What parts of the United States are trying to pass laws against sweetened drinks?

In 2012, in order to counteract the soft drink–obesity connection, New York City mayor Michael Bloomberg, backed by the New York City health department, proposed that the city ban large, oversized sugary drinks, prompted by multiple studies linking sweet beverages and obesity. But after all the advertising and support of the ban—even from the new mayor of the city, Bill de Blasio—in August 2014, the New York Court of Appeals rejected the ban. This was not the first time the city had tried to address the challenge of obesity and especially to get people to stop drinking excessive amounts of sweets. A major ad campaign in 2009 presented commercials of people drinking sweetened drinks, and in an interesting visualization twist, showed just how much fat was associated with consuming the drinks: It showed a stream of a drink coming out of a bottle (representing soda, a "sports drink," and sweetened ice tea) turning into fat as it reaches the glass—with the slogan, "Don't drink yourself fat."

Not to be thought of as unconcerned about people's health, in 2014 the California legislature proposed labeling soda bottles and cans with health warnings, similar to those on cigarette cartons—warning about the drinks' contributions to obesity, diabetes, and tooth decay. Once again, the idea has been scrutinized—with many people pointing out that most people already know the connection between sugary drinks and calories, but still drink the beverages. They also add that it's not only sweet drinks that are responsible for our obesity problems, but other sweets, some processed foods, and even "better-for-you" drinks such as some fruit juices that have just as many calories and sugar as soda.

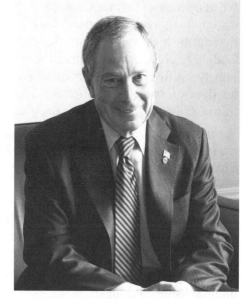

New York City's Mayor Michael Bloomberg made the news for backing a ban on the sale of oversized sugary drinks in his city.

What is the caffeine content of some well-known soft drinks?

Although it seems the opposite of what you would think, there is caffeine in many soft drinks. For example, 12-ounce (355 milliliters) cans of classic Coca-Cola—or Cherry or Diet—hover between about 34 to 46 milligrams of caffeine. Dr Pepper, whether it is regular or diet, has about 40 milligrams; regular Pepsi-Cola has about 38; and ginger ale has 0 milligrams. A regular soft drink that has one of the greatest caffeine contents is Mountain Dew, with about 54 milligrams in a 12-ounce can.

What is caffeine?

Caffeine is considered by many researchers to be an addictive (and the least harmful) drug, and is a stimulant found in coffee, tea, chocolate, soft drinks, and some pills (such as painkillers, cold medications, weigh-loss supplements, and drugs that promote mental alertness). It is readily absorbed by the body: within a few minutes of ingesting, it is absorbed from the small intestine into the bloodstream and carried off to the major organs. As a stimulant, it raises the heart rate, increases the activity of the central nervous system, and increases not only the digestive acids to flow, but also urine (thus it is considered a diuretic). It also causes the smooth muscles (such as those that control our blood vessels and airways) to relax.

Why is too much caffeine a concern—especially in terms of nutrition?

Too much caffeine—and "too much" varies between people—has several drawbacks when it comes to the human body and nutrition. For example, caffeine is mildly addictive; because it's a stimulant, it can cause sleeplessness in many people; it has a diuretic effect, thus often increasing urination; and it has been known to increase blood pressure in some people. Nutritionally, too much can lower the body's ability to absorb calcium—and because caffeine acts as a diuretic, calcium is also lost in the urine. Other than these effects, for most people, caffeine is relatively nontoxic—and it is said that the average adult would have to rapidly consume 80 to 100 cups of coffee in order for the stimulant to prove fatal.

How does caffeine affect humans?

Caffeine is often called "the most-common drug" ingested by people worldwide, the main reason being that it changes our body chemistry in several ways. For example, it stimulates our metabolism and slows the way our body uses glycogen (an

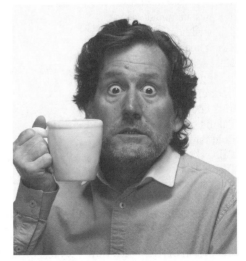

Caffeine—found in coffee, some teas, soft drinks, chocolate, and other foods and drinks—is a popular stimulant. While caffeine can raise our blood pressure, it might also help relieve asthma.

131

energy source), making us more energetic, and stimulates us (which is why many people are wide awake after eating or drinking many foods that contain caffeine). There are also some adverse effects of excessive caffeine intake, such as an upset stomach, headaches, irritability, and even diarrhea.

But many researchers believe that caffeine is not totally bad for us, and may—depending on the dose and food that contains the caffeine—actually be good for our health. For example, many researchers are not sure if caffeine really does cause a rise in our blood pressure as is often mentioned in older studies, and caffeine is often mentioned as being helpful for asthmatics: it has been known to arrest an asthma attack by relaxing the bronchial muscles.

What is the caffeine content of various caffeine sources?

The following chart lists various caffeine sources and the average dose of caffeine in each:

Sources of Caffeine

Source	Average Dose (caffeine in milligrams)
Espresso (2 oz.)	90–100
Coffee, instant	65–120
Coffee (5 oz.) ground, drip	100–180
Coffee (5 oz.) ground, percolated	75–170
Coffee (5 oz.) decaffeinated	1–5
Tea, brewed 1 minute	9–33
Tea, brewed 3 minutes	20–46
Tea, brewed 5 minutes	20–50
Tea, decaffeinated	1–5
Tea, iced (a mix)	22–36
Tea, instant tea	12–28
Most soft drinks (12 oz.)	30–48
Jolting soft drinks (8 to 20 oz.)	50–208
Dark chocolate (1 oz.)	20
Milk chocolate (1 oz.)	6
Baking chocolate (1 oz.)	35
Cold remedies	0–30
Pain relievers	0–30 (aspirin); 65 (Excedrin)
Diet pills	200–280

What are the differences between tea and coffee?

Overall, the differences between tea and coffee are many—especially how they are grown, the origin of the plant, how they are processed, the amounts of caffeine (see below), and especially the health benefits. In general, some of the differences are as follows:

Nonherbal teas—All nonherbal teas come from tea bushes—a warm climate evergreen called *Camellia sinensis*. The tea leaves are gathered, treated (for more about the different teas, see below), and brewed in hot water. It is thought that, after water, tea is the most consumed beverage in the world.

Herbal teas—Teas can also be derived from the leaves, flowers, or roots of plants—such as the drinks made from the flowers of a chamomile or echinacea plant. Most of these teas are consumed for their tastes, while others have long been used for medicinal purposes. For example, it is thought that chamomile and catnip teas help to relax and calm a person.

Coffees—Coffee also comes from bushes, but this beverage is made from coffee beans (also called coffee cherries) that are picked, roasted, and brewed to make various types of coffee. (For more about coffee, see below.)

What are the differences between the various types of nonherbal teas?

There are four types of well-known, nonherbal teas: green, black, white, and oolong (midway between black and green teas). The differences between each—besides the taste, of course—are the ways they are treated after the leaves are harvested. The black teas are fully fermented; oolong teas are usually partially fermented; green teas are not fermented at all, but are "pan-fried" and dried. These three teas come from mature leaves that are allowed to wilt and dry. The white teas are picked just before the buds have fully opened. These leaves are barely processed and are usually the most expensive teas, as they are picked only in early spring.

What are some herbal teas?

There are numerous herbal teas, classified as such because they naturally contain no caffeine; many also have certain health benefits, such as drinking ginger tea for symptoms of motion sickness. These teas include some well-known herbal plants, including chamomile, ginger, peppermint, lemon balm, rosehip, sage, and rosemary. Another tea considered to be herbal is the sweet-flavored rooibos or red bush tea, indigenous to South Africa.

What are thought to be some healthy attributes of certain teas?

Overall, no matter what kind of tea, or how the leaves are processed, all teas are found to have a great deal of nutritional value. They all appear to have many polyphenols, or powerful antioxidants. For example, one study showed that black teas, after fermentation, contain antioxidants that include beneficial biofavonols and theaflavins that help reduce strokes; another study showed that flavonoids (also called bioflavonoids) in black tea may help reduce the production of the "bad" cholesterol LDL that can lead to heart attacks and strokes.

Other teas also have more health value: For example, the antioxidants in green tea may halt the body's allergy response—essentially stopping the allergen before it affects the body; this tea is also thought to block the production of histamines, which are released by your body's immune system when an allergic reaction is triggered. Green teas are also associated with the release of dopamine, the brain chemical that makes us feel good—thanks to a substance in the tea called theanine. Green tea, along with other types of teas such as oolong, apparently helps our bones: Overall, the teas tend to slow down osteoporosis, can help to stop calcium from being leached from your bones, and, with the natural flavonoids in the teas, help to increase bone density. In addition, black and green teas contain catechins, a polyphenol group that is thought to fight cancer.

Coffee beans—such as this plant in Thailand—grow best in tropical areas with rich soil.

What is a coffee bean?

Coffee beans are actually the seeds of the coffee plant's cherries. The coffee cherries are red when they are picked; after processing and before roasting, coffee beans are green. On the average, 100 to 200 pounds of coffee cherries picked will produce about 20 to 40 pounds of coffee beans. Simply put, the coffee is then processed by the dry method (usually dried in the sun for several weeks) or wet method (separating skin and pulp, sent to water-filled fermentation tanks for 12 to 24 hours, then rinsed and dried); both types are then milled, graded, sorted, and exported—and then finally roasted, which brings out the various coffee flavors depending on the roasting method.

Where do coffee beans grow best?

There are some specific conditions needed to grow coffee beans. For example, the coffee plants need rich soil, high altitudes, and a tropical climate—which is so specific that coffee is usually grown only around the Equator between the latitudes 25 degrees north and 30 degrees south. Most places have only one harvest of coffee cherries, whereas some other places, such as Colombia, may have two flowerings a year, and thus two harvests. The quality of the coffee is determined by the type (chemistry) of the soil and the climate in which the beans are grown. The tastes and qualities of a certain coffee are also affected by minute changes, and even beans grown on one side of a plantation (or grown in a different year) can taste different from beans on the other side (or in another year) of the same plantation. Some of the more well-known types of beans include Kona, arabica, and robusta.

What plants have been used in the past to "mimic" the taste of coffee?

Of course, not all coffee has been made from coffee beans in the past—mainly because of scarcity of the product, such as during the American Civil War and World War II. Thus, several types of plants have been used to mimic the taste of coffee, although none seem to be as good as the real thing, including local grains, yams, and roasted nuts, such as acorns.

Is coffee good for you?

The advantages and disadvantages of coffee is a subject that divides researchers—and frustrates many coffee drinkers! Not everyone can drink coffee, but for those who like to have a few cups a day, there is some research that shows there are benefits (although it shouldn't really be considered a "health drink"). For example, it has long been thought that coffee can improve your mood—probably since it acts as a stimulant and gives you energy. Other more recent studies imply that coffee also improves your body's tolerance to insulin and speeds up your metabolism, both of which defend the body against type 2 diabetes; and yet another study confirms that coffee also has some antioxidants—many of which help stop some cell damage and maybe even decrease the risk for dementia.

What plant is most often used as a coffee substitute?

The most favored plant used as a coffee substitute (and it's also been used in certain European ales and beers) is the hardy perennial chicory plant (*Cichorium intybus)*, a purplish-blue flower found almost everywhere along United States roadsides during the late summer. The plant is actually native to Northern Africa, Western Asia, and Europe, and was thought to have originated in Egypt centuries ago; it was first brought to North America in the 1700s. The root is the part of the plant used to make "chicory coffee": it is washed, dried, roasted (which brings out the root's flavor, making it taste more like regular coffee), and cut up (not ground)—then steeped or brewed. Besides being caffeine-free, it is less costly than straight coffee—in other words, because it is more water soluble than coffee, you need less of it when brewing. To make the beverage, use about two parts ground coffee and one part roasted chicory, brewing as you would straight coffee. A couple of warnings: This coffee substitute may trigger reactions from people allergic to ragweed pollen and sensitive to related plants; and because it stimulates the production of bile in the body, it may affect people with gallstones.

What is the connection between inulin and chicory?

Inulin is a carbohydrate fiber, also often referred to as "chicory root fiber." This is why you often see "chicory root" listed as an ingredient in such foods as yogurt, ice cream, salad dressings, and breakfast bars. The inulin—also found in foods such as bananas, onions, and garlic—has a smooth and creamy texture, does not have much of a taste, and is often considered a substitute for fat. Some doctors mention that is also helps the body the same way other high-fiber foods do—by preventing constipation, lowering cholesterol, and helping to maintain the healthy, necessary bacteria in the colon. You don't need much—similar to eating too much of any fiber, too much inulin can cause digestive problems.

What are some effects of alcohol on humans?

Drinking alcohol—especially in excess—can have various effects on the human body. According to the National Institute on Alcohol Abuse and Alcoholism, alcohol can stimulate our brain cells by disrupting the calcium channels within our cell membranes; it can also cause the tissues in our body to become more sensitive to injury. And there is also damage on the small side, for example, to the structures within our cells, and a decrease in the way we synthesize and transport proteins from the liver.

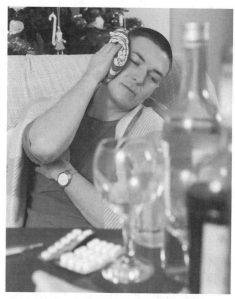

Many adults know the pain of a hangover after imbibing too much alcohol, but it can also adversely affect how your body breaks down food and absorbs nutrients.

Can excessive alcohol consumption affect nutrient intake in our bodies?

Yes, alcoholism can affect not only your family life, job, and personal well-being, but it can also be detrimental to your overall nutrition. In particular, it can lead to malnutrition, mainly because chronic drinkers usually don't eat well. Furthermore, alcohol can alter the digestion of nutrients and the ability to metabolize nutrients. Alcohol inhibits the breakdown of foods in our stomach and intestines by decreasing the amount of digestive enzymes secreted by the pancreas. It can damage the cells that line the stomach and intestines, causing problems with nutrient absorption; and like an endless loop of feedback, such nutrient deficiencies can cause even more absorption problems. For example, if you are deficient in folate because of excessive alcohol consumption, it may alter the cells in the lining of your small intestines; in turn, that can cause problems with water, glucose, and sodium absorption.

And even if a person seems to be eating well and taking in foods that are nutrient-rich, the alcohol can alter the transport and storage (especially in the liver) of nutrients within the body. In fact, many alcoholics get as much as 50 percent of their total daily calories from alcohol, which is nutritionally deficient. The most common result of alcoholism is a deficiency of thiamine; this can cause nausea, muscle cramps, nerve disorders, depression, and appetite loss. Other nutrient losses include vitamin D, folate, riboflavin, several B vitamins, and selenium. Alcohol can also affect protein nutrition; research shows that alcohol can cause impaired digestion of proteins into amino acids, along with other protein deficiencies. Chronic heavy drinking is also associated with deficiency in vitamins and minerals, mainly because the person eats less; the alcohol can also inhibit fat absorption, and thus, the person can be deficient in certain essential vitamins, such as A, E, and D, that are usually readily absorbed when eaten with dietary

Does nonalcoholic red wine help our health?

According to a research study done in 2012, nonalcoholic red wine may help certain people to lower their blood pressure (but of course, more research needs to be done). In this particular all-male study, the men ate a common diet and drank nonalcoholic wine with the meal—about 10 ounces (NA wine is usually less than 0.05 milliliters of alcohol) every day for four weeks. To compare, there were also those who ate the same diet and drank alcoholic red wine (10 ounces) or gin (about 3 ounces) with their meals for four weeks.

Overall, there was no true difference in the blood pressure of those who drank gin; for those drinking alcoholic wine, there was hardly any reduction in blood pressure—even though alcoholic red wines contain polyphenols, including those that decrease a person's blood pressure. The greatest blood pressure changes came from those who drank NA red wine—with a slight lowering of systolic and diastolic blood pressures. It is thought that NA wine, which contains blood pressure-lowering polyphenols similar to alcoholic red wine, also increases a person's level of nitric oxide—a molecule in our bodies that causes the blood vessels to relax and increase blood flow to the brain, heart, and other organs.

fats. And there is a plethora of diseases that can develop from the loss of nutrient absorption and chemical imbalance in the person's system—including diabetes (alcohol stimulates insulin production), obesity (alcohol is high in sugar, and therefore in calories), liver and pancreas damage, and even osteoporosis (calcium loss since vitamin D helps to absorb the mineral).

Why are scientists interested in red wine and its effect on humans?

For those who like the taste of red wine (in moderation), scientists are discovering there may be health benefits to your imbibing: drinking a small amount of the wine, for example, a glass with dinner, may reduce the risk for a heart attack. Researchers don't know the exact reason, but many believe that because red wine contains certain polyphenols that act as antioxidants (for example, resveratrol), they may protect our body's cells from damage during oxidation (or when the body uses oxygen); for instance, it may slow down the oxidation of LDL (the "bad" cholesterol) that causes blood vessels to clog.

WATER AND US

What is water?

Water is composed of two parts hydrogen, one part oxygen, and has no calories or nutrients. It is the most abundant substance in the human body—making up 60 percent of body *weight* for the average healthy adult. To break it down in another way, your body is 83 percent water (*volume*); your muscles are about 75 percent water; the brain, 74 percent water; and your bones are around 22 percent water.

Why is water important to humans?

Water is vital for humans (and most other organisms on Earth, too)—and the list of how water is essential to our bodies is long. For example, it helps with all our bodily functions, including digestion, absorption, and transport of nutrients; it helps us to eliminate body waste (both liquid and solid) by "flushing" the fats and toxins our body doesn't need through the liver and kidneys; it helps keep your skin supple; it allows your muscles and joints to work better; it aids all our body's chemical reactions; and it is necessary for the regulation of our body's temperature. It also cushions cells, limiting any damage (and is also in the amniotic fluid that cushions a developing fetus); is the prime "ingredient" in blood and in fluids that help lubricate our joints and organs; and is the base for our fluid secretions, such as saliva, tears, and gastric fluids.

Does the percentage of water in our system change as we age?

Yes, the percentage of water in our system changes as we age—more than most would think. A newborn infant is about 75 to 80 percent water; by the time a person is 65 to 70, the percent drops to about 50 percent. This drop is seen in many ways, including the wrinkling of the skin, stiffening of the joints (not as much lubrication where the bones join), and less saliva in the mouth.

What is the difference between hard and soft water?

There are differences between hard and soft water—including some differences in nutrient value. Water is considered "hard" when it has high amounts of calcium, magnesium, and other minerals; more minerals means harder water. This water is also notorious for leaving a "mineral film" on washed dishes and utensils, and requires more soap for cleaning purposes than soft water. "Soft" water is hard water that is treated, usually by using a water softener that exchanges calcium and magnesium ions with other ions that do not cause hard water, such as sodium and potassium.

There are some health benefits of hard water over soft water: the calcium and magnesium in hard water give us those specific nutrients; some research also indicates that hard water can help lower cardiovascular disease and/or help reduce blood pressure (although this is often debated, especially depending on just how "hard" the water is). Soft water isn't as helpful, especially for people who have to restrict their intake of sodium, as a water softener's outflow can be a significant source of sodium. In addition, some research seems to indicate that cooking foods in soft water can remove magnesium, calcium, and other essential elements from the foods.

How much water does a person need each day?

Although it has come under scrutiny in the past few years, research seems to indicate that healthy adult females and males should have at least 6 to 8 cups of water per day. Not everyone agrees; for instance, the Institute of Medicine states that adult men need about 13 cups per day, while an adult woman needs about 9 (it also states that we get about 2.5 cups of water a day from our foods); it is also noted that if you want to know if you're drinking enough as an "average adult," your urine should be a light yellow color. And there are specialists who feel that if you are an averaged-sized adult with healthy kidneys in a temperate climate, just about 4 cups (one liter) a day will fulfill a person's water needs (this applies mostly to people who also eat a balanced meal—as the fruits and vegetables consumed are also a source for water). There is no true agreement, and the debate about how much water to consume continues.

What experts do seem to agree on is that the amount of water you drink changes depending on circumstances, from your environment to your age. For example, we need more water when it is hot outside; in dry conditions (a hot or cold desert environment); when we exercise; and when we have a fever, cold, or other illness. And there are also changes in our daily water needs throughout life, from infancy to old age.

What happens if you don't drink enough water?

The average adult human can go without water for only a few days, while a person can usually go without food for about 30 to 40 days (for more about starvation, see this chap-

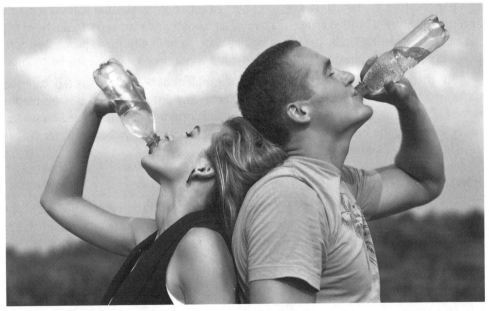

Six to eight cups of water a day are generally recommended to maintain one's health, but some nutritionists say you should consume as many as thirteen cups. Some of that, though, can come from water content in one's food.

ter), as long as they are properly hydrated. If you don't drink enough water, you become dehydrated. In fact, a loss of only 5 to 10 percent of your body water leads to serious dehydration; if the loss is 15 to 20 percent, it is usually fatal.

What are some of the major concerns with bottled water?

There has been a great deal of controversy over bottled water, for example, about whether the water is truly better than other potable (drinkable) water supplies. Some research claims that an estimated 25 percent of bottled water actually comes from a tap; some people also object to the fact that bottled water does not contain the same amounts of fluoride found in tap water (added to protect against cavities); another objection to bottled water is that, if stored for a long period of time, some bottles/jugs may eventually contain harmful bacteria (which is why most bottled water has expiration dates; the labels also suggest storing bottled water in a cool place); another controversy stems from the plastic garbage generated by the use of bottled water; and finally, many people object to the outgassing of the plastic of most bottled water containers, especially the larger jugs.

But there is not a clear-cut answer to the problem of bottled versus tap water, as there are so many different municipal supply areas and dozens of bottled water manufacturers. There are places to check out the possible pros and cons of bottled versus tap water, including the International Bottled Water Association (www.bottledwater.org) or even your local or state Soil and Water Conservation agency.

How much water is in food?

The amount of water in food varies. For example, most fruits and vegetables are about 70 to 95 percent water; an egg is about 75 percent water; meat, poultry, and fish are about 40 to 60 percent water; and bread is about 35 percent water.

FOOD PRESERVATION AND NUTRITION

EARLY FOOD PRESERVATION

What is thought to be the most ancient method of food preservation?

It is thought that drying was one of the most ancient methods of food preservation. According to some studies, there is evidence that Middle Eastern and Asian cultures dried certain foods as early as 12,000 B.C.E.; and of course, because most of those countries are found in hot, less humid climates, the sun was the main source for dehydrating such foods as fish, vegetables, and fruits. The Romans practiced drying fruits in the open air, while during Europe's Middle Ages—because certain areas lacked strong enough drying weather and sunlight—special buildings were constructed to house fruits, vegetables, and herbs that could be dried by fires and fireplaces inside.

Besides drying, what were some other early methods of food preservation?

Food preservation has come a long way, from drying and pickling foods to today's many additives and preservatives. Almost every culture developed various ways to preserve foods, including drying foods in warmer climates or freezing foods in colder regions. Necessity essentially became the mother of invention, and many early peoples learned by trial and error or from other cultures about how to keep various foods preserved. Besides the development of agriculture, food preservation allowed humans to stay in one place and build communities; it also helped people to eat more nutritiously, since certain foods became more available throughout the year.

There were several methods of preserving foods. For example, before refrigeration, fats and oils were used; ingredients such as lard, butter, animal fats, and oils kept out oxygen and sealed in moisture, two factors that caused food to spoil (as long as the layer of fat was thick enough). Another preserving ingredient was lye, a basic (as opposed to acid) substance that makes it hard for bacteria to proliferate. Early on, it was extracted from hardwood ashes and used to cure certain foods; today, it is not used as much for food preservation because of other better and less expensive methods—and because the substance, if not handled correctly, can be dangerous.

Why did North American Indians preserve foods?

Most North American Indian groups preserved foods mainly by drying for the usual reasons—to have foods to eat that were out of season, and even for times of weather extremes and warfare. But they also used some of their preserved foods for trade. One example often cited is of the Pawnee and Wichita peoples who lived in Kansas in the early 1800s: They grew and dried pumpkins, then wove the dried food strips into mats for storage. Many other tribes knew of the dried pumpkin mats—easy to carry and good for flavoring—often trading buffalo meat for the mats with other tribes, such as the Comanche.

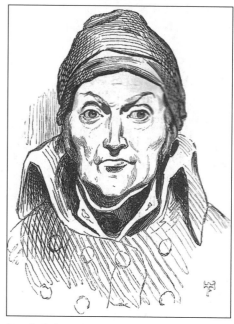

French chef Nicolas Appert developed the method of canning food in 1795.

What were some early advances in food preservation?

There were many advances in food preservation beyond the original methods of drying, salting, and freezing. The following chronology lists the more "modern" steps in food preservation:

Advances in Food Preservation

Year	Event
1765	The Italian Catholic priest, biologist, and physiologist Lazzaro Spallanzani (1729–1799) is the first to suggest preserving food by sealing it in containers that don't let the air penetrate.
1795	Napoleon offers a prize to anyone who develops a practical way to preserve foods, mainly to feed his many far-flung naval troops; it is eventually won by French chef, confectioner, and distiller Nicolas François Appert (1749–1841; for more about Appert and canning, see this chapter).
1806	Nicolas Appert's ideas are tested by the French Navy on such foods as meat, vegetables, fruit, and milk, all successfully and safely sealed in glass jars.
1810	British merchant Peter Durand is the first to use tin cans for preserving foods.

Advances in Food Preservation

Year	Event
1851	Nicolas Appert's son and successor, Raymond Chevalier-Appert, patents the pressure retort, which we now refer to as a pressure canner.
1940	Freeze-drying, mainly used for medicines, is used for food preservation for the first time in the United States.
1955	Deep freezers go on sale in the United States—units capable of freezing fresh food for extended periods.

PRESERVING FOODS BY COLD STORAGE AND FREEZING

Were some foods once preserved by cold storage?

Yes, cold storage of food is probably one of the older ways of keeping foodstuffs—as long as the region was relatively cool. Cold storage usually took place in root cellars, most often small holes dug in the sides of creek banks or in cool cellars where the temperatures stayed around 50 degrees Fahrenheit (10 degrees Celsius), and with high relative humidity from the surrounding soil. But most root cellars could hold only certain fruits and vegetables (meat products were preserved in other ways), and there were many problems keeping pests (animals and insects) away from the stored foods. Not all vegetables and fruits are good for such storage, and must be preserved by freezing, drying, or other methods (for more about the other methods, see this chapter).

Are there certain vegetables that can be kept in the ground over the winters in northern regions?

Yes, there are a few vegetables that can be kept in the ground over the long winters, especially in the northern regions. For example, kale has a good resistance to frost, and usually can be picked all winter as long it is protected with straw during bad freezes; carrots also have a good resistance to frost, and when protected from severe cold with straw, are usually still harvested all winter; and even parsnips and leeks can be overwintered with some protection. But not many people have gardens or keep their vegetables this way. One main reason is that our modern refrigerators keep foods at a certain temperature and relative humidity in order to preserve the original fresh food and its nutrients—so few people find the need to overwinter any produce.

What are some cold storage and/or freezing requirements for certain vegetables?

There are certain storage requirements for various vegetables—especially if you want the foods to keep their nutritional value and original flavors. Not all vegetables are good for cold storing, but many—especially root and hardy vegetables—can be stored for several months under optimum conditions. The following table lists those vegetables (always picked fresh, mature and of good quality, but not cut, bruised, split, or broken) that can be stored, and for how long, and the best conditions (temperature and relative humidity–wise) for storage to keep most of the vegetables' nutritional attributes (from the National Center for Home Food Preservation):

Cold Storage Requirements for Foods

Food	Temperature (Fahrenheit)/ Relative Humidity	Storage Life of Vegetable
Beets	32 degrees/95 percent	1 to 3 months
Cabbage	32 degrees/90–95 percent	3 to 4 months
Carrots	32 degrees/90–95 percent	4 to 6 months
Celery	32 degrees/90–95 percent	2 to 3 months
Dry beans	32–50 degrees/65–70 percent	1 year
Garlic	32 degrees/65–70 percent	6 to 7 months
Kale	32 degrees/90–95 percent	10 to 14 days
Leeks	32 degrees/90–95 percent	1 to 3 months
Onions	32 degrees/65–70 percent	5 to 8 months
Peppers	45–50 degrees/90–95 percent	8 to 10 days
Potatoes	38–40 degrees/90 percent	5 to 8 months
Pumpkins	50–55 degrees/70–75 percent	2 to 3 months
Rutabaga	32 degrees/90–95 percent	2 to 4 months
Sweet potato	55–60 degrees/85–90 percent	4 to 6 months
Tomatoes	55–60 degrees/85–90 percent	2 to 6 weeks
Winter squash	50–55 degrees/70–75 percent	3 to 6 months

What is blanching?

Blanching is often used to loosen the skin of fruits and vegetables by dipping them first in boiling water, then in ice-cold water. But it is used in the process of freezing fruits and vegetables: blanching a fruit or vegetable—or dipping them for a short time in boiling water or in steam, then into ice-cold water—helps to stop the activity of the plants' enzymes that cause decay.

What happens when food is refrigerated—or when it freezes?

Under refrigeration (most experts say your refrigerator should be at 35 to 40 degrees Fahrenheit [1.7 to 4.4 degrees Celsius]), certain foods are affected in various ways. For example, when fruits such as peaches are stored below a certain temperature, the activity of certain enzymes that contribute to ripening becomes inhibited in this case, too, it can also change the texture of the peach, making it mealy when the fruit warms to room temperature. Other foods benefit from the cold; for example, at 40 degrees Fahrenheit, dairy products and meat spoilage slows, as the foods' natural bacteria activities are suppressed.

For frozen foods, the water within food freezes below 32 degrees Fahrenheit (0 degrees Celsius). This causes ice crystals to literally cut through the food's cell walls and internal cell structures; in fruits and vegetables, this causes certain enzymes to be released, and when thawed, the foods become soft and mushy. This is why frozen food companies and people who preserve at home blanch and then freeze fruits and vegetables, as the blanching stops this enzyme activity.

How long can certain meats remain in the refrigerator or freezer and still be nutritious?

Various meats can be refrigerated or frozen for a certain amount of time and still be nutritious. The following table lists some meats and their storage times in the refrigerator (stored in the coldest part of a refrigerator that is set at 40 degrees Fahrenheit [4.4 degrees Celsius]) and freezer (0 degrees Fahrenheit [−17.7 degrees Celsius]) (from the U.S. Department of Agriculture):

Maximum Refrigeration Time for Meats

Meat	Refrigerator	Freezer
Bacon	7 days	1 month
Chicken, whole	1 to 2 days	1 year
Turkey, whole	1 to 2 days	1 year
Ground meat (beef, lamb, veal, turkey, chicken, or pork)	1 to 2 days	3 to 4 months
Cold cuts	2 weeks (unopened)	1 to 2 months

Does freezing vegetables affect the nutritional content?

Most research shows that vegetables that are frozen have *almost* the same nutritional value as fresh; this is because most frozen vegetables are picked, blanched, and frozen within hours of being picked (although some studies indicate that you can lose vitamins E and B_6 in frozen foods). In most cases, this quick-freeze helps retain many of the nutrients because lower temperatures slow down the actions of natural enzymes that can destroy some vegetables' nutrients, although there will always be some loss right after a vegetable is picked. Some vegetables are also affected by the ac-

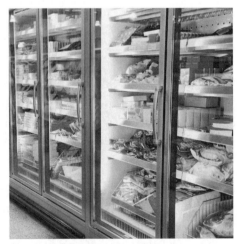

After fresh foods, the best option for buying food that still maintains much of its vitamin content is to get it from the frozen foods aisle.

tual freezing. For example, frozen broccoli will lack the enzyme myrosinase, which helps form an antioxidant to fight inflammation and, some say, cancer If you do freeze your broccoli, don't worry—you can always pair it with other foods that contain myrosinase, such as arugula, mustards (the greens, not the condiment), and radishes.

Which are more nutritious—fresh or frozen vegetables?

This is actually a "trick" question because the answer depends on how the fresh and frozen foods are treated—from picking to your plate. In general, fresh foods you grow in your gardens or buy at a local farmer's market are usually the most nutritious. And while fresh produce at the grocery store is usually nutritious, it depends on many factors: For example, how long it took to truck the vegetables to the store; how long they have been sitting in the produce section of the store; how the store maintains its produce refrigerators or displays; and even the temperature the vegetables have been exposed to from farm to your grocery bag (including how long you leave the vegetables in your hot car).

This is why many nutritionists say that fresh is best, but frozen vegetables are sometimes more nutritious than those from the grocery bins. But there is one caveat: Be careful that the frozen food has not been refrozen, which means that it is not as fresh and nutritious. You can determine this by making sure the vegetables are not clumped together, and that there are no signs of ice crystals inside (if the bag is clear) or outside the bag.

Can you freeze milk and egg products?

Yes, depending on the type of food, you can freeze some milk and egg products. For example, you can freeze egg whites and some products, such as some cookie dough; but you should not freeze eggs in the shell. You can also freeze milk for about three months, but it will often not have the same consistency as fresh milk from your refrigerator.

Does freezing destroy bacteria in various foods?

No, freezing does not destroy bacteria in or on food—but it usually stops the bacteria from increasing in number. But some still survive; thus, if your food is not safe to eat because of bacteria before freezing, it won't be safe after it thaws. The only true way to kill bacteria is to cook the food, as heat destroys the microbes—and it depends on the food what temperature and cooking time is needed to eliminate the bacteria.

PRESERVING FOODS BY DRYING, SMOKING, AND SALTING

How do you preserve food by drying?

Humans have been drying foods for centuries, from fish, game, and other meats to squash, apricots, and other vegetables and fruits. Simply put, drying—usually by controlled heat or sunlight—removes the water from the foodstuff, making it less prone to the growth of organisms, including molds and bacteria (although if the dried food is not dried enough, or not stored well, it can still develop molds or become contaminated with bacteria). Not all foods can be dried, but many can, and once the food is dried, it must be protected from condensation or any other types of moisture.

Does drying maintain nutrients of a food?

In most cases, the nutrient content depends on the food. When it comes to meat, drying does concentrate some nutrients, especially minerals, but it can have a detrimental effect on the vitamins within the meat. Drying vegetables often causes them to lose a great deal of their flavor and much of the vitamin content (except in the case of tomatoes); fruits usually keep much of their flavor when dried, but can lose some vitamins—but not as many as dried vegetables (the acidity of the fruits preserves the vitamins more).

What are some familiar dried foods?

There are many familiar dried foods, especially dried fruits. In fact, fruits are one of the easiest foods to dry, and even after drying, most retain their nutrients and flavor. There are some familiar dried meats—including beef jerky, chipped beef (a very old preservation method, a throwback to the U.S.'s pioneer past), and the Italian ham called prosciutto. Although these dried meats keep well, most people use refrigeration to keep meat fresh—especially so that it retains its original flavors and textures.

What are some familiar dried fruits, mushrooms, herbs, and vegetables?

There are definitely more dried fruits, mushrooms, herbs, and some vegetables, than dried meats. This is because meats have to be treated before drying so the food won't decay or become contaminated with harmful microorganisms. Plants don't decay like meats; thus, depending on the food, they are often dried for consumption later. For example, most fruits—such as

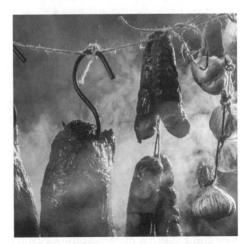

Ham, sausage, and garlic hang in a homemade smokehouse. Smoking meat is an ancient method for preserving it for long periods.

147

apples, apricots, berries, peaches, and grapes—can be dried; not as many vegetables can
be dried, but those that can include green beans, onions, spinach, beet greens, peppers,
and tomatoes. Many types of mushrooms are dried, including those used in many Chinese dishes, such as oyster or shiitake and most herbs can be dried, such as oregano,
sage, savory, and garlic—although some, such as basil and parsley, can lose much of
their flavor, oils, and color when dried.

Is it more nutritious to use dried or canned beans in a recipe?

In general, similar types of dried and canned beans will have relatively the same nutrients—it's what you do with the beans that can change the food's nutritional value. For
example, because many beans contain vitamin C, which is sensitive to heat, you may lose
much of that vitamin in your cooked dish. But you'll still be ingesting protein, fiber,
and other healthy nutrients that are not affected by cooking. (Not everyone agrees about
beans—see more in "Appendix 3: Comparing Diets," under the Paleo diet.)

How does smoking preserve a food, and does it retain its nutritional value?

Smoking is another "older" way of preserving certain foods, usually meats such as pork
(which is why most of us have heard of smoked ham). The smoking of fish and meats preserves the food by slowly lowering its moisture content; the smoke also leaves compounds
on the meat that help destroy many microorganisms. Most meats that are smoked still contain the protein content of the original meat; some nutrients can be lost, but because there
are not as many nutrients as in fruits and vegetables to begin with, it is not a true concern.

How is a food smoked?

Meat or fish to be smoked is usually soaked in a brine (salt water) or rubbed in salt before smoking (mainly to discourage insects, inhibit the growth of bacteria, and help
speed up the removal of moisture); it is then rinsed with warm water and allowed to dry
before smoking. Foods are most often smoked in a special building (often referred to as

a "smokehouse"), or in a closed box or barrel; a firebox containing chips of various types of wood or corn cobs (all of which can impart certain flavors) provides the smoke and some heat (but not enough to cook the meat). In general, the meat may be smoked up to three weeks before it is ready for storing.

Is there a controversy about eating smoked foods?

As with many foods that undergo certain processes to change their overall characteristics, there are controversies about eating foods that are smoked. In particular, most research indicates that there are many chemicals in the smokehouse smoke—more than 200 components so far identified, such as acids, phenols, and toxic substances. The chemicals may stop the meat from spoiling, but they are also coating the meat—meaning a person who eats the smoked foods will also ingest many of these possibly harmful chemicals.

Why and how were (and are) foods preserved with salt?

Preserving food by salting, like many other methods, has been around for centuries. It was once used on long ocean voyages, mainly to preserve meat, fish, and butter; and almost every rural household had a salt tub for preservation of foods (often called salt curing). Today it is still used for fish (for example, anchovies and cod), as well as for pork and butter. Occasionally, it is also used to preserve such vegetables as green beans, some herbs, and vegetable mixes used for soup stock. There are two methods, depending on the time needed to preserve the foods—either by soaking the meat in brine or rubbing dry salt into the meat. The main reason for using salt is obvious: Salt dries foods out and makes them last longer. This is because at a certain concentration of salt, microorganisms cannot grow and foods do not decay—mainly because, along with the meat, the salt also draws water from the molds and bacteria.

Is it good to eat foods cured with salt?

Many people enjoy foods cured with salt, including ham and bacon products, but overall, preserving with salt and salt curing are not in favor anymore; a great deal of research indicates that salt can increase blood pressure, and it also promotes fluid retention. For some people with salt-sensitivity or on low-salt diets, foods containing too much salt can result in a major health problem. Plus, although salt may mean a meat will keep better, the more salt used in curing, the more nutrients that are lost. And if salted meat is soaked to get rid of some of the salt, even more vitamins and minerals can be lost.

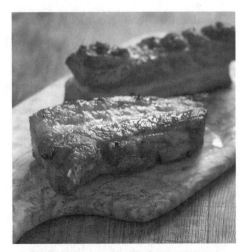

Using salt to preserve this pork belly works by drying the meat so that microorgamisms cannot grow in it.

149

What is mincemeat?

Mincemeat is usually thought of as a filling for a certain type of pie. Originally, mincemeat (or mince meat) was a means of preserving meat without smoking or salting, and was developed about 500 years ago in England. Medieval cooks realized that sugar was a powerful preservative—as was the alcohol that would often go into the mincemeat mix. The older version of mincemeat included meats such as goose, beef, venison, or the meat available, dried fruit, cider, molasses, candied peel (such as orange), all doused in brandy or other alcohol. Suet was also added—mostly beef or mutton fat from around the kidneys and loins—which was shredded and stirred into the pot. Eventually, after the Crusaders brought back many new spices (such as nutmeg and cinnamon), these, too, were added to the mincemeat mix. The concoction was then placed in a jar, and sealed with wax—a good way to preserve meats during the long winter months in Europe.

Since that time, the term has gone through some changes: In the early twentieth century, *mincemeat* usually pertained to everything on the list above but the meat and suet; modern mincemeat usually has no meat, thanks to the overabundance of fat in the recipe, and people have even used vegetarian "suet" (usually a soy-based product) in their recipes.

And history has not been exactly pleasant for those people who like mincemeat pies. In 1657, during the reign of Oliver Cromwell, traditional mincemeat pies were banned, as they were associated with Christmas, a fete that Cromwell thought of as a pagan holiday. The ban spread to the American British colonies, and by 1659, many towns in New England—including Boston (a town that banned Christmas from 1659 to 1681)—banned not only Christmas, but the mincemeat pies associated with the holiday.

PRESERVING FOODS BY AGING, FERMENTATION, YEASTS, PICKLING, AND CURDLING

What does penicillin have to do with cheese?

The unique flavors of certain well-known cheeses are produced by members of the genus *Penicillium*, or what we call penicillin—the same mold that is used to create the familiar antibiotic. Here are some of the cheeses associated with this mold:

Roquefort—This rich, creamy cheese with blue veins (called a "blue cheese") is often referred to as "the king of cheeses" and it is one of the oldest and best known in the world. Made from sheep's milk that has been exposed to the mold *Penicillium roqueforti*, it has been around since Roman times and was a favorite of Charlemagne, king of the Franks and emperor of the Holy Roman Empire (742–814). It is aged for three months or more in the limestone caverns of Mount Combalou, near the village of Roquefort in southwestern France—the only place where true Roquefort can be made.

Camembert and Brie—The mold called *Penicillium camemberti* gives Camembert and Brie cheeses their special flavors and qualities. Napoleon is said to have christened Camembert cheese with its name; supposedly the name comes from the Norman village where a farmer's wife first served it to Napoleon. This cheese is formed of cow's milk and has a white, downy rind and a smooth, creamy interior. When perfectly ripe and served at room temperature, the cheese should ooze thickly. Although Brie is made in many places, Brie from the region of the same name east of

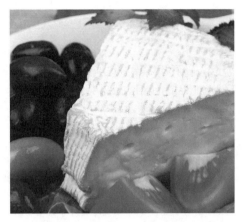

The mold called *Penicillium camemberti* gives Brie cheese its special flavor and qualities.

Paris is considered one of the world's finest cheeses by connoisseurs. Similar to Camembert, it has a white, surface-ripened rind and smooth, buttery interior.

What bacteria are necessary for the production of certain food products?

There are many bacteria that help humans produce some very well-loved foods. The following chart lists some of those foods, and the bacteria that are responsible:

Bacteria in Food Production

Food	Microorganism
Buttermilk and sour cream	*Streptococcus cremoris* and *Leuconostoc citrovorum*
Pickles	*Enterobacter aerogenes*, *Leuconostoc* spp.* and *Lactobacillus brevis*
Sauerkraut	*Leuconostoc* spp. and *Lactobacillus brevis*
Swiss cheese	*Lactobacillus* spp. and *Propionibacterium* spp.
Vinegar	*Acetobacter aceti*
Yogurt	*Streptococcus thermophilus* and *Lactobacillus bulgaricus* (and many others that are often seen on a container of yogurt)

*spp. = unspecified species

What is fermentation?

Fermentation has been around for 2.5 billion years—and maybe even longer—a process scientists believe was the way early organic compounds (and thus organisms) gathered their energy. Centuries ago, various fermentation processes were developed to produce such foods as vinegar, wine, bread, and beer. And today we use fermentation to produce a multitude of "old" and new foods—most using a combination of bacteria and fungi in the fermentation process. For example, fermented foods include cheese, sour cream, yogurt, sauerkraut and kimchi (both types of fermented cabbage), vinegar, cer-

151

tain baked products, olives, pickles, soy sauce, miso, tempeh, chocolate, coffee, and most alcoholic beverages.

What is crème fraîche?

Crème fraîche is French for "fresh cream," and it is actually made from the cream that rises to the top of whole milk. The crème fraîche is actually a cultured cream and a product of fermentation; the "starter culture" (some people start their own from surrounding natural bacteria; others use buttermilk as a starter) used to ferment the crème fraîche is actually good bacteria that cause the cream to get thicker. The process to make crème fraîche is easy, but takes time: A starter culture is added to a certain amount of fresh cream (some people use pasteurized heavy cream, but not ultra-pasteurized); it is then allowed to sit for about 24 to 48 hours in a relatively warm spot (65 to 75 degrees Fahrenheit [18.3 to 23.9 degrees Celsius]). The cream and the starter culture act together to make a thick, glossy cream that tastes tangy with a rich, creamy butter-like flavor. It can keep in your refrigerator for up to about a month.

What was Louis Pasteur's theory of fermentation?

In the mid-1800s, most scientists believed that fermentation was just a chemical process in which the microorganisms involved were just a byproduct, not the catalyst for the process. It was French chemist and microbiologist Louis Pasteur (1822–1895)—one of the founders of medical microbiology—who proposed that fermentation was a process carried out by what he referred to as "living ferments"—what we now know as microorganisms such as yeasts and bacteria.

What is lacto-fermentation?

Lacto-fermentation has been around for centuries. The ancient Greeks knew about the types of chemical changes that took place during this fermentation, which they labeled "alchemy." The lactic acid is a natural preservative that inhibits bacteria that decay foods; and vegetable and fruit starches and sugars are converted into lactic acid by lactic-acid-producing bacteria called lactobacilli. They are everywhere—and their main byproduct of lactic acid helps to promote the good bacteria in our digestive tract. In addition, using lacto-fermentation for certain vegetables not only preserves the foods, but also enhances the

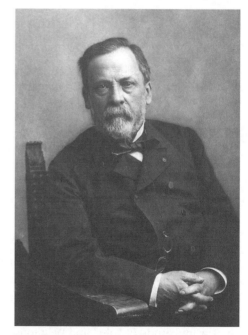

Louis Pasteur was a nineteenth-century microbiologist who figured out that fermentation was caused by what we now call microorganisms.

vegetables digestibility, and, for some, helps increase the absorption of the food's vitamins in our systems.

And there are many examples. Perhaps the most popular one is the lacto-fermented European favorite, sauerkraut; other pickled vegetables include beets, cucumbers, and even pickled lettuces, green tomatoes, eggplant, onions, and carrots. Interestingly enough, this type of fermentation has never been popular with industrial food sources—it takes too long and the results are not always predictable. Thus, when pickling became industrialized, changes were made to the traditional "formula." This often means that it's easier to make a uniform product. But the resulting foods usually don't have as many nutrients—and the pasteurization kills off the good bacteria that help our digestive tract.

What are some fermented drinks?

There are several fermented drinks that seem to be popping up all over—a trend that seems to have started in California in what are called "fermentation bars." The drinks vary from teas to milk products; all are fermented to bring out their flavor, and to add some health benefits, such as gut-friendly bacteria and yeasts that help your digestion and some B vitamins. For example, kefir (found in most health food stores) is a fermented milk drink that is rich in calcium and is formed as certain bacteria break down the milk's lactose into the more digestible lactic acid and lactate. (A study also found that drinking kefir may improve lactose digestion in lactose-intolerant people; for more about lactose intolerance, see the chapter "Nutrition and Allergies, Illnesses, and Diseases.") Yet another fermented drink is kefir water, or a mix of fruit and water brewed with a probiotic cocktail of bacteria and yeast—called water kefir grain—that has more of an intense (and creamy) taste than just fruit-flavored water.

What's an example of a fermented tea?

There are several ways in which teas are treated before they are used for drinking. For example, Kombucha is a sweet tea (either black or green) that is fermented with bacteria and yeast. As an already prepared drink, it can be flavored with herbs or fruit. There can also be a small amount of alcohol produced during fermentation (less than 0.5 percent by volume, similar to what are classified as nonalcoholic beers and wines—so read the label because sometimes fermentation can create a Kombucha drink with up to 3 percent alcohol). In addition, other teas are infused with various herbs, spices, or fruit to obtain various flavors. (For more about teas, see the chapter "Nutrition in Eating and Drinking Choices.")

How are alcoholic beverages produced?

The alcohol found in alcoholic beverages is known as ethanol; it is produced by yeast through the process known as alcoholic fermentation. During the breakdown of glucose in order to obtain energy, the yeast cells generate ethanol as a way to recycle a molecule that is crucial to their metabolism. But this process eventually stops, as yeast can survive only in a beverage like beer or wine that contains less than 10 percent alcohol by volume. Thus, if you find a beverage with an alcoholic content greater than 10 percent, additional alcohol has been added or the beverage has been distilled.

What is used in beer production?

Beer is made by fermenting water, malt, sugar, hops, yeast (*Saccharomyces* spp.), salt, and citric acid, with each ingredient having a specific role in the process. For example, hops is the herb *Humulus lupulus* (a member of the mulberry family); the fruit is picked when ripe and is then dried—an ingredient that gives beer its slightly bitter flavor. Malt is from a grain—usually barley—that has been sprouted, dried in a kiln, and ground into a powder; it gives beer its characteristic body and flavor.

Is there a difference between active and instant yeasts?

Yes, there is a difference between active and instant yeasts—mainly in how you use them in a recipe. Active dry yeast usually has more inactive yeast cells, and when making, for example, yeast muffins, you have to dissolve the yeast in a portion of water from the recipe and heat it to 110 degrees Fahrenheit (43.3 degrees Celsius) and let it stand for five minutes; but note that fermentation of the yeast slows above 120 degrees (48.9 degrees Celsius) and yeast cells die at 140 degrees (60 degrees Celsius). With instant yeast, or rapid-rise, you don't have to let it activate, but can usually add it directly to the other ingredients.

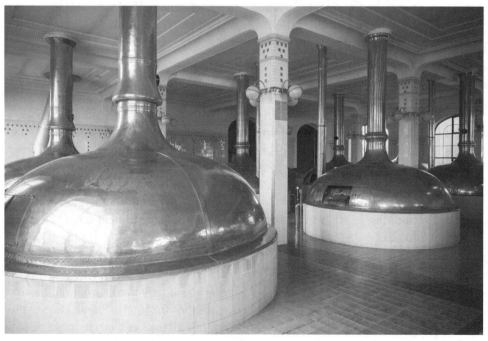

A brewery building interior, container cooking pots. Beer is made by combining malt, sugar, hops, and water and fermenting it all with yeast.

What are yeasts?

Yeasts are single-celled organisms that are actually fungi, with about 600 different species known to date. It has often been called the first "domesticated animal," as various yeasts have been used in wine making, beer making, and bread making for centuries. Most yeast species reproduce rapidly, and their main purpose is to serve as a catalyst in the process of fermentation; it converts food into alcohol and carbon dioxide during the process. You can see this in the kitchen when you add dry yeast to water containing sugar—and especially when you make bread. Yeasts feed on the sugars that are in the flour, and/or that you add, releasing carbon dioxide in the process.

How is bread made?

Breads have been made for centuries—and although the contents may change, the idea behind how bread is made has not changed: it's all about fermentation. Simply put, breads contain water, flour, and yeast (for more about flours, see the chapter "The Basics of Nutrition: Macronutrients and Non-nutrients"). But after the mixing and kneading, one of the most important steps is the fermentation—also called "letting the bread rise." This fermentation process not only allows the yeast to help the dough rise, but also helps produce many aromatic molecules that give bread that wonderful aroma you smell as you walk past a bakery (although if bread rises too fast, it may produce some sour-smelling volatile acids). During this fermentation, the gluten will relax and become more supple, the yeast cells will react with the sugars (from the breaking down of starch, the sugars in the flour, and/or if you add sugars to the recipes) and release carbon dioxide and ethyl alcohol—which causes the bread to "rise." Most recipes call for a second rise or proofing; the third and last "rise" (chefs call it "oven spring") from the heat of the oven keeps the bread "growing" until the last of the yeast is killed off.

What is cool fermentation?

It may seem just the opposite from what most of us know about baking bread—that the yeast causes the bread to rise in warmer temperatures. But another good fermentation method is called cool fermentation, and it is just as the words imply; the cool fermentation of dough that often contains a preferment (also called a starter culture or sponge; for more information, see below). Bakers who use this baking method let dough (breads, rolls, waffles, pizza, etc.) rise in the refrigerator so the yeast can develop more flavor in the dough—and more slowly.

What is a starter or sponge?

When making artisan breads, many bakers use either a sponge or starter as their "yeast"—made before the bread is even started—and use it to boost the flavor of the bread. A sponge is made from yeast, water, and flour, then allowed to ferment for several hours, usually at room temperature, then added to the final bread dough. A starter, or starter culture, takes longer—it is, initially, a part of the dough that is saved in a refrigerated crock. Every so many days, part of the starter is removed (and used in various baked goods as a starter culture); more water and flour are "fed" to the starter, then it is allowed to sit and ferment for a few hours, or immediately put back into the refrigerator again (especially on hot summer days when the starter can become so active, it will overflow the crock). Some starter cultures have been in bakeries (or if a person makes his or her own bread, in homes) for years, with some bakers claiming the original "ancestor" of their starter is over a hundred years old.

What are baker's yeast and brewer's yeast?

Baker's yeast is a leavening agent and is used to increase the volume of baked goods such as bread. It comes as active dry and compressed fresh yeast: Active dry yeast is made up of tiny, dehydrated granules of yeast and it becomes active when added to a warm liquid. (Although the yeast granules are alive, the cells are dormant because of a lack of moisture—and thus dry yeast has a long shelf life.) Compressed fresh yeast is more moist, extremely perishable, and has to be stored in the refrigerator (use it in one to two weeks). Brewer's yeast is much different—it is a special nonleavening agent used in beer making, converting the sugars in malted barley into alcohol. And because it is a rich source of B vitamins, brewer's yeast is also used as a food supplement.

What is pickling?

According to people who preserve fruit, meat, or vegetables by the pickling process, these foods are most often preserved by either fermentation in brine (salt) or packed in vinegar. Heat is also used in the processing to destroy microorganisms and stop the activity of enzymes in the foods that can affect the flavors, colors, and textures. For example, brined pickles are usually made with vegetables such as cucumbers (dill pickles are a favorite), with additional flavors from herbs, such as dill or garlic; they are submerged and fermented or cured in a salt solution for several weeks. Fresh packed pickles are canned in a spicy vinegar solution, but not usually brined. They are processed, then allowed to sit for a few weeks to cure and develop more flavor.

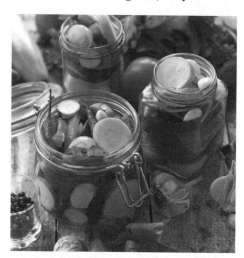

How is tofu made?

Tofu is a soybean product, often referred to as "soybean curd." It is usually sold in most grocery stores, or you can make it at home. For vegetarians, tofu is a rich source of protein and iron, a good source of B vitamins, potassium, zinc, and other minerals, and, if treated with nigari or gypsum (calcium sulfate), a source of calcium. It is also low in calories and saturated fats.

Pickling—like salting and smoking—works by creating an inhospitable environment for organisms that would spoil food.

Simply put, to make a "cake" of tofu (there are several good tofu recipes available in books or on the Internet), you need soybeans, either dried or raw. If dried, the soybeans need to be soaked in water overnight; the raw soybeans do not need to be soaked. The soybeans and water are measured (depending on how much tofu is being made), then blended together. This slurry is then heated to a certain point, and drained through cheesecloth, catching and squeezing out most of the liquid from the soybean coatings (this is called okara and can also be used in cooking). The liquid (soybean milk) is then heated again; after a certain time, a coagulant is added (the usual choices are food-grade gypsum, nigari, and even lemon juice), and the liquid is allowed to sit, covered, for a certain amount of time. The result is the formation of soybean curds and whey. The curds are scooped out of the pot, put into a container with holes, and allowed to drain for a certain amount of time (depending on if you want softer or firmer tofu). The block of tofu is then kept in water in a refrigerator until needed; freshly made tofu usually lasts for about a week to ten days, as long as the water is changed each day. (For more about tofu, see the chapter "Nutrition in Eating and Drinking Choices.")

Is yeast used in the "old way" of making soy sauce?

Yes, yeasts are used to make soy sauce—the dark brown, salty liquid; it was first produced in Japan to make unpalatable soybeans more palatable. Although there are newer methods to make soy sauce, many modern soy sauce makers still use the older fermenting process methods: First, the soybeans are soaked and cooked, then the results are mixed with roasted wheat. *Aspergillus oryzae* (a fungus) is added and kept active for up to 40 hours. When a paste forms, it is put in a deep vat with the yeast *Saccharomyes rouxii* and *lactobacilli*—both of which stop the growth of the *A oryzae*. A month later, a liquid forms—complete with large concentrations of amino acids, simple sugars, and some vitamins—or what we call soy sauce.

How is paneer made?

Paneer is mostly associated with Indian cuisine, and is actually curdled milk, made by squeezing the liquid from the curds. It can be simply made by heating whole milk (or 2 percent) to the boiling point, then adding lemon juice. The result will be milk curds and liquid whey; the curds are then scooped from the whey, wrapped in cheesecloth, and pressed, releasing more of the whey. The result is paneer, which can be used almost as a cheese in certain dishes.

PRESERVING FOODS BY CANNING

What is canning and why has it been so important to food preservation?

Canning is one of the "newest" ways to preserve foods. It is a method of putting various foods in cans or jars and heating them under special processing conditions to kill off microorganisms. As the foods cool in a container, the lid hermetically seals because of the

Although canning was known in the United States in the mid-1800s, it was not until the Civil War (1860–1865) that the use of canned foods became most popular. The reason during the war was obvious: The troops needed to eat, and canned foods were one of the best ways to carry certain foods. And from that experience, the word spread and canned foods became more in demand, as it was one of the best ways to carry (especially for traveling settlers) foods without worrying about spoilage.

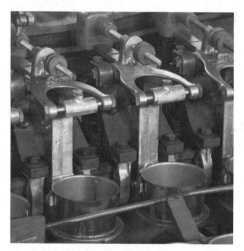

The process for storing and shipping food in cans first became widespread in the United States during the Civil War.

resulting vacuum, keeping out other microorganisms and allowing the foods to be stored until needed for a meal.

Steps to today's canning processes began in the 1790s when French chef, confectioner, and distiller Nicolas François Appert (1749–1841) discovered that food would not deteriorate as fast if it was heated in sealed glass bottles. Appert's ideas were tested by the French Navy; such foods as meat, vegetables, fruit, and milk were all successfully "canned" in glass jars and carried on long voyages. Glass jars were replaced by tinned iron canisters; and those were eventually replaced by even lighter canning materials (today, cans are said to weigh about 30 percent less than they did even two decades ago). Appert had no idea why his preservation technique worked—he believed air caused spoilage and heating the container's air would solve the problem (plus, the germ theory had not been discovered). A few decades later, researchers would find that the heat from the canning process killed the microorganisms that caused foods to decay.

Do many people home can in the United States?

Because of the availability of canning equipment in the past century, home canning grew for many years, especially before, during, and for a while after World War II. When canned goods became more available in grocery stores after the war, home canning was not as popular. But with the demand for more access to fruits and vegetables, the rise in home gardens, and the concern about what goes into processed, industrialized canned goods, there has been a resurgence in home canning. (*Note:* The USDA warns us to be cautious about using any canning recipes published before 1990; before then, all canning recipes were based on research done in 1942, before today's safer methods were developed.)

At what temperatures do microorganisms grow or die off, especially in terms of canning?

Microorganisms such as molds, yeasts, and some bacteria, are usually destroyed in the canning process. This is because, at certain temperatures, microorganisms flourish—or die. The following chart shows what temperatures are important for growth and destruction of microorganisms in the canning processes:

Temperatures for Food Preservation

Temperature(s)	Effect
240°F to 250°F	Canning temperatures for low acid vegetables, meat, and poultry in a pressure canner
212°F	Temperature water boils at sea level. Canning temperature for acid fruits, tomatoes, pickles, and jellied products in a boiling-water canner
180°F to 250°F	Canning temperatures are used to destroy most bacteria, yeasts, and molds in acid foods. Time required to kill these decreases as temperatures increase
140°F to 165°F	Warming temperatures prevent growth, but may allow survival of some microorganisms
40°F to 140°F	DANGER ZONE. Temperatures between 40°F and 140°F allow rapid growth of bacteria, yeast, and molds
95°F	Maximum storage temperature for canned foods
50°F to 70°F	Best storage temperatures for canned and dried foods
32°F	Temperature water freezes
32°F to 40°F	Cold temperatures permit slow growth of some bacteria, yeasts, and molds
−10°F to 32°F	Freezing temperatures stop growth of microorganisms, but may allow some to survive
0°F to −10°F	Best storage temperatures for frozen foods

This data was extracted from the "Complete Guide to Home Canning," Agriculture Information Bulletin No. 539, USDA (Revised 2009).

What are low- and high-acid foods?

When discussing what vegetables or fruits to can, it's necessary to know whether the food is considered "low-acid" or "high-acid"; this, then, determines whether you use a water bath or a pressure cooker canning method. Low-acid foods have very little natural acid, and include many vegetables, meats, stews, and soups; they include such foods as carrots, beets, green beans, peas, and corn. Low acid means that the foods must be heat-processed in a pressure canner—with temperatures reaching 240 degrees Fahrenheit (116 degrees Celsius) for a certain time in order to destroy toxin-producing bacterial spores.

High-acid foods are those that can be heat-processed in a boiling water bath—where the temperatures reach 212 degrees Fahrenheit (100 degrees Celsius) in order to kill off molds, yeasts, and some bacteria found in these types of foods. They include some fruits and vegetables, jams, jellies, and fruit spreads; some examples include pickles, apricots, plums, apples, peaches, pears, and tomatoes (see below for more about these canning methods.)

What is water bath canning?

Water bath canning is just as the name implies: The food is canned in a jar that is immersed in boiling water (temperature at 212 degrees Fahrenheit [100 degrees Celsius]). The large kettle, called a boiling-water or water bath canner, is filled with enough boiling water to immerse and fully surround the capped canning jars, with two inches of water above the top of the cap. Water bath canning should be used only for processing high-acid foods, such as tomatoes and applesauce. The amount of time each food should be processed varies; but because the times are relatively short, many of the nutrients are preserved within the canned foods. One of the best references for this information is the *Ball Blue Book of Preserving*, first published in 1909, but still referenced today in its 2005 edition.

What is pressure cooker/canner processing?

A pressure cooker/canner processor (or steam-pressure canner) is a heavy kettle with a lockable lid and outside pressure gauge. Heating up a small amount of water inside the kettle with the lid closed creates pressures and temperatures that destroy harmful bacteria in low-acid foods, such as beets, carrots, or corn. The temperatures in this type of canner can reach above 240 degrees Fahrenheit (115.6 degrees Celsius); the steam under ten pounds of pressure at this temperature helps destroy bacteria—but the higher heat and pressure may also cut down on certain nutrients within the foods, such as heat-sensitive vitamin C. In addition, incorrect processing (temperatures too low and/or not enough processing time) of low-acid foods—or the unseen breaking of a canning jar seal containing low-acid food—can result in botulism, a toxin from the spores of a bacteria that thrive on poorly processed low-acid foods (for more about botulism, see this chapter).

Does canning affect the nutrient value of the canned foods?

Yes and no—when you can, some foods lose their nutrients during the canning process, while others actually have some of their nutrients enhanced. Almost all canned foods lose some nutrients to the heating process, sometimes between 50 and 80 percent of their nutrients, while other foods release antioxidants and make them more available to our digestive systems. The following list describes a few of those vegetables and some of the possible nutritional effects from canning:

Tomatoes—When exposed to the heat of canning, usually in a water bath, the heat causes the release of antioxidants.

Carrots—When carrots are canned in a pressure cooker/canner, the beta carotene increases, but because of the high heat, some other vitamins may be lost.

Corn—When corn is canned, it has the same amount of dietary fiber as fresh corn and releases its antioxidants—but the heat from canning also causes this vegetable to lose vitamin C.

Pumpkin—Canning pumpkin concentrates the vegetable, making calcium, iron, magnesium, and vitamin K available; and heat also causes the pumpkin's carotenoids to be more available.

Beans—The heat from canning beans—from black and kidney to pinto—does not affect the nutritional calcium and iron of the beans, nor the fiber and protein; but canning does cause some loss of folate.

In canning, what is usually the meaning of the term *antioxidant*?

The term *antioxidant* has a slightly different meaning in canning than when using the word in terms of nutrition. In canning, an antioxidant usually refers to citric acid (such as lemon juice), ascorbic acid (vitamin C), or a combination of both. These substances are used to inhibit the oxidation, and thus browning (such as when you cut open a pear or apple), of light-colored fruits and vegetables, especially to make the food look more appealing. Antioxidants also mean the same when talking about the nutrition of canned goods—they are believed to neutralize free radicals that can cause long-term damage to our cells (for more about antioxidants and nutrition, see the chapter "The Basics of Nutrition: Macronutrients and Non-nutrients").

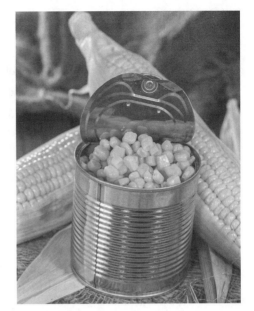

Canned corn has the same fiber—but fewer vitamins—than fresh.

How does pickling or canning salt differ from table salt?

Pickling or canning salt is usually a fined-grained salt, although it's still sodium chloride, the same chemical composition as table salt. But they differ in two important ways: Pickling salt has no anticaking agents like table salt, which can cause the pickling liquid to brown or become cloudy; and it has no iodine that can turn the pickles dark.

What are some concerns with store-sold canned food?

There are concerns with canned foods—in particular, the processing of the food and even the can that holds the food. For example, processing canned fruit often reduces the vitamins, particularly vitamins A and C. Most fruit is also peeled, which means it has less fiber—and even vitamins—than fresh fruit. If the fruit is canned in syrup, even if it is so-called "light syrup," it means the canned fruit has more calories. Another example is canned vegetables, in which vitamins are reduced because of the processing, and salt is often added to help with the preservation. More recently, canned fruits and vegetables have also been under attack because of the cans themselves—especially the cans coated with BPA (bisphenol A), a plastic additive (for more about BPA and cans, see the chapter "Controversies with Food, Beverages, and Nutrition").

What is a major concern when home canning—or with any canned food—especially regarding a toxin called botulinum?

Bacteria called *Clostridium botulinum* are dangerous, as they produce a toxin called botulinum—one that is considered one of the most deadly toxic substances known. They can grow in food products, producing the botulinum that can cause a condition called botulism; the toxin is so potent that it is said that one gram can kill 14 million adults! The spores of this bacteria are usually present in dust, wind, and soil; thus, they can cling to fresh, raw vegetables. But they cannot thrive in the presence of air, or in high-acid foods, which is why high-acid foods can be processed with a boiling water bath. But in the case of low-acid foods, the bacteria can survive if the food is not processed correctly; processing them over a temperature of 248 degrees Fahrenheit (120 degrees Celsius) can kill off the bacteria within five minutes—which is why it is imperative to can such foods at the correct temperature and pressure for a specific amount of time (depending on the low-acid food).

This makes *C botulinum* a serious concern for people who preserve certain low-acid vegetables and fruits at home. If the home canning process is not done properly, the bacteria will grow in the no-oxygen (anaerobic) environment of the sealed container, creating an extremely poisonous food. The toxin is produced in poorly prepared canned goods, such as a leaking seal around the rim of the jar. That is why you should never eat food from a swollen can or a can in which the lid is not depressed in the middle (or if the lid is easily opened). More often than not, this is a sign that the can has become filled with gas released during germination of the bacteria. Consuming such food can lead to nerve paralysis, severe vomiting, and even death. And although there are two major antiserums for botulism, their effectiveness depends on how much and how long the toxin has been in a person's body.

OTHER FOOD PRESERVATION METHODS

What is freeze-drying?

Freeze-drying is a technique that preserves foods (vegetables, fruits, and meats), allowing them to be very shelf stable. Most also retain their flavor and most of their nutritional value; for example, one study found that freeze-dried berries retained about 90 percent of their anthocyanins, compounds that give the berries their color and are thought to help prevent certain cancers. Although often thought to be similar, freeze-drying differs from dehydration in several ways—in particular, drying foods tends to change the color and texture of the food, and does not always remove all the water, which means it can go bad faster.

The ancient Incas, about 1200 C.E., practiced a type of freeze-drying technique, allowing foods to be frozen at high elevations overnight—then allowed to dry in the sun the next day. Today, freeze-dried foods are manufactured, and are used by people who need lightweight (less water means less weight), easily packable, and tasty foods that can be stored at various temperatures without spoilage. The list includes backpackers and hikers, service personnel overseas, and even the astronauts on the International Space Station.

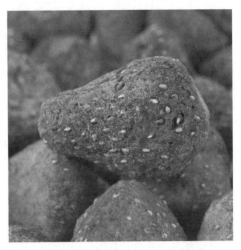

These strawberries were flash-frozen to dehydrate them. Adding water and warming them up makes them taste pretty good, but not as good as fresh.

How does freeze-drying work?

In general, the process of freeze-drying is as follows: First the food is flash-frozen. It is then put into a vacuum, which causes the frozen liquid in the product to vaporize without going through the liquid phase (called sublimation); about 98 percent of the food's moisture is drawn off (temperatures can be as low as about –50 degrees Fahrenheit [–45.6 degrees Celsius] during the process). Finally, the food is nitrogen-sealed in packaging to prevent contamination by water or oxygen. When a person wants to eat a certain freeze-dried food, he or she just adds water. In most cases, the food actually keeps its original color, form, size, taste, and texture. Of course, there are a few drawbacks: environmentally speaking, freeze-drying foods requires a great deal of energy—much more than canning or freezing.

How is sugar used to preserve food?

Sugar is one substance most of us ignore when it comes to preserving foods, but it truly is an amazing substance. For example, sugar has strong antiseptic qualities, and in sufficient quantities resists spoiling. In addition, fruits—with their mostly water content—do not have to be fully dried for this preservation technique; instead, fruit can be preserved in its whole state and dried so that 65 percent of its weight is composed of sugar—what is often called candied fruit.

The introduction of sugar cane to Europe came during the surge of trading with countries in Asia. For northern climates that could not use drying as an alternative to preserving, foods such as fruit could be immersed in a syrup made of water and sugar.

What are jams and jellies, and are their nutrients preserved after processing?

Jams are a soft spread made by combining chopped or mashed fruit with sugar, and cooking it until it forms a thick gelatinous substance. They can be made with one fruit or a combination of fruits; and they often contain added pectin or use certain fruits'

No, in fact honey and table sugar are almost indistinguishable chemically, and once in our system, they are also identical. Sugar and honey are both without nutritional value other than calories; and measure for measure, sugar actually has fewer calories than honey—around 16 versus 22, respectively. The reason has to do with the consistency of both sweeteners: The dissolved sugars in a teaspoon of honey take up less space than a teaspoon of the dry table sugar crystals.

natural pectins to make them more spreadable, but not firm. Jellies are firmer than jams, but are made in almost the same fashion: this soft spread is made by taking the fruit of the juice (the juice is strained from crushed fruit pulp), adding sugar (and sometimes pectin), and cooking it to form a more solid gel than a jam. And yes, for the most part, nutrients are preserved in jams and jellies, but some are lost since both processes involve the heating of the fruits.

Has honey ever been used to preserve food?

Yes, early civilizations used honey to preserve foods—mostly fruits. In the warmer regions of Greece, the process included soaking the fruit in honey, then drying and packing the results into tightly sealed jars.

How is alcohol used to preserve foods?

Alcohol is often used to preserve certain foods, mainly as an additional ingredient in pickling or with sugar to preserve jams and jellies. Because alcohol is known as a "toxic inhibitor," it prevents the spoilage of preserved foods. Almost any type of drinking alcohol (not alcohols such as wood alcohol, of course) can be used, and because no bacteria can grow in the liquid, it is considered an all-around preservation ingredient.

How is meat aged before cooking?

Meat is often aged in order to either tenderize it or to keep in the moisture. There are two usual methods of aging meat: wet-aged and dry-aged. In the United States, wet-aging is the most dominant method, in which the meat (most often beef) is aged in a vacuum-sealed bag to retain its moisture. It is quick—it usually takes only a few days to age—and the meat does not lose any weight or volume.

Dry-aged meats (again, most often beef) usually means a higher grade of meat, as the drying process needs meat in which the fat content is evenly distributed. The process takes place under refrigeration and can take from two to three weeks. The meat is first dried, concentrating the flavor; as it dries, the meat's natural enzymes break down the connective tissues in the muscle, making it more tender. Fungi also form on the exterior of the meat (this form of natural "crust" is cut off before cooking), and their natural enzymes also help to tenderize the piece. The piece of meat does lose weight during this aging process—by around a third—but many people believe such meats' flavor and tenderness are well worth the time and expense. Because of the intensity of this method, it is usually found only in better butcher stores and restaurants. (For more about the chemistry of meats, see the chapter "Food Chemistry and Nutrition.")

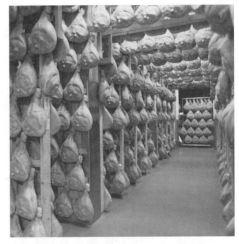

Aging meat, usually beef, is done to make the meat more tender.

What are nitrites and nitrates?

Nitrites and nitrates are chemicals that are added to preserve foods, especially meats. In particular, they are found in processed meats such as hot dogs, bacon, ham, sausages, luncheon meats, and smoked fish. They are added to extend a food's shelf life and to protect the foods from fungi and bacteria; this practice is also why the meats you usually find in the grocery store have such a pink color, and why few fruits lose their color, even after being on the shelf for many days.

There is a great deal of controversy surrounding nitrites and nitrates, and many products no longer contain them. But there are still foods—highly processed, and some pickled and salt-cured foods—that contain, for example, nitrates, which are thought to be converted to cancer-causing nitrosamines during digestion. (For more about food additives, see the chapter "Modern Nutrition"; for controversies surrounding food additives, see the chapter "Controversies with Food, Beverages, and Nutrition.")

What are some of the best ways to preserve various foods?

There are several ways to best preserve certain foods—from meats and herbs to fruits and vegetables. The following chart lists some of them—and the overall best preservation methods for each (all methods are mentioned earlier in this chapter):

Preserving Foods

Food	Best Preservation Methods
Anchovies	vinegar; salt
Apricot	drying; sugar; alcohol
Banana	drying
Basil	oil; vinegar; freezing (loses color); drying (loses some oil and flavor)
Blueberries	store whole; drying; freezing
Carrot	store whole; lactic fermentation (pickling)
Cherries	drying; vinegar; alcohol

Preserving Foods

Food	Best Preservation Methods
Cucumber	lactic fermentation (pickling)
Eggplant	drying; lactic fermentation (pickling); oil
Garlic	store whole; vinegar; drying
Green beans	drying; lactic fermentation (pickling)
Lemon	salting
Mushroom	drying; oil; vinegar
Onion	store whole; drying; lactic fermentation (pickling); vinegar
Peach	drying
Pear	store whole; drying; sugar
Prune	store whole; alcohol
Raspberries	drying; sugar; alcohol
Spinach	drying
Swiss chard	drying; lactic fermentation (pickling)
Tomato	store whole; drying; lactic fermentation (pickling); oil; vinegar; salting
Zucchini	drying; lactic fermentation (pickling); oil

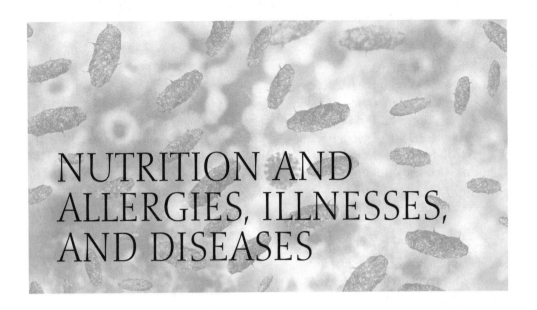

NUTRITION AND ALLERGIES, ILLNESSES, AND DISEASES

NUTRITION AND THE IMMUNE SYSTEM

Why do we have an immune system?

Our immune system protects our bodies from attacks by microorganisms, abnormal cells in our body, and some chemicals and toxins. The outside invaders include viruses, bacteria, and fungi; internally, even our own body can "turn" on us, producing abnormal or cancerous cells.

What are allergens?

An allergen, or antigen, is a substance that our bodies believe is a harmful foreign invader, and thus, the immune system tries to eliminate the "bad" substance. At first, there is usually no reaction. But if a person is exposed to the allergen again, the immune system starts its job: attacking the foreign body, which results in an allergic reaction.

How does the human immune system work?

One of the main reasons for eating well is to stay as healthy as possible, and that means keeping our immune system in good working order. The immune system has two main components: white blood cells and antibodies circulating in the blood. Simply put, when an antigen—either a harmful bacterium, virus, fungus, parasite, or other foreign substance—invades a person's body, a specific antibody is generated by the body's system to attack the antigen (called the "immune response"). These antibodies are produced by B cells (lymphocytes) in the spleen or lymph nodes. Often thought of as our natural "antibiotics," the antibodies can either destroy the antigen, or "label" it so that a white blood cell (called a macrophage or scavenger cell) can engulf the foreign intruder. After a person has been exposed to an antigen, a later exposure to the same antigen will produce a faster immune system reaction, and thus, the necessary antibodies will be produced more rapidly and in larger amounts—a process that protects us from harm. (*Note*: This is a general description and it doesn't always work for all antigens, or if a person has a compromised immune system.)

What are T cells and B cells?

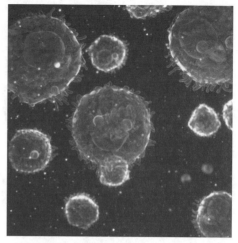

Lymphocytes (white blood cells) are the body's defense mechanism against antigens; they also help activate the immune system.

Simply put, there are several types of white blood cells (lymphocytes), including the T and B cells, that are a major part of our immune system. The T lymphocytes, or T cells, make up about 60 to 80 percent of the lymphocytes circulating in the blood, whereas B cells make up about 10 to 15 percent of the lymphocytes. Both keep intruding antigens from invading the body and, in tandem, help the immune system to activate much faster.

Why are nutrients important to our immune system?

Nutrients play an extremely important part in keeping our immune systems in shape. According to experts, the amount of energy we get from nutrients has an important influence on our immune activity; this is readily seen in people who are undernourished—they are at a greater risk for infections. In addition, some research indicates that if a person takes in too much fat, it can influence how well the immune system works. This is because a high-fat diet appears to depress the immune response, and increases the risk for infection. And it's not just the amount of fat, but the type—some research shows that a good balance of different fatty acids (such as those from oily fish or nuts) can also help to strengthen the immune system. Finally, a great deal of research has shown that vitamin and mineral supplements do not stimulate the immune response in healthy adults; however, among the elderly, nutritional supplements are often prescribed to help boost immunity.

Are there certain foods that boost your immune system?

Yes, there are many foods that can boost your immune system, especially if you eat a balanced diet of vegetables, fruits, nuts, seeds, and whole grains. There are specific foods that can help, too. For example, flax, either as a supplement, oils, or seeds, can boost immunity; drinking smoothies that contain immune-building fruits (such as strawberries, papaya, and cantaloupe) and yogurt can help; and eating more "colorful" vegetables can assist your immune system, as researchers have discovered that in most cases, the deeper the vegetable color, the more healthful nutrients are in the food.

Do "quick fix" diets boost our immune system?

Contrary to some advertising claims, there are truly no "quick fix" diets that will boost our immune system. Many of these diets claim that cleansing the body (usually meaning days of not eating or just drinking liquids), then taking mega-doses of supplements will quickly boost the immune system. But so far, most research shows such methods do not work as efficiently—or effectively—as claimed, and may even be harmful to many people.

What is the Inflammatory Factor (IF)?

The Inflammation Factor (IF) Rating was described almost a decade ago, and is a way of rating foods based on their potential ability to increase or decrease inflammation in the body. The numbers in the range vary widely (there are no upper or lower limits), and each rating is considered to be dependent on serving size. Most studies on the IF have shown a mixed result—some say there is no way to control the inflammation in our systems based on this method; others believe eating foods with the IF in mind will help decrease inflammation in the body.

How is our immune system affected by nutrition?

Our immune system is directly affected by what we eat—and thus, the right, balanced diet for a person is critical to a strong immune system. Most nutritionists suggest eating foods rich in vitamins, minerals, and antioxidants—especially those foods that naturally stimulate the fighting power of your body's natural defense system. They include garlic (the sulfur compounds may help our white blood cells), probiotics (the friendly bacteria for our intestinal tract that are helped by good-bacteria-rich foods such as yogurt and kefir), and "darker" berries, such as blueberries and blackberries (they contain powerful antioxidants that improve the fight against bacteria and viruses).

How does stress affect our immune system?

As most humans know, stress can cause many mental and physical problems. It also can directly affect our immune system—no matter what our age or sex—and even our nu-

---

Why can't antibiotics treat viral infections?

Antibiotics are not used to treat viral infections for a good reason: Viruses lack the specific structures, such as certain cell walls, that an antibiotic attacks. In fact, it is important to note that because a virus sets up in a healthy host cell in order to replicate, antiviral medications can also affect that host cell. Therefore, even though there are some antiviral medicines available for certain viruses, the best way to fight a virus is to keep your immune system healthy—which means eating healthy, too.

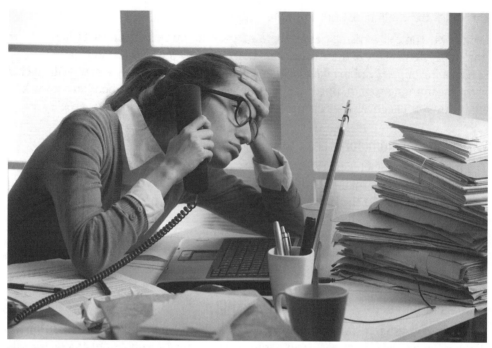

Stress is one of the worst things that can happen to a person's health. Stress compromises the immune system and makes it more likely that we will become ill.

tritional health. For example, some disorders related to stress are not from the stress itself, but because of nutrient deficiencies from an increase in your body's metabolic rate during stress. Vitamin C is one example: This vitamin is used by the adrenal gland during stressful conditions, and thus, any prolonged stress could mean a depletion of the vitamin. In addition, the increase in the body's metabolism can lead to an increase in several minerals, such as potassium and phosphorus, and proteins in the body—which also helps to decrease calcium.

Another response that affects our immune system is how your gut responds to stress—it actually has its own nervous system (called the enteric nervous system) that governs our digestion. When you are tense, your brain sends messages to a nerve that runs from around the base of the brain to the abdomen; your body responds by diverting some of your blood flow from the digestive tract to the brain and limbs, so that you can be ready for the "fight or flight" reaction to the "danger" of the stress. This can cause cramping, diarrhea, and other symptoms—and if you are under a great deal of stress for a long time, it can create even more gastrointestinal chaos, such as irritable bowel syndrome and nutrient deficiencies. (For more about our "gut brain," see the chapter "Nutrition in Eating and Drinking Choices.") For these reasons (and many others), nutritionists recommend people experiencing stress should eat a well-balanced, nutritious diet—whole grains, fruits, and vegetables—with an emphasis on the nutrients that become depleted because of stress.

FOOD ALLERGIES
AND INTOLERANCES

What's the difference between an intolerance and an allergy?

There is a big difference between an allergy and an intolerance. An allergy is caused by your immune system's reaction to a food or allergen; for example, you may have an allergy to ragweed that causes you to sneeze, have a runny nose, or watery eyes—in other words, an immune system response. (For more about allergies, see below.)

An intolerance is usually used in terms of food; it is caused by the inability to absorb or digest certain foods, and involves your gastrointestinal tract but not any other specific organ. For example, if you have lactose intolerance and you eat a dairy product, such as ice cream, your gastrointestinal tract can react with bloating, gas, diarrhea, or vomiting. Such food intolerances are usually caused by an enzyme deficiency; for example, lactose-intolerant people lack the enzyme lactase. In other cases, they are caused by the intestines being supersensitive to certain foods—and is most often a reaction to the protein content of the food. (For more about the human digestive tract, see the chapter "Nutrition in Eating and Drinking Choices.")

How do our bodies often respond to the allergens surrounding us?

In general, many researchers consider allergic reactions to be a disorder of the immune system—the part of our body that protects us from attacks by foreign substances. When an allergen-sensitive person is exposed to an allergen, the immune system sends signals to special cells that make antibodies (called immunoglobulins) to fight off the invader— for instance, tomatoes. The body mistakenly sends out the antibodies (what scientists call IgE) to fight off the ingested tomato—but nothing usually happens at this point.

But the next time a tomato is eaten, or a person comes in contact with a tomato (even just touching the skin), the immune system kicks into gear again, creating histamines and other substances in the body to "fight" against the food. This rush of natural body chemicals can cause a variety of symptoms in the now-food-sensitive person, depending on where in the body the substances are released. For example, those released in our upper respiratory system can cause a sneezing attack; if they are released in the digestive tract (as would be the case with an ingested tomato), they can cause vomiting and diarrhea within minutes to a couple hours of eating the food.

What allergies can a human develop?

There are a huge number of allergens that can affect humans. The most common allergens are various foods, pollen, chemicals in cosmetics, medications, fungal spores, insect venom, various microorganisms, and even our own body's cells that develop abnormally. If a person is sensitive to one of these foods, creatures, substances, or abnormal cells, allergies can develop. In people who are not sensitive, there will be no response.

171

How many humans have food allergies?

Humans—and certain other animals—can have plenty of food allergies. And although it seems as if many people have an allergy to some type of food, in reality, only 2 to 8 percent of children, and 1 to 2 percent of adults, have a definite allergic reaction to foods. But those percentages still translate into a large number of people: According to Harvard Medical School, to date, about 15 million people in the United States alone suffer with some type of food allergy.

What are some allergic responses to foods?

There are many allergic responses to certain foods. For example, your skin may break out in hives, a red rash, or become dry and itchy; your hands and feet may swell; you may begin to sneeze, get a runny or stuffy nose, watery eyes, and you may cough or wheeze; or your intestines may respond with bloating, gassiness, or diarrhea. And even your behavior can be affected, including fatigue, migraine headaches, irritability, and anxiety.

What are some foods that can trigger allergies?

There are many foods that can trigger an allergic response—either all year long, or depending on the season. For example, year-round allergies can be triggered by such foods as apples, cucumbers—almost any food you can buy from the grocery store throughout the year; while seasonal allergies can be triggered by foods that are associated with certain times of the year, such as strawberries.

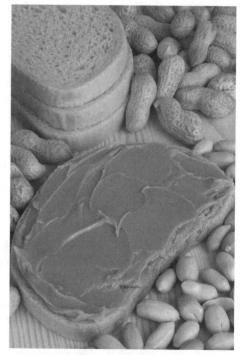

Why are peanut allergies thought to be so dangerous?

There is one food allergy that has received a great deal of media attention in the past—and rightly so—peanut allergies. This is one of the most dangerous forms of food allergies: It can stop a person from breathing as the windpipe goes into spasms, or the cardiovascular system goes into shock (called anaphylaxis). The reasons for concern are many. For example, peanuts may show up in the processing of various foods; some facilities not only process one food, but may have also processed a food containing peanuts in the same manufacturing plant. For some peo-

An allergic reaction to peanuts can cause death by restricting breathing or inducing shock, which is why peanut allergies are no laughing matter.

ple with peanut allergies, any exposure to peanut pieces, or even peanut dust, can cause a violent allergic reaction.

Because of this, if you have a peanut allergy, check the labels of all foods—food production companies are required to list all the ingredients in their foods, and also mention if the food has been processed anywhere near peanuts. And to help others know what to do if you are exposed, wear a medical alert bracelet, and talk to your doctor about carrying special allergy medicines with you for emergencies.

Can some people be allergic to vegetables, fruits, and legumes?

Yes, there are many people with allergies to vegetables, fruits, and legumes—and many such reactions are often overlooked because they don't seem as common as other allergies. For example, some people are allergic to members of the rosaceae family (apple, pear, cherry, peach, and plum), members of the cucurbitaceae family (including cucumber, melon, watermelon, zucchini, and pumpkin), and, more rarely, to kiwi fruit (people with this allergy will often also be allergic to bananas and avocados). Although not as common as vegetable or fruit allergies, some people are allergic to legumes, including lentils, green beans, soybeans, peas, and dried beans.

Most people with fruit and vegetable allergies have a reaction to proteins called profilins, most often in association with pollen allergies, and called pollen-food syndrome (PFS). Thus, many people who are allergic to profilins and associated certain pollens will react: for example, a person with hay fever may also have allergic reactions to watermelons, tomatoes, bananas, and citrus fruits, all of which contains profilins. (For more about pollen-related allergies, see Sidebar.)

What is oral allergy syndrome, or pollen-food syndrome?

Oral allergy syndrome, or OAS (also pollen-food syndrome, or PFS), is a food allergy and occurs when a food-sensitive person eats (or is even exposed to) certain foods, such as fruits, vegetables, nuts, and spices. It is also called PFS because it usually occurs in people who are allergic to pollens from trees, grasses, and weeds—pollens that contain proteins quite similar to those found in some fruits, vegetables, nuts, and spices. Some of the most common of these foods include apples, peaches, kiwi, carrots, celery, tomatoes, walnuts, hazelnuts, almonds, coriander, cumin, and mustard. After eating such foods, a person with OAS can experience an allergic reaction, including such symptoms as itching, tingling, and sometimes swelling of the tongue, lips, and/or upper palate. When OAS is caused by a vegetable and/or fruit, it usually occurs when the person is exposed to the fresh or raw versus the cooked food.

Do certain age groups have allergies to fruits and vegetables?

Yes, in some cases, there are certain age groups that seem to have a specific allergy. For example, young children tend to have potato allergies (although this type disappears over time). And allergies to fruits and vegetables are most commonly found in older children and young adults, with many of these allergies affecting them throughout their entire life.

Can a person be allergic to milk?

Yes, not only is there lactose intolerance, there is also a possibility of being allergic to milk—but it is not as common as most people believe. It is estimated that around five percent of children and adults have either a milk allergy or lactose intolerance (for more about lactose intolerance, see below).

Most milk allergies are associated with young children. In one study, it was shown that 75 percent of infants less than one year old had an allergy to cow's milk—but the majority outgrew the allergy by the time they were two or three years old. The reason for the allergic reaction seems to be the protein in the cow's milk; when a person is allergic to the milk, it usually means his or her digestive tract cannot tolerate the cow's protein. And in children, this allergy to milk has often been cited as the underlying cause of repeated colds and ear infections.

How can your doctor tell if you have a food allergy?

Besides the obvious—that is, you react within minutes to a certain food—one way doctors usually tell if you have a food allergy is by a skin prick test. In this skin test, certain food allergens are pricked onto your skin, usually on your back or arms; the results are usually quick, with the allergen causing a bump where you were pricked if you are allergic. From there, your doctor will give you advice as to how to handle any possible future allergic reaction to the food or foods; you can also help yourself and others by wearing a medical-alert or similar bracelet specifying what foods cause you to have an allergic reaction.

What is lactose intolerance?

Lactose intolerance occurs when a person's system cannot produce lactase, the enzyme that breaks down milk sugar (lactose) in most dairy products. Because of this, if any

---

What does latex have to do with some food allergies?

There are many people who are allergic to the natural rubber called latex, with symptoms ranging from rashes to sneezing. Researchers also know that if you are allergic to latex, there is a good chance you will be allergic to certain specific foods, too—mainly because proteins in certain fruits, vegetables, and nuts are similar to those found in natural rubber. These foods include chestnuts, bananas, melons, avocados, kiwi, and tomatoes.

dairy is eaten, the milk sugar cannot be broken down, and it affects digestion—resulting in bloating, gas pains, and, if severe, vomiting and/or diarrhea. While this condition is not life-threatening for most adults, it can have severe consequences for infants, children, and the elderly. For most lactose-intolerant people, the best "remedy" is to stay away from all dairy products, including those made from the milk of goats and sheep. For others, experimenting with what affects you sometimes works—as some people are not as lactose-intolerant as others. For those people, too, sometimes certain aged hard cheeses, yogurts, or products made from goats or sheep are more tolerable.

What is gluten?

Gluten is a substance found in wheat; as flour, it is most often used to make (mainly yeast) breads. When the flour is mixed or kneaded with a liquid, the gluten proteins absorb the liquid to form an elastic dough; this traps gas from the fermenting yeast and gives us the air bubbles that make breads lighter. (For more about bread, see the chapter "Food Chemistry and Nutrition.")

What is "gluten intolerance"?

Some people have a slight to moderate intolerance to grain products—especially wheat—a condition called gluten intolerance or gluten sensitivity. It usually becomes apparent when a person eats foods containing gluten—mainly cereal grains, such as wheat, rye, and barley. The major culprit is one of the proteins found in gluten called gliadin; it combines with antibodies in the digestive tract. Once this happens, sometimes gradually, the gliadin causes damage to the intestinal walls, which, in turn, interferes with the absorption of many necessary nutrients. (For more about disease and gluten intolerance, see this chapter.)

Is there a connection between allergies and the bacteria in our digestive tract?

Yes, some research indicates that the health of our digestive tract can be linked to some allergies. In one study, it was found that too few "good" or beneficial bacteria in our guts can throw the immune system off balance—and increase the chances for having such allergies as hay fever. Another study showed that infants who had fewer diverse colonies of

Can some foods actually cause dandruff, hair loss, or baldness?

Yes, it is thought that some foods can actually cause dandruff—along with baldness and hair loss. Although most of these problems have to do with various types of illnesses or a normal genetic response (for example, pattern baldness in men and women is usually hereditary), sometimes these "heady" problems can be caused by the foods we eat, or don't eat.

bacteria in their gut were also more prone to allergies as they became older. (For more about the digestive tract, see the chapter "Nutrition in Eating and Drinking Choices.")

OVERWEIGHT PROBLEMS AND OBESITY

What are triglycerides?

Triglycerides are a type of fat (lipid) found in your blood. When you consume a meal or snack, the body converts any calories it doesn't need to use right away to triglycerides, storing it in your fat cells. If you eventually need energy, hormones cause the triglycerides to be released. Because, like cholesterol, triglycerides cannot dissolve in the blood, they circulate throughout your body with the help of proteins called lipoproteins. (For more information about fats, lipoproteins, and triglycerides, see the chapter "The Basics of Nutrition: Macronutrients and Non-nutrients.")

How do triglycerides affect your health?

Triglycerides are the most common fat in your body, and if you eat more calories than you burn, you may be a candidate for high triglycerides, called hypertriglyceridemia. According to the American Heart Association, the normal range for triglycerides is less than 150 milligrams per deciliter (or mg/dL, the standard unit when measuring triglycerides); borderline high is 150 to 199; high is 200 to 499; and very high is 500 mg/dL or above.

If you have a higher than normal triglyceride reading—and even though levels vary by age and sex—it may be a sign of several medical conditions. For example, high levels are often found in obese people, and in people who have what is called the metabolic syndrome (also sometimes called Syndrome X; for more, see this chapter)—a cluster of conditions, including too much fat around the waist, high blood pressure, high triglycerides, high blood sugar, and abnormal cholesterol levels (especially lower than average HDL, the "good" cholesterol). In addition, high triglycerides are often seen in people who have heart disease or diabetes; if it is combined with low "good" HDL cholesterol and high "bad" LDL cholesterol levels, it seems to speed up the buildup of fatty acids in artery walls (called atherosclerosis); and high triglycerides are often associated with low thyroid hormones (hypothyroidism) or liver or kidney disease.

Can a person lower his or her triglycerides without taking medication?

Yes, it is possible to lower your triglyceride levels naturally—but don't forget to talk to your doctor about trying some of the following: lose weight, cut back on daily calories (eat plenty of low-calorie fruits and vegetables), avoid sugary and refined foods, choose healthier fats, eliminate trans fats, and exercise regularly (at least 30 minutes a day if possible). These recommendations will also help if you have high cholesterol.

What are some effects in the body from excessive trans fats?

There are several effects from ingesting too many trans fats. For example, there is an increase in triglycerides, which may contribute to the thickening or hardening (atherosclerosis) of the artery walls, and is associated with a risk for stroke, diabetes, and heart disease. Trans fats can also increase your Lp(a) lipoprotein (a type of LDL "bad" cholesterol in your blood); the trans fats make the Lp(a) into smaller and denser particles, also contributing to the buildup of plaque in your arteries. And trans fats can increase inflammation; these fats contribute to blockages in the heart's blood vessels by damaging cells lining the vessels, which leads to inflammation. (For more about trans fats, see the chapter "The Basics of Nutrition: Macronutrients and Non-nutrients.")

What are the two types of cholesterol?

Most of us have heard from our health-care providers about two main types of cholesterol: LDL, or low-density lipoprotein (also known as the "bad" cholesterol) and HDL, or high-density lipoprotein (also known as the "good" cholesterol). These two types are known to greatly affect our circulatory system—in particular, our hearts: the LDL circulates in your blood, building up a material called plaque on the inner walls of the arteries that supply blood to your heart and brain; and at the same time, HDL cholesterol carries away cholesterol from the arteries and to the liver, where it is passed from the body.

Not all cholesterols in our bodies are alike—in fact, if your LDL levels are too high, and HDL too low, it can cause an increase in plaque, which, in turn, can cause your ar-

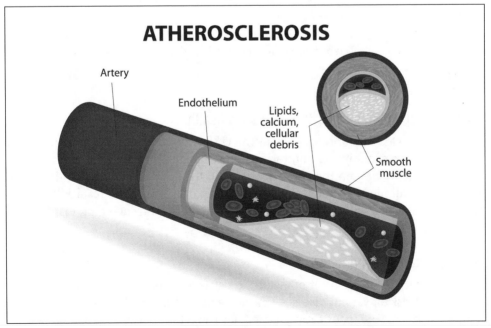

ATHEROSCLEROSIS

Artery

Endothelium

Lipids, calcium, cellular debris

Smooth muscle

Atherosclerosis is a thickening or hardening of the artery walls, which restricts blood flow and can lead to heart attacks and strokes.

teries to narrow, become more inflexible, and eventually lead to a heart attack (the arteries become blocked with plaque) or stroke (especially if the plaque is dislodged). There is also another type of cholesterol called Lp(a)—a genetic variation of your LDL cholesterol. Although not much is known about Lp(a) at this time, higher levels of Lp(a) may be connected to an excess of the fatty deposits in your arteries.

What is the connection between trans fats and cholesterol?

Doctors believe there is a definite connection between trans fats and cholesterol: The more trans fats you eat, the more your LDL cholesterol levels increase and your HDL cholesterol decrease. Trans fats, or trans fatty acids, are usually found in processed foods as "partially hydrogenated oil" (hydrogen is added to an oil to make it more solid at room temperature, and to increase the oil's shelf life).

What are the best cholesterol levels for an adult human?

There are many factors that affect the overall health of our body—and one of them has to do with our cholesterol levels—especially in terms of our heart health. To date, the following chart from the American Heart Association lists what is currently thought to be the best cholesterol levels for an adult (although this has recently been debated; see below):

Cholesterol Levels for Adults

Total Cholesterol Level	Category
< 200 mg/dL	Desirable level; lower risk for heart disease
200–239 mg/dL	Borderline high
> 240 mg/dL	High cholesterol. Studies show people with high levels of cholesterol can be twice as likely of getting coronary heart disease as someone with desirable levels

How does eating too much affect a person's health?

There is a medical term for eating too much: A *nutritional disorder* is actually a disease that results from excessive (or contrarily, an inadequate) intake of food and nutrients. Over time—depending on the amount eaten and the body's constitution—this often leads to harmful medical conditions; for example, obesity and the resulting medical problems associated with carrying around too much weight, including diabetes and heart problems.

What is metabolic syndrome?

Metabolic syndrome is a cluster of metabolic risk factors that a person has, all making the person at risk for various diseases. One of the major traits is obesity—or being overweight, either through poor eating habits, not enough exercise, or other factors. According to the National Heart, Lung, and Blood Institute (NHLBI) and the American

Heart Association (AHA), any three of the following traits in the same person meet the criteria for the metabolic syndrome—many of which are related to nutrition and the foods we eat (*Note:* the term *mg/dL* means milligrams per deciliter, a unit of measure):

Abdominal obesity—This means a waist circumference of 40 inches (102 centimeters) or more in men and 35 inches (88 centimeters) or more in women (there are also different criteria for various ethnic groups, for example, for Asian Americans, the values are greater than or equal to 35 inches [90 centimeters] in men and greater than or equal to 32 inches [80 centimeters] in women).

Triglycerides—If your triglyceride level measures 150 mg/dL or above.

Cholesterol—If your level of HDL cholesterol (the "good" cholesterol) is 40 mg/dL or lower in men, and 50 mg/dL or lower in women. (For more about cholesterol, see this chapter and the chapter "Nutrition Basics: Macronutrients and Non-nutrients.")

Blood pressure—If you have a (usually resting) blood pressure reading of 130/85 or more, also seen as a systolic of 130 over diastolic of 85 (although this reading is often debated, more recently in favor of a bit higher reading).

Blood glucose—If you have a fasting blood glucose reading of 100 mg/dL or above.

What is considered underweight for humans?

For the average human, there really is no such thing as a "perfect weight." Everyone has certain conditions—whether height, shape, genetics, or health—that together make us a certain weight. That being said, there are still desirable ranges based on a person's age, height, and build that usually mean a lower chance of disease or death.

Health-care professionals most often define underweight—or people who are excessively thin (but not anorexic) to the point of being unhealthy—as 15 percent or more under the low end of that person's range. There are multiple problems with being underweight; in particular, most underweight people lack energy to do most activities, have a difficult time obtaining healthy nutrients from foods, are usually cold because they don't have any excess fat, and are very vulnerable to infections and other diseases.

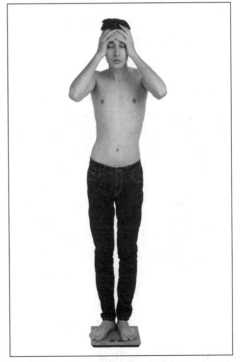

Being underweight is unhealthy because a person's body then lacks the nutrients to maintain an immune system that can fend off diseases and infections.

What recent study connected flame retardants and weight gain?

A recent study from the National Institutes of Health suggested that common flame retardants found in everything from electronics to furniture—called brominated flame retardants, or BFRs—may be responsible for some people gaining weight. The researchers believe that the BFRs bind to and inhibit an enzyme in a person's body that metabolizes estrogen, raising levels of the hormone and causing weight gain. Other research points to BFRs as chemicals that can disrupt the body's metabolic processes—and possibly cause fat and weight gain in many people.

What are some statistics concerning Americans' weight overall?

According to the National Health and Nutrition Examination Survey 2009-2010, there are some troubling statistics about all Americans' overall weights. The following list offers the findings:

- More than 2 in 3 adults are considered to be overweight or obese
- More than 1 in 3 adults are considered to be obese
- More than 1 in 20 adults are considered to have extreme obesity
- About one-third of children and adolescents ages 6 to 19 are considered to be overweight or obese
- More than 1 in 6 children and adolescents ages 6 to 19 are considered to be obese

According to the Centers for Disease Control and Prevention, what is obesity?

According to the Centers for Disease Control and Prevention, a person becomes obese when his or her body fat accumulates over time—mainly as a result of what is called a chronic energy imbalance. Said in more familiar terms—when the calories you consume are more than calories you expend in such activities as exercise, the result is often obesity. Obesity is thought to be a major health hazard worldwide; in fact, in the United States alone, it is estimated that around 27 percent of adults are obese (or close to one in three); and it is estimated that about 86 percent of Americans will be obese by the year 2030. This trend toward obesity is becoming costly—mainly because of all the diseases associated with obesity (diabetes, hypertension, heart disease, some cancers, etc.) and the resulting medical costs to everyone.

FOODBORNE ILLNESSES

What is foodborne illness, also called food poisoning?

Foodborne illnesses, or what is usually referred to as food poisoning, are gastrointestinal ailments that are usually caused by bacterial contamination of a food, most often meats (such as undercooked meat), old leftovers, foods long past their expiration dates, or food that is left out for too long, especially meats or foods containing dairy, eggs, or mayonnaise. (For more about foodborne illnesses, past and present, see the chapter "Nutrition throughout the Centuries.")

There are a few precautions you can take so you don't contract food poisoning. For example, if the food you're about to cook smells bad, throw it away. It's not worth contracting food poisoning—and since you can't "smell" bacteria, if the food looks bad or discolored, toss it out. Don't eat a canned food if the can is bulging—that often means botulism. And if you're not going to eat a food right away—especially meat, dairy, eggs, or other such products—keep it refrigerated (or freeze it, in the case of meat).

What is *Salmonella*?

One of the most common pathogens associated with foodborne illnesses is *Salmonella*, a family of bacteria that can cause such food-poisoning symptoms as diarrhea, nausea, fever, or abdominal cramps within about 12 to 48 hours after eating an infected food. It is caused when animals become infected, then are eaten for their meat; through raw milk and egg products; and by undercooked poultry. For a healthy adult, the symptoms do not last long—usually about one to four days. But for those who have compromised immune systems, gastrointestinal problems, or young children and frail or elderly people, the effects may last longer and be harsher, with secondary medical problems.

What is *Listeria*?

Listeria monocytogenes is a foodborne illness from a bacterium that causes listeriosis; the resulting infection may cause short-term symptoms in healthy adults, but for people who are at high risk for food poisoning the symptoms can be much more intense, such as in young children, pregnant women, the elderly, and people with weak immune systems. Unlike many other foodborne bacteria, *Listeria* can live and grow at temperatures associated with refrigeration and they are found on raw vegetables, contaminated dairy products, and in refrigerated, ready-to-eat foods, such as hot dogs, deli meats, and raw or undercooked meats, poultry, and seafoods. The contamination can cause headaches, high fever, a stiff neck, nausea, adnominal pain and diarrhea, eye inflammation, and even swollen lymph nodes, with the symptoms usually appearing within 8 to 24 hours after ingesting the food. The best way to counteract *Listeria* is to keep your refrigerator and kitchen clean, wash all raw vegetables, keep meats refrigerated, and follow cooking instructions for all meats.

What is *Campylobacter*?

Campylobacter is one of the most common causes of diarrhea—the major symptom of this illness—in the United States. It is usually associated with eating raw or undercooked poultry and meat, and raw, unwashed fruits and vegetables, along with drinking contaminated water; it can also be contracted by cross-contamination of other foods that are near the contaminated meats (such as if the bacteria are on your hands, or a knife). The best way to prevent these bacteria from spreading is to cook all foods thoroughly; don't drink untreated water (for example, from a stream); wash your hands before eating; and wash all raw fruits and vegetables before eating.

What is *Staphylococcus aureus*?

Staphylococcus aureus (also called staph) is usually found on the skin and also in the throats and nostrils of organisms—from healthy people to animals. Most of the time, these bacteria do not bother us, but if a person transmits the bacteria to a food product, it can multiply. It is most often found in association with unpasteurized dairy products, salty foods (such as ham and "deli meats"), and foods that don't require cooking (such as some foods associated with parties and picnics—like egg,

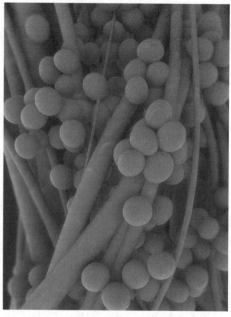

Staphylococcus aureus is a bacteria that is common and that lives on and in us, usually causing no harm. If it proliferates on food you consume, however, they can make you ill.

tuna, potato, and chicken salads, or even puddings). In fact, you cannot destroy the staph bacteria by cooking, as they are heat resistant. The symptoms of staph are similar to those of *Salmonella* foodborne illness, including nausea, stomach cramps, vomiting, or diarrhea. Once again, to keep the staph at bay, always wash your hands; and don't prepare any foods if you have a wound (especially on your hands or arms), or an eye, nose, or skin infection.

What is *Cyclospora*?

According to the Centers for Disease Control and Prevention, *Cyclospora* is a somewhat rare parasite that is spread by people ingesting something (such as food or water) that is contaminated with feces (stool). (In the United States, such outbreaks of *cyclosporia (set rom)* have been often associated with imported fresh produce.) It takes about a week after infection before a person becomes sick. Cyclosporia (the name of the disease associated with *Cyclospora*) doesn't always cause symptoms, especially in healthy adults; if contracted, it can cause flu-like symptoms, including stomach cramps, gas, bloating, nausea, frequent, watery (and sometimes explosive) diarrhea, headaches, appetite loss, and in some people, it can often lead to a lengthy gastrointestinal illness. *Cyclospora* needs time (days to weeks) after being passed in a bowel movement to become infectious for another person, so it is unlikely that *Cyclospora* is passed directly from one person to another.

How soon and at what temperature will microorganisms begin to grow on a food that is left out?

This is a question everyone who has ever been to a picnic asks: How long can I keep the food out on the table? According to government food safety groups, in general, you should not leave *most* foods out for longer than 2 hours at temperatures between 45 degrees Fahrenheit (7 degrees Celsius) and 140 degrees Fahrenheit (60 degrees Celsius; not that you'll picnic in such heat, but it is in reference to keeping the food in such places as a hot car). This is the ideal range of temperatures for microorganisms to grow and is often the cause of food poisoning at picnics and parties, especially during the warmest months of the year. Of course, there are ways to avoid spoilage by using common sense, such as putting most meats away after less than an hour, or not letting the mayonnaise-rich potato salad sit in the hot sun all that time.

Can you contract a foodborne illness if you drink milk?

The majority of milk you buy in the store is treated to rid the beverage of harmful pathogens. But what most health-care professionals worry about is raw milk—or milk that has not been pasteurized. This process takes the milk to a temperature of 161 degrees Fahrenheit (71.7 degrees Celsius) for about 20 seconds; this temperature kills off the disease-causing bacteria, such as *Salmonella*, *Listeria*, and *Escherichia coli*—all while not affecting the taste or nutritional value of the milk. On the other hand, raw milk is not heated; and it can be contaminated by bacteria that thrive on a cow's skin, in the dirt, and the surrounding environment. And even a small amount of contamination can spread, as the bacteria often quickly grow and multiply.

The reactions to the possible contamination range from diarrhea and vomiting to gastrointestinal bloating and fever. Depending on a person's health—especially if the immune system is weak—and age, results might be even more severe. Thus, most nutritionists believe drinking pasteurized milk is best to limit the chances of becoming sick.

What is ultra-high temperature (UHT) pasteurization?

If milk is ultra-pasteurized, it is heated to a higher temperature in order to kill off harmful bacteria—and also to extend the shelf life of the product. Not only does this process cause a loss of nutrients—they usually have to be added artificially—but there is a wide gap between the good taste of pasteurized milk and often-described "watery" taste of ultra-pasteurized milk. (For more about milk, see the chapter "Nutrition in Eating and Drinking Choices.")

Why do some foods get "recalled"?

Nothing seems to be immune to recalls—from cars and trucks to chicken and spinach. In the case of food, harmful pathogens are often detected in a certain food, usually at the processing plant; at other times, if there is an outbreak of food poisoning after people eat at a certain place, or all bought the same food, the offending foods are quickly recalled. For example, in February 2014, the U.S. Food and Drug Administration listed a hummus recall on their food safety-recalls page, because of contamination with *Listeria monocytogenes*, and a fresh tomato recall, because of potential contamination with *Salmonella* (a list of recent and archived recalls can be found at www.fda.gov/Safety/Recalls/default.htm).

What is a norovirus?

In the past few years, the term *norovirus* has been in the news, especially in reference to cruise ships. But cruise ships aren't the only places affected—it can also strike people in any type of crowded conditions, such as airplanes and trains. According to the Centers for Disease Control and Prevention, the norovirus is one of the leading causes of food poisoning and results in something similar to the "stomach flu" (for more about the flu, see below). The virus spreads by coming in contact with someone who is infected, which is why it spreads rapidly in crowded conditions—through foods, drinks, and even surfaces. It is most often associated with such foods as fresh produce, shellfish, ice, fruit, and salads—especially those foods prepared by an infected person. It is difficult to prevent if you are exposed, but the warning should be for infected people—don't cook, prepare, or serve foods if you are infected. Otherwise, frequently washing your hands is one of the best deterrents for those who are not infected.

What recent study points to a fast way of finding certain harmful bacteria in foods?

With so many food recalls due to bacteria in the past decade, scientists are endeavoring to find harmful food bacteria on your food before it gets to your plate. In one recent study, scientists examined *Salmonella*—one of the most common microbes that cause foodborne illnesses—and found that tests to detect the bacteria in food are actually inexpensive and reliable. But there was a problem: The tests are complicated and take a long time to complete, and thus, the damage may already be done in the form of sickening some people. Their solution was to catch the microbes before this could happen by using an array of what they call "nanomechanical cantilevers" with peptides attached to the ends of the cantilevers; when the peptides bind to the *Salmonella*, the cantilever "bends," creating a signal. A special screening system allows the researchers to receive the signals and rapidly tell the difference between *Salmonella* and other types of bacteria—and even differences between various types of bacteria in the *Salmonella* family.

What is the difference between the flu and food poisoning?

According to the Centers for Disease Control and Prevention, around one in six Americans suffers from food poisoning each year; many people end up in the hospital, and it is estimated that about 3,000 die from food poisoning each year, many of them infants and the elderly. But how do you tell the difference between the flu—also called influenza, and which seems to have similar symptoms—from foodborne illnesses, often referred to as food poisoning? According to the Academy of Nutrition and Dietetics there are differences, as seen in the following chart of the flu versus food poisoning:

The Flu vs. Food Poisoning

Symptom	The Flu	Food Poisoning
Body aches and pains	Common: headache and muscle aches	Common: headache, backache, and stomach cramps
Fatigue	Common (and often extreme)	Common (and often extreme)
Fever	Common	Common
Gastrointestinal	Rarely prominent*	Common (often severe)
Nausea	Rarely prominent*	Common
Diarrhea	Rarely prominent*	Common
Respiratory		
Chest discomfort and cough	Common (often extreme, can become severe)	Rare
Nasal congestion, sore throat, runny or stuffy nose	Common	Rare

*Although nausea, vomiting, and diarrhea can sometimes accompany influenza infection, especially in children, gastrointestinal symptoms are rarely prominent.

What are foodborne zoonotic diseases?

Foodborne zoonotic diseases—also considered infections—are those that are transmitted directly or indirectly between animals and humans. In particular, they are caused by consuming food or drinking water that is contaminated with the microorganism responsible for certain diseases. Because we eat certain contaminated foods, the first place we usually feel the effects is in the gastrointestinal tract—with the resulting infections varying depending on exposure and type of microorganism. The most common microorganisms that cause such disease include the following:

- Bacteria—These include *Salmonella*, *Campylobacter*, *Listeria*, pathogenic *Escherichia coli* (more well-known as *E coli*), and *Yersinia*

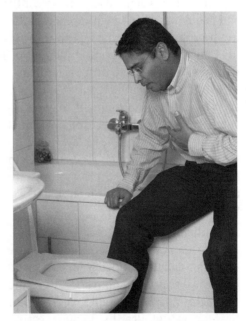

Symptoms of food poisoning include stomache-, back-, and headaches, fever, nausea, diarrhea, and fatigue.

- Viruses—The viruses include *Calcivirus* (including norovirus), hepatitis A virus, and hepatitis E virus
- Parasites—These include *Trichinella*, *Toxoplasma* (also often contracted by cats), *Cryptosporidium*, and *Giardia* (also often contracted by dogs)
- Bacterial toxins—This includes the toxins from *S aureus*, *Clostridium botulinum* (causes botulism), and *Bacillus cereus*

How do foods become contaminated?

When it comes to food, there are many ways a product can become contaminated at different stages of the food cycle. For example, animals on a farm can eat animal feed that is contaminated with bacteria, such as *Salmonella*; from there, the products from those animals can end up in other food products. In addition, parasites can infect food-producing animals, also leading to contamination of foods. And infected humans handling the food can contaminate the food products, which can occur even in your own kitchen if you don't pay attention to how you handle foods.

DIGESTIVE ILLNESSES AND DISEASES

What is Crohn disease?

Crohn disease is defined as a chronic inflammation and irritation of the digestive tract and is often associated with inflammatory bowel disease, or IBD (see below), an often frustrating condition that has no known true cause. According to the Crohn's and Colitis Foundation of America, hundreds of thousands of Americans have the disease, although it is thought that there are many more who are undiagnosed. The condition is known to run in families, and research has shown that a person's immune system and even his or her environment may be involved. The symptoms include abdominal pain, diarrhea, weight loss, fever, and fatigue; the most common foods that seem to be associated with the symptoms are dairy, high-fiber grains, alcohol, and extremely spicy foods.

Although it is thought of as a digestive disease, it is known that foods do not cause Crohn's—and unfortunately for those who have the disease, so far, no known specific diet helps allay the symptoms. The best tips for eating healthy include eating smaller meals many times a day; eating many fresh fruits and vegetables (although

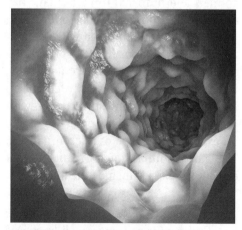

This is what the inside of a human intestine looks like when the person is suffering from Crohn disease.

in small amounts to first see any reaction) to get needed nutrients; and consult your physician or a nutritionist for help in working out the best food plan for you.

What is ulcerative colitis?

Similar to Crohn disease, ulcerative colitis involves the gastrointestinal tract and an abnormal response by the body's immune system. It is limited to the large bowel (colon) and affects only the top layers of the colon. For half the people with ulcerative colitis, the symptoms are mild. Others may suffer from symptoms such as the progressive loosening of the stool: it is generally bloody and may be accompanied by abdominal cramping and urgency to have a bowel movement, with diarrhea beginning slowly or quickly.

What is inflammatory bowel disease (IBD)?

Inflammatory bowel disease (IBD) is often confused with irritable bowel syndrome (IBS; see below)—but they are two distinct gastrointestinal disorders. According to the Centers for Disease Control and Prevention, *IBD* is actually a broad term that describes conditions with recurring or chronic immune response, and the inflammation of the gastrointestinal tract. Thus, the two most common forms of IBD are Crohn disease and ulcerative colitis (see above). On the average, the peak age for the onset for IBD is about 15 to 30 years old; more men have ulcerative colitis, whereas more women suffer from Crohn disease. It is thought that there is a strong genetic connection for those who have IBD; more smokers have IBD; and some studies have shown that rates of IBD may be higher in northern than in southern states, and higher in urban than in rural areas.

What is irritable bowel syndrome—or IBS?

It is estimated that 10 to 20 percent of adult Americans have the disease, although it is thought that there are many more people who are undiagnosed. That means that about one in five Americans has experienced symptoms of IBS—with twice as many women as men reporting the disease (this may be because women are more likely to report the symptoms to their doctors). IBS is called a functional gastrointestinal disorder (meaning there is some type of disturbance in bowel function) that affects the muscle contractions in the colon, often called spastic colon, mucous or nervous colitis—but those terms are inaccurate and lead to confusion.

In general, for IBS, unlike IBDs (Crohn or ulcerative colitis), there is no destructive intestinal inflammation. The symptoms—which usually come and go—include bloating, abdominal pain and cramping, constipation or diarrhea, and gas pains. The only similarity to Crohn disease and ulcerative colitis is that no real cause is known, although it seems to be connected to heredity, allergies, infections, lifestyle, and even the type of bacteria that live in a person's intestines. There also seem to be some triggers that start IBS, with stress and diet at the top of the list. Most doctors and nutritionists recommend that people with IBS eat small frequent meals; eat whole grains, vegetables, and fruits, if possible; drink plenty of water (and watch the intake of alcohol, caffeine, and sugary drinks); and take note of the foods that can trigger an attack, and try to avoid them.

Will eating nutritious foods help with chronic fatigue syndrome?

Chronic fatigue syndrome (CFS) is often confused with irritable bowel syndrome and inflammatory bowel disease (IBS and IBD; see above), but there are definite differences. First, CFS is a syndrome, not a disease. According to the Centers for Disease Control and Prevention, CFS is "a debilitating and complex disorder characterized by profound fatigue that is not improved by bed rest and that may be worsened by physical or mental activity." The symptoms can vary depending on the person, but in general, they include weakness, some muscular pain, difficulty concentrating, and insomnia. So far, there is no known reason for the syndrome, and it is thought that it is not caused by what we eat or a nutritional imbalance. But even so, most doctors agree that a well-balanced diet can help alleviate the symptoms of the syndrome.

What are the differences between gluten sensitivity, celiac disease, and wheat intolerance?

Many people have reactions to wheat products, ranging from celiac disease to wheat allergy to gluten sensitivity. The following list describes some of the differences between these three conditions:

Celiac disease—This is a severe intolerance to grain/gluten products and is also known as celiac sprue or nontropical sprue. It is considered an autoimmune disease in which the protein gliadin—found in many grains, especially wheat—causes mostly gastrointestinal health problems. (For more about celiac disease, see below.)

Wheat allergy (sometimes called baker's asthma)—This condition is thought to be because of a wheat-specific antibody in the body called IgE. When a person eats a product containing gluten, it can often lead to hives, sudden anaphylaxis, sneezing, and/or wheezing. But a true wheat allergy is believed to be very rare, because while symptoms are similar to several other conditions involving food, there is no good test for a wheat allergy. And even the blood test for IgE (called a radioallergosorbent test, or RAST) to determine the substances a person is allergic to, is often unreliable.

Gluten sensitivity (or gluten intolerance)—Gluten intolerance may be one of the most frustrating conditions for health-care providers to identify. This condition is not an autoimmune disease, like celiac disease, nor an allergy, like a true wheat allergy—but seems to be a mostly gastrointestinal response in some people to gluten products. (For more about gluten intolerance, see this chapter; and for the controversies surrounding gluten intolerance and sensitivity, see the chapter "Controversies Food, Beverages, and Nutrition.")

How does celiac disease affect a person?

Celiac disease often causes severe symptoms such as diarrhea, bloating, constipation, and abdominal pain (which is why is it difficult to diagnose, and is often incorrectly labeled as irritable bowel syndrome, a vitamin deficiency, or an eating disorder). The disease is often apparent in children when they start eating gluten-rich foods early in life;

some research indicates that symptoms occur in infancy between six months and two years of age. The symptoms in children range from stomach upsets and bloating to diarrhea, mouth sores, and a decreased ability to fight off infections. Later in life, usually between the ages of 30 and 50 years, people—more often women than men—who develop celiac (they may have had a mild to symptomless sensitivity in childhood) may also experience these same symptoms. The "solution" is usually a gluten-free diet; and for a person starting such a diet, it may take from several weeks to a few months to feel better.

How many people have celiac disease?

To date, this disease affects about 1 in 130 people in the United States—almost 3 million Americans—and the numbers have been rising in the past few years since the condition has become more well known. Worldwide, it is estimated that about 1 percent of the population has celiac disease. It is also interesting to note that many recent research papers have reported an "overdiagnosis" of celiac disease, so just how prevalent this disease is in the United States alone is still debated.

What does a gluten-free diet entail?

As people who have been diagnosed with celiac disease will mention—and even those who think they have an intolerance to gluten—maintaining a gluten-free diet is a challenge. In the United States, there are so many foods that contain gluten—from breads and baked goods to sauces, soups, and even some candies, ice creams, and puddings—that gluten-sensitive people have to pay close attention to foods they purchase and consume.

Gluten-sensitive people can eat pastas, breads, and other baked products—but only if they are gluten free (*Note:* some labels do mention what type of facilities were used to manufacture the food and sometimes mention wheat, which is a food to stay away from if you need to be gluten free). But overall, most gluten-sensitive people have to read food product labels no matter what they buy; at parties, they either have to eat only what they know contains no gluten or bring their own food; and when at restaurants, they must order only "plain" foods, such as steamed vegetables or broiled fish (although some restaurants are becoming more aware of the needs of gluten-sensitive customers; just ask the server if there are any gluten-free items on the menu).

What is diverticulitis?

In yet another digestive tract disease, small pockets or pouches called diverticula form throughout a person's large intestines. Pain and discomfort occurs when the waste products naturally flowing through your intestines get caught and impacted in a pouch (or several), causing a condition called diverticulitis, in which the pouches become infected or inflamed. Although no one knows what actually causes diverticulitis, it usually occurs in people sixty years or older—especially if they are overweight. If the lining of the intestinal wall weakens, which usually happens as we age, and the intestines are stressed (for example, if you have diarrhea or constipation), it "stretches" the intestinal wall, creating a pouch.

Studies have also shown that diverticulitis is most often found in the industrialized Western cultures, in which diets are often high in fat and low in fiber. Thus, doctors and nutritionists often suggest a diet high in fiber (vegetables, fruits, and whole grains), and plenty of fluids, especially water. And although it is often said that eating seeds, corn, and nuts causes a flare-up of diverticulitis, not everyone agrees, and many people who eat seeds and nuts in a balanced diet show fewer bouts of diverticulitis. Of course, that does not pertain to

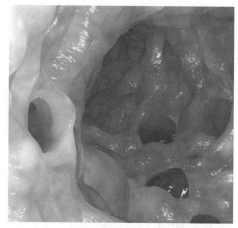

Diverticulitis is a condition in which deep pockets appear in the intestine that can easily become infected.

everyone—and those who do have diverticulitis should be aware of what foods do cause them to have an attack—and avoid such foods.

CANCER, DIABETES, AND OTHER DISEASES

Is there a connection between cancer and nutrition?

Although there is a wide discrepancy of percentages between studies—from 30 to 50 percent—most researchers agree that there are some connections between diet and cancers. In particular, there is a general agreement that a diet high in fat and processed foods (especially those foods that are salt-cured, smoked, charcoal-grilled, or prepared with certain fermentation processes can lead to some types of cancer, and this could be avoided with proper nutrition. Besides cutting back on fats and processed foods, and along with eating more fiber, proper nutrition also means eating more whole grains, fruits, and vegetables that have cancer-fighting benefits. For example, broccoli contains beta carotene, vitamin C, fiber, and phytochemicals—all of which help to fight cancers. Nutritionists advocate eating whole grains (especially for fiber) and a variety of various vegetables and fruits that have either one or several such nutrients to help your system fight off cancers. (And, of course, along with eating well, you can fight cancers if you stop smoking and limit your alcohol intake.)

What are some of the best "cancer-fighting" foods?

There are some cancer-fighting foods that nutritionists point to when it comes to diet. The following list describes only a few of those foods, and why they are important in keeping cancers away:

Buckwheat—This seed is nutrition rich, with magnesium, iron, and plenty of protein and fiber. It is also known to lower cholesterol levels, help build and strengthen blood vessels throughout the entire body, and to lower blood pressure. As for cancer, buckwheat contains a known cancer-fighter, called rutin.

Tomatoes—Tomatoes, and their products such as sauces, contain lycopene—a known fighter against such cancers as prostate cancer.

Green tea—Green tea has long been known for its healthy benefits, especially in Chinese medicine. It is thought that a catechin called epigallocatechin gallate (EGCG) can help fight cancer by reducing the formation of carcinogens in the body, and boosting our immune systems. In fact, many researchers believe that EGCG may be one of the most potent cancer-fighting compounds yet discovered in foods.

Alliums—The allium family of plants—primarily garlic, onions, and shallots—are thought to contain cancer-fighting sulfur compounds. These substances may help to boost a person's immune system—and thus keep certain cancers away.

Fresh fruits and vegetables, legumes, and whole grains—And as most nutritionists agree, the top way to fight cancer—and of course to be healthy—is to eat fresh fruits and vegetables, especially those rich in flavonoids (such as broccoli and apples); legumes (such as lentils and kidney beans) that have high fiber and many cancer-fighting minerals and vitamins; and whole grains (such as whole wheat and oats) that are rich in selenium—a mineral associated with fighting off cancers.

What foods are associated with certain cancers?

There are many foods that have been associated with certain types of cancer. One of the most well known are processed foods. For example, people who eat large amounts of smoked, fried, cured, pickled, or processed meats are often found to have a higher incidence of stomach and esophageal tumors. Nitrites, such as those found in many processed hams, hot dogs, and bacon, have long been associated with certain types of cancer, especially since they can form nitrosamines, compounds that are known carcinogens. (For more about cancers and meat, see the chapter "Food Chemistry and Nutrition.")

What is diabetes?

Diabetes is a metabolic disorder that is caused by the decreased ability (or the complete inability) of the body to use carbohydrates. For people without diabetes, the body breaks down carbohydrates into glucose—one of the energy sources for our systems. In order to convert this glucose into energy, we rely on insulin, a hormone produced in the pancreas. If a person is a diabetic, he or she cannot convert the glucose into energy; instead it accumulates in the blood, causing a rise in glucose in the body, what is often referred to as "blood sugar." The results range from constant infections to mental confusion—and even coma if the blood sugar levels go too high.

There are two forms of diabetes: type I and type II (also seen as type 1 and type 2). Type 1 is also called insulin-dependent diabetes and usually begins in childhood; type II

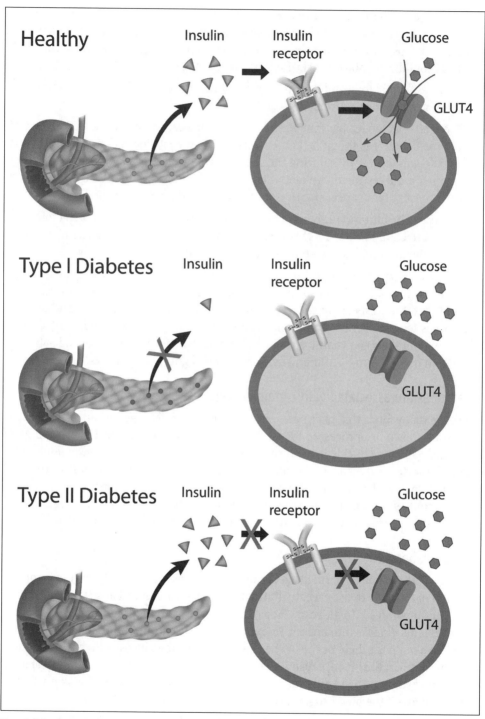

Type 1 diabetes results from the pancreas making too little insulin, while type 2 occurs when your body makes enough insulin but is unable to use it.

diabetes is also called adult-onset or noninsulin-dependent diabetes, and is usually found in people from adulthood to old age. Diabetes can seem to start slowly (many people have "prediabetes" in which their fasting glucose readings are high, but not over the recommended number for a diabetic); this is because the symptoms—from fatigue, increased appetite, thirst, and frequent urination—are often ignored, and usually attributed to "getting older," or to other illnesses or diseases.

Is there a connection between nutrition and diabetes?

Yes, there is a connection between diabetes and nutrition—especially that you should pay close attention to your nutrition if you are a diabetic! But there is another connection: Although the tendency to develop diabetes seems to be hereditary, triggered by pregnancy (although this type of diabetes often disappears after the baby is born), surgery, or physical and emotional stress, one of the biggest reasons (especially for type 2 diabetics) is obesity, or being overweight because of eating an unhealthy diet that contains too many foods rich in fats, salts, and sugars. In fact, many people who are prediabetic or have type 2 diabetes have been known to reverse their condition by weight control, proper nutrition, and exercise.

What is a glycemic index?

The glycemic index (GI) is an important tool for diabetics, as it gives a numerical ranking to foods based on the rate of their conversion to glucose in the body. The scale is from 1 to 100, with pure glucose (sugar) being the standard at 100. The lower numbers represent a low rise in blood sugar after a certain food is consumed; the higher numbers represent a more rapid rise in blood sugar after a certain food is consumed.

Although the GI is a useful tool, it is not a perfect system. One reason is that the GI ranking applies only when you eat something on an empty stomach—and most people eat many foods at a meal. Another reason is that the GI doesn't take into consideration how much you actually consume, but is based instead on a serving of food that contains 50 grams of carbohydrates minus the fiber, then measuring the person's blood sugar levels over the next two hours. Because of these inherent problems, the glycemic load (GL) method was developed.

Does eating too much sugar cause diabetes?

No, if you don't have diabetes, eating sugar will not cause you to get the disease, especially type 2 diabetes. This disease is most often caused by a diet high in calories, little or no exercise, and becoming overweight or obese. People who have type 1 diabetes do have to watch their sugar intake—not because the sugars will give them "more" diabetes, but because sugar will adversely affect their blood sugar levels.

What is a glycemic load?

Not all foods will immediately give you a boost—even if the item has a high glycemic index. What also becomes important to a diabetic is the glycemic load, or the body's response based on the glycemic index and the amount of whatever carbohydrate you consume. For example, even though a piece of candy has a high glycemic index, if it is small, it will have a relatively small glycemic response. According to the Harvard School of Public Health, where the idea of the glycemic load was developed, the glycemic load is equal to the glycemic index over 100, then multiplied by the net carbohydrates (that is, equal to the total carbohydrates minus the dietary fiber). Thus, diabetics use both low glycemic index foods and restricts their carbohydrates in order to control their diabetes.

What are the glycemic indexes and loads of some common foods?

GI and GL for Common Foods

Food	GI	Serving Size	Net Carbs	GL
Apples	38	1 medium (138g)	16	6
Baked potato	85	1 medium (173g)	33	28
Bananas	52	1 large (136g)	27	14
Bean sprouts	25	1 cup (104g)	4	1
Brown rice	55	1 cup (195g)	42	23
Carrots	47	1 large (72g)	5	2
Glucose	100	(50g)	50	50
Grapefruit	25	1/2 large (166g)	11	3
Honey	55	1 tbsp (21g)	17	9
Ice cream	61	1 cup (72g)	16	10
Lowfat yogurt	33	1 cup (245g)	47	16
Macaroni and cheese	64	1 serving (166g)	47	30
Oatmeal	58	1 cup (234g)	21	12
Oranges	48	1 medium (131g)	12	6
Peanuts	14	4 oz (113g)	15	2
Pizza	30	2 slices (260g)	42	13
Popcorn	72	2 cups (16g)	10	7
Potato chips	54	4 oz (114g)	55	30
Raisins	64	1 small box (43g)	32	20
Snickers Bar	55	1 bar (113g)	64	35
Spaghetti	42	1 cup (140g)	38	16
Sugar (sucrose)	68	1 tbsp (12g)	12	8
Watermelon	72	1 cup (154g)	11	8
White bread	70	1 slice (30g)	14	10
White rice	64	1 cup (186g)	52	33

Is Parkinson's disease associated with a certain nutrient?

Parkinson's disease—also called shaking palsy or *paralysis agitans*—is a slow-progressing disease of the nervous system that occurs when a special type of nerve cell located in the brain is destroyed. Although there is still speculation as to what causes the disease, some research indicates that it may be a deficiency of vitamin E in early life. The disease seems to start when there is an imbalance of two brain chemicals, dopamine and acetylcholine, both of which transfer messages between nerve cells that control muscles. Initial symptoms include rigid muscles in the legs and arms, cramping, and tremors; the disease eventually affects speech, walking ability, and even appetite.

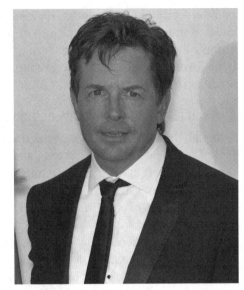

Television and film star Michael J. Fox created a foundation to raise money for Parkinson's disease research after he discovered he had the illness in the early 1990s.

Is there an association between the ingestion of aluminum and Alzheimer's disease?

According to the Alzheimer's Association, this disease is a type of dementia that creates problems with memory, thinking, and behavior. The symptoms seem to develop slowly, and get worse over time, eventually interfering with simple daily tasks. To date, little is known about what causes this disease, although there seems to be a very strong genetic component. The idea that Alzheimer's disease was caused by the ingestion of aluminum started during the 1960s and 1970s: some research indicated that this disease could be caused by the use of aluminum pots and pans, and even aluminum foil and antacids. Since that time, there has been no scientific proof that aluminum can cause—or even exacerbate—the disease.

How has calcium been linked to certain diseases?

Calcium—or the lack of it—has been linked to many human diseases (for more about calcium, see the chapter "The Basics of Nutrition: Micronutrients"). For example, the National Cancer Institute found that the more calcium in your diet, the lower your risk for colon cancer; it suggests that a person not take more than 1,300 milligrams (mg) per day, as higher amounts don't seem to help. In other studies, researchers found that oxalic acid—found in soybeans, almonds, kale, and rhubarb—when combined with calcium can create an insoluble compound that can form stones in the kidney or gallbladder (a typical diet should not cause this condition).

What happens if a person's calcium level is too high or low?

For a healthy person, if the concentration of calcium is too high (calcium rigor), the body's hormones and vitamin D make sure the excess is deposited and stored in the bones. If the calcium is too low (calcium tetany), the imbalance can be corrected in the body, especially in the kidneys (it slows down excretion, so you don't go to the bathroom as much and lose the calcium in your urine). It's interesting to note, too, that a chronic dietary deficiency in calcium will help to lower the amount of calcium in your bones, which could affect their strength and eventually lead to osteoporosis, or weakening of the bone structure.

Can you test your blood for its nutrition content?

Although there are some laboratories that promise to analyze the entire nutritional content of your blood, it is not that easy, and the results can be difficult to interpret. In fact, most researchers agree that laboratory testing of your blood for nutrients is less precise (and often more expensive) than many other fields of medicine, such as testing your blood for TSH (thyroid stimulating hormone). Thus, to date, there are no true routine screening tests that can be conducted to show everything about your blood's nutrient balance. Furthermore, many nutrients are stored or produced in sites other than your blood—your bone marrow, for example. This means that laboratories that promise an entire nutrient scan of your blood may be fooling you—at least to this date.

Even so, there are some specific tests to determine a specific deficiency; other tests can also determine the functional effects of a certain nutrient deficiency, not the nutrient concentration. For example, doctors can measure hemoglobin in a person's blood to determine the iron content (and to determine if the person is iron deficient, called iron-deficiency anemia; for more, see below). Another test is the red cell enzyme reactivation assay, which measures certain nutrients in the body (such as the B-complex vitamins) by testing just how well a certain enzyme that is dependent on the nutrient functions in the red blood cells. But there is a caveat to such testing: Patients need to reveal what they have eaten or what medications or supplements they are taking. This is because certain tests, for example, that for serum iron, are strongly influenced by the iron content of whatever meal has been recently eaten; or the serum B_{12} tests, which can show a lower amount of the vitamin in people who take vitamin C supplements.

What is anemia?

A person who is anemic (the condition is called anemia) does not have enough healthy red blood cells, or hemoglobin, the oxygen-carrying, iron- and protein-based red pigment in the blood, in his or her body. There are many types of anemia, and all differ greatly in terms of cause and treatments. Overall, it can cause general weakness, fatigue, and even brittle nails; more severe anemia can result in shortness of breath, cardiac arrhythmias ("fluttering" heartbeats), and sometimes fainting.

How much iron does a person need?

Because the human body needs iron to make new red blood cells—cells that carry oxygen to all the organs and tissues in the body—there are some recommended standard amounts of iron intake. Because only a small amount of iron is absorbed into our systems, the Recommended Daily Requirements (RDA) for iron are as follows: 8 milligrams per day for men and postmenopausal women; 18 milligrams for women under 50; and 27 milligrams for pregnant women. In the case of iron, more is not necessarily better—excess iron in your blood can cause hemochromatosis, what many call "iron overload" disease. And beware of "iron grabbers," or eating an excessive amount of certain foods that can bind with iron and make it unavailable for absorption; this includes the natural compounds in tea called tannins, phytates found in nuts, and oxalates in spinach, Swiss chard, and chocolate.

What is iron-deficiency anemia?

Certain types of anemia are thought to be caused by a specific nutritional deficiency, and the most common of these is iron-deficiency anemia. It occurs when there are low levels of iron (a micronutrient classified under minerals) in the blood. As the center of our bones (bone marrow) creates hemoglobin, it uses the iron in our system to create red blood cells; those cells, in turn, carry oxygen all over the body. If there is a deficiency of iron in the blood, the bone marrow cannot produce the hemoglobin, resulting in iron-deficiency anemia. Most often, iron-deficiency anemia can be caused by an iron-poor diet (which happens most often in infants, children, vegans, vegetarians, and those with gastrointestinal illnesses that often suppress appetites); depletion of iron in pregnant and lactating women; menstruating women; people who give blood frequently; certain drugs, foods, and caffeinated drinks (to susceptible people); people who have digestive conditions such as Crohn disease; or even people who have to have their stomach or small intestines surgically removed because of disease. Most deficiencies can be treated with iron supplements, or by eating iron-rich foods, such as liver and seafoods, eggs, legumes, leafy greens, whole grains, nuts, seeds, and some fortified cereals.

What is vitamin-deficiency anemia?

Vitamin-deficiency anemia is caused by the deficiency of vitamin B_{12} and folate—both nutrients needed to make red blood cells. There are several reasons for the development of a vitamin-deficiency anemia, including the following subtypes of this anemia:

Megaloblastic anemia—This occurs when vitamin B_{12} or folate or both, are deficient.

Pernicious anemia—This occurs when a person can't absorb vitamin B_{12} because of illnesses such as Crohn disease, an intestinal parasite infection, surgical removal of part of the stomach or intestine, or an infection with HIV.

Dietary deficiency—As the name implies, this deficiency is based on a lack of a certain nutrient because of a person's diet. For example, often thought of as a vegetarian or vegan condition, a vitamin-deficient anemia occurs when someone eats little or no meat; thus, he or she can lack vitamin B_{12}; in addition, it can also be when someone cooks at too high a heat or overcooks vegetables, or eats very few vegetables, creating a folate deficiency.

Other causes—There are other reasons for a vitamin deficiency, including pregnancy (especially not eating well during and after pregnancy); certain medications that can interfere with the absorption of vitamins; severe alcohol abuse (which also interferes

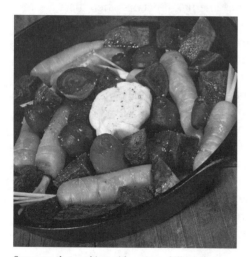

Some say that cooking with an iron skillet adds iron to one's diet.

with the intake and absorption of nutrients); and gastrointestinal diseases such as celiac disease.

What foods affect your blood pressure?

Overall, there are numerous reasons behind each person's blood pressure, including their habits (for example, if they smoke or drink); but health-care professionals agree that it is also what you eat, if you are heavy, and if you eat certain foods. According to the Cleveland Clinic, there are many food-based reasons for high blood pressure—especially if you eat many of the following foods: butter, margarine, regular salad dressings, fatty meats, whole dairy products, baked goods (especially with shortening), processed meats, salty snacks, canned soups, fast foods, and deli meats—all of which have an abundance of fats, sugars, and salt. Instead, the Clinic suggests eating such foods as those with lower fat (skim or 1 percent milk, for instance), low salt (cook with a variety of spices instead and read package labels to determine the overall salt content of certain foods), and fresh vegetables, fruits, and whole grained baked goods—all of which will help control your blood pressure. (For more about blood pressure, see the chapter "Nutrition and You.")

NUTRITION AND YOUR ORGANS

What foods should you eat if you have chronic kidney disease?

According to the National Kidney and Urologic Diseases Information Clearinghouse (part of the U.S. Department of Health and Human Services), you can prevent or delay health problems from chronic kidney disease (CKD) through your diet. In particular, you should eat foods that are high in phosphorus, potassium, and sodium. You should not eat much protein—it can burden the function of your kidneys and speed up the progression of CKD. With healthy kidneys, high-protein foods like meat and dairy products are broken down into the waste products of nitrogen and creatinine, and are removed from the blood. But diseased kidneys cannot stop these waste products from building up in the blood, and thus resulting in the health problems that accompany CKD.

How do kidney stones form?

Kidney stones are small "stones," or hard deposits of minerals and acid salts (most often calcium phosphate or oxalate) that form inside the kidneys and often travel through the urinary tract. They can form in several places from the kidney to the bladder, and can also be found in both or only one kidney. The movement of the stones—which range in size from a grain of sand to a bird's egg—is the reason for the pain, which can be concentrated in the middle back to the groin area. The stones form for a variety of reasons, including an increase in calcium in the blood caused by an overactive parathyroid gland; an increase in uric acid that cannot be diluted by the fluid in the urine; stress (which draws out minerals from the bones and thus increases calcium excretion); dehydration (which concentrates the urine); and some infections. The types of stones include calcium (the most common), uric acid, struvite, and cystine stones—all of which form depending on the amount of the various minerals and acids in your urine.

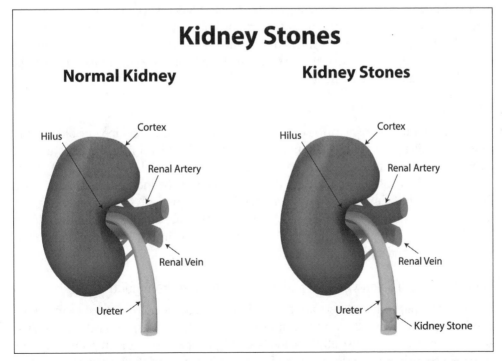

Kidney Stones

Normal Kidney

Hilus
Cortex
Renal Artery
Renal Vein
Ureter

Kidney Stones

Hilus
Cortex
Renal Artery
Renal Vein
Ureter
Kidney Stone

Kidney stones are painful, hard deposits of minerals in the kidneys and ureter. They can be caused by a diet too low in potassium or too high in salt.

Is there a connection between kidney stones and nutrition?

Yes, nutrition may be a factor in the formation of some kidney stones. For example, a deficiency of magnesium can increase the alkalinity of urine, thus forming calcium phosphate stones; if there is a decrease in vitamin B_6, it will increase the oxalic acid in the urine, thus forming calcium oxalate stones. In addition, it is thought that various dietary factors may contribute to stones. For example, too much salt; too little potassium (often a problem in refined-food diets); and not enough fruits and vegetables in a diet make the urine too alkaline, and thus create stones.

What foods are best to eat if you have kidney stones?

People with the various types of kidney stones should manage their weight as much as possible, and eat as many nutritious foods as possible. For example, it is best to choose a diet low in oxalates, especially if you tend to form calcium oxalate stones; thus, you should stay away from rhubarb, beets, spinach, Swiss chard, sweet potatoes, nuts, soy products, and chocolate. Your diet should be low in salt and animal proteins, with more of an emphasis on the proteins from legume products. It is also interesting to note that eating more calcium-rich foods may help: the calcium is thought to bind with oxalates in the gastrointestinal tract, stopping the oxalates from entering the bloodstream.

What is in normal human urine?

Normal human urine has, on average, water (about 95 percent), organic wastes (urea, creatinine, uric acid, and some enzymes, carbohydrates, and hormones from our body), and salts. But the composition varies depending on several daily factors; for example, how much water, tea, coffee, soft drinks, or any liquid you have consumed, the time of day, what you ate that day, and if you have any illness or disease.

What is gout?

Gout is a painful form of arthritis caused by high levels of uric acid in your blood. This causes crystals to form and accumulate around a joint—often in the fingers and toes, although it can occur in any joint in the body—and in the heel, knee, or even the ear. The reasons for contracting gout are thought to be obesity, increasing age, improper diet, and even heredity. It is often recommended to people with gout to lose weight if possible (but not to lose weight too fast, as that can promote a gout attack), drink plenty of fluids, and avoid high-protein weight-loss diets (in which your body would make too much uric acid and suffer a gout attack).

What foods should you watch—and eat—if you suffer from gout?

In terms of food, gout sufferers are often advised to stay away from dried beans, peas, lentils, and other legumes, as well as mushrooms, anchovies, organ meats, asparagus, and herring. This is because all these foods are high in purines—and in people who are susceptible, purines increase the level of uric acid in the blood that can cause a painful gout attack. In addition, nutritionists suggest that you cut back on fats, especially saturated (they tend to lower the body's ability to eliminate uric acid); limit or avoid alcohol that can interfere with the elimination of uric acid from the body; eat more complex carbohydrates, such as whole grains, and fresh fruits and vegetables; avoid foods sweetened with high-fructose corn syrup (fructose tends to increase uric acid in the body); and drink plenty of water to help flush the uric acid from your system.

What is the connection between food and the liver?

We should all be thankful for our livers. According to the National Liver Foundation, everything we consume and absorb has to be refined, processed, and detoxified by the liver; in addition, about 85 to 90 percent of the nutrient-rich blood that leaves the stomach and intestines reaches the liver, which then converts the nutrients into substances the body can use.

Each important food substance—carbohydrates, proteins, and fats—has some connection to the liver. Carbohydrates (sugars) are stored as glycogen in the liver, then released as energy between meals or when the body has high energy demands. Proteins reach the liver as amino acids, and once there, are released to muscles as energy, converted to urea and excreted in the urine, or stored as energy for later use. Fats cannot be digested without the bile made in the liver (which is then stored in the gallbladder and used as needed, released into the small intestines during digestion). This bile is necessary in many ways: it breaks up fat into smaller particles to allow for better absorption in the intestines; helps with the absorption of fat-soluble vitamins (A, D, E, and K); and as one of the ways our body recycles—as after digestion—bile acids can be reabsorbed by the intestines, returned to the liver, and recycled as bile again.

What disease is associated with liver and nutrition?

One of the major diseases associated with the liver is cirrhosis—when damaged liver cells are replaced by fibrous scar tissue that slows down (and can eventually stop) the functioning of this organ. It is most commonly caused by excessive alcohol consumption, viral hepatitis, ingestion of certain drugs, exposure to certain toxic chemicals, or an obstruction in the bile ducts associated with the liver. But if detected early enough, eating a balanced diet with enough calories, proteins, fats, and carbohydrates can help a damaged liver to regenerate new liver cells—which is why many people with some liver disease can be treated with a nutritional diet prescribed by their doctor.

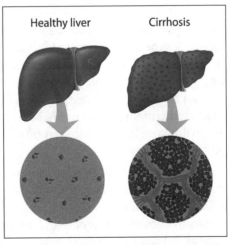

Cirrhosis of the liver refers to the damage caused to the liver that then leads to scar tissue, hampering the liver's normal functions.

Can bacteria in your digestive tract affect your liver?

Although it needs more research, there is an indication that the bacteria in your digestive tract—beneficial and not beneficial—can affect your liver. This is because about 70 percent of the blood that flows into the liver comes from the intestines, the organs in which your natural bacteria live. When researchers examined patients with chronic fatty liver disease—or diseased livers from certain illnesses, not alcoholism—they discovered that between 20 and 75 percent of these people had an overabundance of gut bacteria. Some scientists believe the presence of excessive amounts of bacteria in the digestive tract could be responsible for some types of chronic liver disease.

What are hyperthyroidism and hypothyroidism?

Hyperthyroidism is when the thyroid gland puts out too much of the thyroid hormone; symptoms include nervousness, fatigue, loss of weight and hair, insomnia, intolerance of heat, and fluctuating moods. Hypothyroidism occurs when there is an abnormally low rate of thyroid hormone secretion from the thyroid gland—often resulting in a goiter, an enlargement of the thyroid gland. Symptoms include obesity, sluggish metabolism, being cold most of the time, slow mental reactions, dry hair and nails, palpitations of the heart, and restlessness. In children, it can also result in cretinism, or slow physical and mental growth.

Is there a connection between hyperthyroidism, hypothyroidism, and nutrition?

Yes, there are several connections between problems with the thyroid gland and nutrition. For example, the excessive amount of thyroid hormone of a hyperthyroid person causes the body processes to speed up. As a result, all the nutrients in the body are "chewed up" at a more rapid rate than for a person with a normal thyroid—which is why nutritionists suggest that people with hyperthyroidism should increase the amount of nutrients in their diet. And for those who have lost weight from the disease, additional protein may be needed to replace lost muscle tissue (this often includes additional B-complex vitamins—needed for metabolism of the extra carbohydrates and proteins).

For a hypothyroid person, the underproduction of thyroid hormones causes the metabolism to slow down. Nutritionists suggest that people with this disease should eat a diet rich in all nutrients—including vitamins A, C, and E, along with riboflavin, niacin, pyridoxine, and zinc—and for some people, the addition of foods rich in iodine, such as iodized salt, seafood, and seaweed is recommended. (But be aware that some foods can inhibit the absorption of iodine, including peanuts, cabbage, soybeans, mustard, and turnips.)

NUTRITION AND THE MOUTH

Is there a connection between tooth decay and nutrition?

Yes, in many cases, there is a connection between tooth decay, gum disease, and nutrition. Tooth decay—what we all know of as cavities or dental caries—is the primary dental problem in the United States and in many countries around the world. It is most often caused by the persistent eating of refined sugars and starches, all of which mix with our saliva, forming an acid that erodes our tooth enamel. It is often suggested that people susceptible to tooth decay—besides improving their dental hygiene habits, such as brushing and flossing—cut back on eating refined carbohydrate foods, sweet drinks, and snacks, and especially to eat nutritionally balanced meals.

In addition, some people also suggest that you can protect your teeth at the end of some meals with certain foods; for example, eating aged cheeses, such as cheddar, may help prevent cavities if eaten at the end of a meal. Still another study suggests that chewing sugarless gum can increase the flow of saliva—and that not only gets rid of food particles, but also cuts back on the acids in your mouth (but be aware that for some

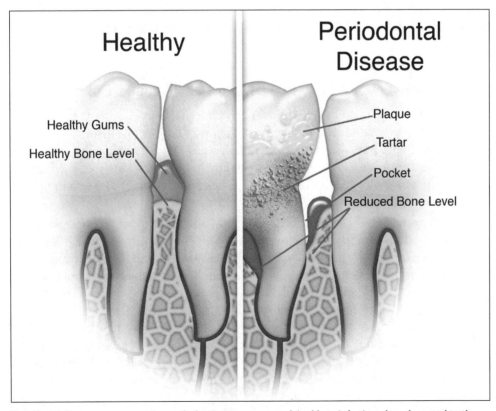

Periodontal disease causes gums to recede, leaving gums more vulnerable to infections, bone loss, and teeth more likely to decay.

people, sugarless gum may increase the amount of gas in your system). And of course, rinsing out your mouth after every meal (especially if you can't brush right away) can also help cut down on cavities.

Is there a connection between gum disease and nutrition?

Yes, there seems to be a connection between gum disease and nutrition. This disease usually starts out as gingivitis, in which the gums are sensitive or bleeding a bit; gingivitis usually begins when plaque—a mix of food, bacteria, and mucus—attaches to the spaces between the teeth and gums. If not promptly and properly removed (which is why visiting the dentist regularly is necessary), this can harden into calculus—a hard substance that looks like whitish plaster that can irritate and eventually infect the gums. This can lead to periodontitis, an irreversible disease that is often thought to account for more tooth loss than dental cavities.

When it comes to nutrition and periodontitis, there are several recommendations. For example, bioflavonoids found in vitamin C foods may help bleeding gums; vitamin A helps with the general health of the gums; important minerals are sodium, potassium, calcium (including vitamin D to help absorption of the calcium), phosphorus, iron, and magnesium. Many of these vitamins and minerals can be obtained by eating a well-balanced diet of vitamin C-rich fruits, green leafy vegetables, and whole grains.

What does licorice root have to do with gum disease?

Gum disease is often associated with certain bacteria in our mouths that can eventually lead to such problems as gingivitis or periodontal disease. A recent study has found that two substances in licorice can kill the major bacteria responsible for gum disease and even tooth decay. This is not the usual licorice found most often in the United States—which has been replaced with anise oil in most "licorice" candies—but the actual licorice plant.

In this study, the researchers examined the dried root of the licorice plant—known to be a common treatment in Chinese traditional medicine, which is used to enhance the activity of other herbs, or as a flavoring, and to treat such ailments as respiratory and digestive problems. The researchers examined two licorice compounds—licoricidin and licorisoflavan A—both very effective antibacterial substances. The two compounds actually helped to kill off the major bacteria that cause dental cavities, and two of the bacteria that can lead to gum disease; in addition, the licoricidin also killed off a third bacteria that causes gum disease. But don't rush out and start chewing on licorice roots—more studies need to be conducted on just how extensive licorice treatments would have to be to curtail, or even prevent, these dental diseases.

FOODS AND CERTAIN INTERACTIONS

What foods can interfere with medications?

There are several foods that can interfere with medications—too many to mention here (and they change as newer drugs are developed). It is best to ask your doctor or pharmacist, along with reading the information listed with your medicine, to determine what you can and cannot eat if you take certain medicines. Two of the more common interactions with medications are the following:

Green Leafy Vegetables—Although you should eat your greens, sometimes these vegetables can interfere with your body's ability to clot. This is because vegetables are high in vitamin K, which can decrease the ability of some blood-thinning medications to prevent clotting. What researchers are truly warning about are people who eat an exorbitant amount of greens and take blood-thinning drugs such as warfarin. So check with your doctor if you are concerned about interactions with your greens.

Grapefruit—Most people who take cholesterol-lowering drugs are warned not to eat grapefruit or drink grapefruit drinks, and there are numerous other prescription and over-the-counter medicines that react with this fruit, too. There are many ways in which the fruit interacts with the drugs; for example, it often increases the absorption of drugs, such as certain cholesterol-lowering statins; can cause you to metabolize a drug differently; or, because grapefruit contains compounds called furanocoumarins, it may cause your body to alter the characteristic of a medicine. So if you love grapefruit, ask your doctor if there is a way you can still enjoy this fruit without the side effects. (*Note:* There are also fruits called tangelos, which are a grapefruit and tangerine hybrid. Most research indicates that although the tangelos have genetic material from the grapefruit, there are few, if any, furanocoumarins in the fruit. Even so, it may be best to contact your doctor to discuss whether you can eat tangelos, based on the amount you eat, and the amount of statins you take.)

Do some drugs deplete certain nutrients?

Yes, there are many drugs that can affect the nutrients you eat. For example, if you take over-the-counter or prescription antacids, these can interfere with the absorption of many minerals; thus, many doctors suggest taking an antacid about an hour after eating. Another are the tetracycline antibiotics—they can lessen your ability to absorb vitamin C. Thus, if you are taking any type of drug, ask your doctor or pharmacist if there are any nutrients that are affected—and the best way to make sure you still are getting enough of that nutrient (or nutrients) while you are taking the medication.

How do laxatives affect your body's nutrient balance?

Laxatives—not including natural laxatives such as prune juice, but specifically the powder, pill, or liquid forms—are often used to start the bowels moving. People use laxatives most often if they are constipated, or for such procedures as a colonoscopy. Contrary to

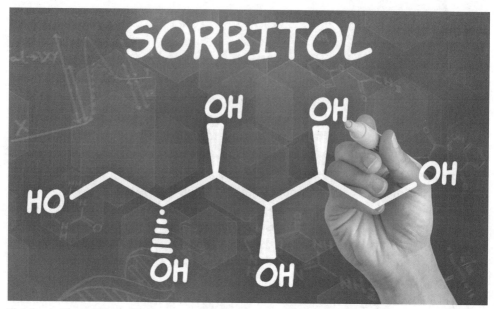

The chemical formula for sorbitol, a sugar substitute often used in candies, baked treats, and fruit juices. Eating or drinking too much sorbitol, however, can lead to diarrhea and gastrointestinal distress.

what most people think, laxatives work by causing water to be sucked into the large intestines in order to bulk up the waste (stool); this also stimulates the muscles of the large intestines, allowing the digestive tract at this point to contract and eliminate the waste. Because most of the effects are in the large intestine, a laxative usually does not cause a nutritional imbalance—the food waste has already gone through the small intestines where nutrients and calories are absorbed.

There can be a major problem with nutrition if someone abuses laxatives, taking too many, not following directions (on the bottle or your physician's recommendations), or abusing the reason for taking laxatives. For example, they can be harmful to people who believe they can use laxatives to lose weight. This can slow down a person's metabolism, prevent the absorption of certain nutrients, and thus cause a deficiency; it can also cause dehydration and an electrolyte (important minerals in the body) imbalance, and even make a person dependent on laxatives. If fact, using laxatives to lose weight is a fallacy: what you are actually doing is losing water weight, which will return once you hydrate.

What "sugar" can act like a laxative?

There is a common sugar substitute, called sorbitol, that can act like a laxative, a sugar alcohol in the same league as maltitol and lactitol. It is often found in baked goods, "sugar-free" candies, chewing gum, some fruit juices, and is the sugar substitute many people find in tiny packets on tables at the local café. But sobitol can be hard on the intestines—especially if you ingest large amounts of it—and can lead to gastrointestinal bloating, cramping, and sometimes diarrhea.

NUTRITION THROUGHOUT THE CENTURIES

THE FOOD CHAIN

What is a food chain?

A food chain follows how animals eat and find their food—especially those animals that are interconnected. For example, a simple food chain in the oceans includes a small fish eating smaller plankton; the small fish is eaten by a larger fish; and so on. On land, an example of a food chain would be a grasshopper eating grass, then being eaten by a frog; the frog is eaten by a snake, and the snake eaten by a hawk.

What are the various functions of species in an ecosystem's food chain?

In an ecosystem's food chain, species are often divided into several groups. The most common roles are: Producers—which are considered mostly plants—take energy (food) from one source and convert it to another so others in the ecosystem can use it. The consumers in an ecosystem are those organisms that use what the producers produce—in other words, mostly animals. They are further divided into primary consumers, in which an organism relies heavily on the producers, and secondary consumers, or organisms that use other consumers (and sometimes producers) for their source of energy. (Some research breaks down consumers further, into tertiary and quaternary consumers; still other studies divide consumers into upper and lower, or basal.) To translate into natural terms, for example, a lion (primary consumer) eats a zebra (secondary consumer) that eats grasses (producers). Humans, as one can imagine, are primary consumers—which is a good thing for us.

What is a food web?

A food web is much broader than a food chain (see above) and represents several food chains together; in other words, it is how plants and animals are interconnected (often called ecological interactions), usually in a certain region or ecosystem. It was first detailed by English zoologist and animal ecologist Charles S. Elton (1900–1991; also called by some the "father of animal ecology") around the late 1920s to describe the feeding and food relationships between all species—plants and animals—on Bear Island, just off the north coast of Norway in the Arctic.

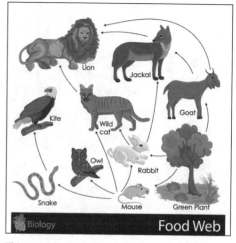

This example of a food web illustrates how plants and animals are all connected and dependent upon one another.

What are some of the general eating characteristics of animals called omnivores, herbivores, and carnivores?

Animals' eating habits fall into three general categories: omnivores (those that eat meat and vegetation), herbivores (those that eat only vegetation; *Note:* this term is also used in a different way, to describe grazing animals, such as cattle and sheep), and carnivores (those that eat only the meat or flesh of other animals). The following list describes some of the general characteristics—based on anatomy and physiology, or their adaptations for eating—of these divisions:

Carnivores—These animals swallow their food whole, and do not usually chew (their teeth are not made for chewing, but tearing and shredding, with sharp, well-developed canine teeth); they have no digestive enzymes; their stomach volumes are usually 60 to 70 percent of their digestive tract; their small intestines are only about three to six times their body length; and their colon is short.

Herbivores—These animals chew extensively and out of necessity in order to help break down vegetation, and they have wide molars for grinding (and no canine teeth); they have carbohydrate-digesting enzymes; their stomach volume takes up less than 30 percent of their digestive tract; their small intestines are around ten to twelve times their body length; and their colon is very long.

Omnivores—These animals swallow their foods whole, or just simply crush their foods; their saliva usually has no digestive enzymes; their stomach volume is about 60 to 70 percent of their digestive tract; their small intestines are about four to six times the length of their body; and their colon is short.

Are there other divisions based on what animals eat?

There are, of course, animals that cross over into the three categories of omnivore, herbivore, and carnivore. For example, a carnivore may also eat some vegetation at times, or may eat another animal that consumes vegetation. In addition, there are other subcategories, such as frugivorous animals, or those that primarily eat fruit; or carnivores

Why is it difficult to classify humans in terms of their anatomy and physiology?

Humans are almost an enigma in the animal world when it comes to what we eat, and based on our anatomy and physiological characteristics, it is difficult to classify humans as herbivore, carnivore, or omnivore (although *omnivore* is the term most often used). There are several reasons for this confusion. For example, in terms of teeth, humans have broad wide molars for grinding, a long and complex colon, carbohydrate-digesting enzymes, and very long small intestines (around ten to eleven times their body length)—all similar to the herbivores. But humans also have differences in their teeth when compared to herbivores—humans have canines (short and blunted), more flattened molar teeth—and have a simple stomach (in comparison to many herbivores that have many stomach chambers). Thus, overall, when you use these general comparisons, humans resemble herbivores more than carnivores and omnivores.

that are often classified as piscivores, or animals that eat mostly fish. And although modern humans are often thought of as "omnivores" (eating meat and plant material), this is too much of a generalization. In fact, depending on culture, custom, and training, humans are very difficult to classify!

What are some representative omnivores, carnivores, and herbivores?

There are many animals in this world, and in general, many of them are categorized as omnivores, carnivores, or herbivores. The following chart lists some of those animals:

Animals and Their Diet Types

Animal	Type
Cattle	Herbivore
Cow	Herbivore
Camel	Herbivore
Elephant	Herbivore
Horse	Herbivore; although some list horses as omnivores
Tiger	Carnivore
Cat, domestic	Carnivore
American Alligator	Carnivore
Lion	Carnivore
Dolphin	Carnivore—actually a piscivore
Sea Lion	Carnivore—actually a piscivore
Penguin	Carnivore—actually a piscivore
Bear	Omnivore; not including polar or giant panda bears
Cockroach	Omnivore

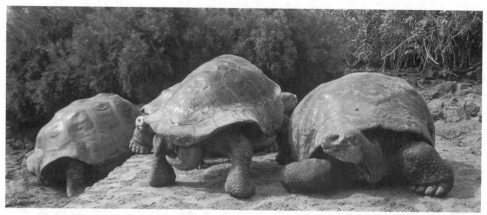

These Galapagos tortoises can live to be over two hundred years old, but it's not because they are vegetarians. Genetics are why some species live longer than others.

Animals and Their Diet Types

Animal	Type
Chipmunk	Omnivore
Mice	Omnivore
Human	Omnivore, but this is highly debated (see above); and they can choose to be an herbivore (vegetarian)

Which animals live longer, carnivores, herbivores, or omnivores?

This is a highly debated subject, as are most ideas about nutrition! If you take the average lifespan of some animals, it seems as if the herbivores live longer than the carnivores. For example, the camel and elephant live for around 50 and 70 years, respectively (some herbivores can even live to be 200 years old, such as the Galápagos Land Tortoise); whereas the tiger and lion live an average of 22 and 35 years, respectively. Humans, often said to be omnivores, can live up to 122 years—but other omnivores, such as coyotes and mountain gorillas, live only 14 and 35 years, respectively. Thus, in nature, there is no real proof that animals that eat a plant-based diet live longer. In fact, there are often other factors that are not taken into account when discussing longevity of animals, such as where the creatures live, their "genetics," an increase or decrease of other animals in their territory, and even the climate conditions in which they live.

EARLY HUMAN ANCESTORS AND FOOD

Why has it been so difficult to determine what ancient humans ate?

Humans (like most living creatures) were definitely built to eat certain foods as they traveled (and continue to travel) along their evolutionary path. But what ancient humans ate over time is often a highly debated mystery. Overall, researchers are trying to piece together different ancient human diets, taking into account many factors. For example, what was the climate like, and thus what were the available foods; what were the hunting abilities of certain human groups; how did they process, cook, or use their foods; and even what were the differences in ancient humans' teeth and what does that tell us about their eating habits?

What recent study examines a two-million-year-old hominin diet?

A recent University of Arkansas study of two-million-year-old hominin remains has revealed what some ancient peoples ate, especially what plants. The fossil bone remains of an elderly female and young male had their skulls intact, with teeth; the pristine condition of the skulls indicated that the two hominins probably were rapidly buried, thus the decay was less. The researchers examined the teeth, discovering plaque and tartar buildup, much like what dentists tell us today to eliminate with flossing and brushing. In this case, it was a boon for the researchers. They found phytoliths, or bodies of silica from plants, in the tartar and plaque; they also found evidence of bark, leaves, sedges, grasses, palm, and fruits eaten by the hominins. Not all hominin remains have evidence of the same foods; but researchers do know that these two individuals enjoyed a plant-based bounty from a nearby forest.

What is the difference between hominid and hominin?

There is a difference between these two definitions when discussing human evolution: The hominids are a group of all modern and extinct Great Apes—that includes modern humans, chimpanzees, gorillas, and orangutans (and their immediate ancestors), whereas hominin is the group that includes modern humans, extinct humans species, and all of our immediate ancestors, such as the members of the genera *Homo*, *Australopithecus*, *Paranthropus*, and *Ardipithecus*.

Who was the "Nutcracker Man"?

In 2014, researchers at Oxford University in England concluded that our ancient human ancestors from East Africa ate quite a different diet than today's humans—mostly tiger nuts (also called grass bulbs), with the odd grasshopper and worm thrown in at times. The discovery was based on the skull of a *Paranthropus boisei*—an individual they nicknamed "Nutcracker Man" because of his big flat molar teeth and powerful jaws—found at Olduvai Gorge, Tanzania. The researchers determined that hominins who lived in East Africa between 2.4 and 1.4 million years ago survived mostly on tiger nuts—bulbs that are grown and even eaten today in various parts of the world. The bulbs are high in vitamins, minerals, and fatty acids—and were nutritionally perfect for the development of the hominin brain.

Scientific reference to humans in evolution once used the word "hominid" to define the lineage leading to modern humans; today, scientists now use the term *hominin* in the same way. As seen above, the term *hominid* now has a broader meaning, referring to the all the Great Apes and their ancestors. These changes have been made because of the way humans, chimpanzees, gorillas, and orangutans are now classified on the primate evolutionary tree.

Why was the discovery of fire so important to humans?

In terms of human evolution, one of the most important discoveries was fire. Not only did fire protect humans from predators and keep them relatively warm, it also allowed our ancestors to cook their food. Before fire, our hominin ancestors were much like other animals, eating and chewing (and chewing) tough plant foods long enough to make the food small enough to swallow and digest.

Researchers believe the human use of fire began around 1.8 million years ago—a time that also coincides with an increase in human brain size. Because food was cooked, it was much easier for humans to chew and digest—after all, ancient humans had small teeth, weak jaws, and their digestive systems couldn't handle certain foods (such as raw meat and the cellulose fiber in plants) if it was not for cooking. And because it took less time to chew foods, some researchers believe the "extra" time was used for hunting, building, and exploring—which helped the human race to evolve.

What plants did early humans eat?

It appears that our early human ancestors did not have a very varied diet. In 2013, researchers compared various early human teeth from Africa to determine our ancestral diets. Since plants are divided into three categories—C3 for trees, shrubs, and herbs, and C4/CAM plants for grasses, sedges, and succulents—the researchers essentially looked at what was "stuck in the teeth" of the ancient humans. Using carbon-13 dating techniques on the tooth enamel, they were able to determine the type of foods the early humans ate (C4/CAM plants have higher amounts of carbon-13 in their tissues).

They discovered that before 3.5 million years ago, early humans ate mostly leaves and fruits from trees, shrubs, and herbs (C3 plants); after 3.5 million years, early humans—such as *Australopithecus afarensis*

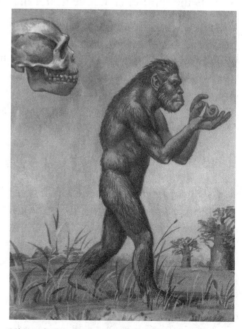

Like early *Homo sapiens* this relative of humans, *Australopithecus*, ate a lot of roughage. The jaw bone and muscles and teeth were well developed to eat uncooked meats and fibrous plants.

and *Kenyanthropus platyops*—began to eat grasses, sedges, and succulents (C4/CAM plants). And, although still debated, these early ancestors may also have eaten the animals that ate the C4/CAM plants. (In fact, a study from 2010 showed evidence that early humans began using tools around 3.4 million years ago, and also began eating meat.)

What are some differences between primates' and humans' digestive tracts?

Some of the more recent research into what primates eat—and have eaten in the past—has led into the world of the gastrointestinal tract. Even though humans' and other primates' gastrointestinal systems seem to be similar when developing, once in adulthood, humans develop a shorter large intestine tract than those of other living primates, relative to the overall size of our gut. For example, most human colons are around 25 percent of the whole digestive tract versus around 50 percent of the whole in primates such as chimpanzees and gorillas. (Even so, there are still some mysteries of the human colon, including why certain people, depending on their country or culture, can differ in the length of their colon, with some saying it may be genetic.)

Our "shorter" colons don't break down or absorb plant material as well as our primate cousins' colons. Because of their mostly plant-based diets, nonhuman primates need a longer colon for the fermentation of the plant foods. In fact, the human colon absorbs few nutrients, but is used mostly for water absorption that helps to recycle fluids we use up in digestion. In addition, the human colon supplies only about 10 percent of the energy our body needs; in contrast, nonhuman primates' larger colons provide a great deal of energy—for example, about 65 percent of apes' energy for their body comes from the processes that take place in their colon. In fact, if an ape's colon is removed, it will not survive; whereas, if a human has his or her colon removed, he or she can still live just fine.

Is there a connection between a primate's brain size and energy demand?

Research has shown that nonhuman primates cannot meet the energy demand of a human-sized brain. For example, a human brain uses more than 25 percent of the calories (which give us energy) a person ingests; an ape brain uses only about 8 percent of the food calories ingested. Thus, it can be said that a nonhuman primate's (such as an ape's) smaller brain size is a good match with its long colon, low-nutrient diet of vegetation, and slower metabolic rate, and may suggest how our human physiology supports our larger brain size.

Why is the human colon shorter than other primates' colons?

There are probably many evolutionary reasons why humans have a shorter colon than other primates, and the topic is highly debated. Some researchers believe our colon became shorter because of our eating habits over the past hundreds of thousands of years: eating less vegetation and more meat meant the colon didn't have to be of a length that would process and absorb nutrients from plant material or meat. Still other researchers believe that early humans needed more energy to develop a larger brain, not to serve the digestive tract, and thus, more energy was "rerouted" to the growing brain. But in a way, humans make up for the lack of a long colon that nonhuman primates have to absorb nutrients: We have a much longer small intestine tract than nonhuman primates that allows us to absorb nutrients.

Why are there so many debates about ancient humans' eating habits?

Most studies of early human eating habits are highly debated because one discovery leads to ten more questions! For example, Stone Age humans (the Paleolithic age, or the time between when stone tools were used and the first stages of agriculture took hold) are often studied in terms of eating habits. Some researchers say these early humans ate only fruits, vegetables, and nuts, with the occasional piece of meat; still others believe early human ancestors were great hunters who dragged back plenty of meat and ate a few berries along the way. There are even debates as to the types of meat and how the hominins found the meat. For example, some say the meat was in the form of the occasional insect or small animal, such as a lizard; others say early humans were scavengers that lived off other animals' killings.

Many of these highly debated topics come down to several factors: for instance, what is the time period studied (is the study based on ancient humans a thousand, ten thousand, or a million or more years ago); the interpretation of very few ancient human fossil remains; and even how the climate has changed, forcing ancient humans to change their eating habits over the past million or so years.

What do scientists know about the diets of the Neanderthals?

Neanderthal—a human species (possibly a subspecies of *Homo sapiens*) that lived around 150,000 to 30,000 B.C.E.—was thought to be an animal-hunting, cold-climate group that lived in a wide area, from Germany and France, east to Russia and the Middle East, and down to North Africa. They had even larger brains than today's humans, and were thought to ritually bury their dead and even take care of their crippled and elderly. Their diet was thought to include a great deal of meat, especially big game such as horses and reindeer. For some reason (and some scientists believe it had to do with a too-focused diet), the Neanderthal eventually died out as a species.

Whether the species disappeared because of diet, no one really knows—and part of the problem is that the true Neanderthal diet is highly debated. One recent study looked at the teeth of several Neanderthal remains, examining the tooth tartar, and concluded that the ancient humans ate not only meat, but also cooked vegetables (the researchers found evidence of grass seeds and legumes), and even ingested medicinal plants such as yarrow and chamomile. But not everyone agrees: Some researchers suggest that the plant material in the teeth exists because Neanderthals ate the stomach contents of their kill—especially herbivores such as deer and bison. They further cite some modern peoples—such as the Inuit who also live in a colder climate—who eat the stomach contents of animals they kill because it's a good source of vitamin C and other nutrients.

LATER FOODS AND NUTRITION

How did agriculture bring a different type of nutrition to humans?

Although it did not happen "overnight," ancient human groups eventually changed some of their eating habits after the development of agriculture. The rise of agriculture is often cited as one of the major reasons for the establishment of settlements and civilizations.

Some researchers believe that many ancient human groups changed their diets as agriculture became more prevalent. For example, some hominins were hunters of wild game or scavenged kills from other animals. With the introduction of grains—and especially of cereal agriculture—the amount of animal protein in the diet diminished. (One study stated that this decrease in animal protein for several ancient human groups also meant a decrease in their body sizes.)

Why was scurvy so prevalent at one time?

Scurvy is caused by a dietary deficiency of vitamin C (and B), and was a major problem for maritime explorers—especially those on long voyages of discovery. For example, Vasco da Gama lost two-thirds of his crew to scurvy as he made his way to India in 1499; Magellan, in 1520, lost more than 80 percent of his crew while crossing the Pacific Ocean. The disease was horrific: Physically, it caused a blackening of the skin, ulcers, res-

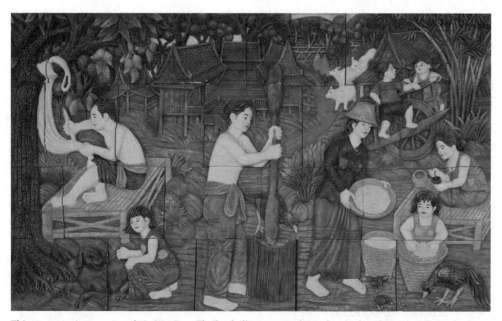

This stone carving on a temple in Wat Dan, Thailand, illustrates traditional agricultural practices dating back centuries. The development of agriculture put an end to the nomadic life and led to the establishment of permanent settlements.

How did humans develop a taste for cereal grains?

Grains—either "new" or ancient—come in a wide assortment, with many high in protein, minerals, and vitamins. But in 1999, a study about the original human diet was conducted at Colorado State University that made everyone think twice about grains and human health: The head author was Dr. Loren Cordain, who published the paper called "Cereal Grains: Humanity's Double-Edged Sword" in *World Review of Nutrition and Dietetics*. Cordain believed that humans' genetic constitution has remained virtually unaltered over in the past 40,000 years, and that their early diet did not include grains. In particular, humans would hunt, gather, or fish for their meals, as seen with some of the more ancient cultures (such as the Inuit above the Arctic Circle, whose meals consist of what they fish). It was only in the past 10,000 years that humans embraced grains—when civilization spread and agriculture was born. The "double-edged sword" is so labeled because civilization grew with agriculture, and eating cereal grains became somewhat of a necessity to keep those civilizations growing and nutritiously fed.

piration problems, stiffness in the limbs, teeth to fall out, and rotting of gum tissue. Sensorial and psychological problems included difficulty tasting, smelling, and hearing, along with hopelessness. By the early eighteenth century, they still did not know what caused scurvy, and it was often mistaken for other diseases such as leprosy, syphilis, and even insanity. By then, too, scurvy killed more British sailors than any enemy action. Today, we know that scurvy on those ships was most often caused by a deficiency of mainly vitamins C and B, and was sometimes compounded by an overdose of vitamin A from eating such meats as seals' livers.

When did they finally discover the reasons for scurvy?

It was not until the late eighteenth century that scurvy was not as much of a problem on maritime vessels. Even as early as the mid-1700s, some scientists, such as British scientist James Lind (1716–1794), claimed that citrus fruits would be beneficial to stave off scurvy, but carrying and keeping fresh such fruits as lemons and oranges was not practical or possible for most long voyages. Some captains preferred to try other means; for example, Captain James Cook (1728–1779) insisted that his crew eat malt and sauerkraut—along with vinegar, mustard, and wheat—on his voyage around New Zealand and Australia. Not only that, he stopped frequently for fresh foods and kept everything on his ship as clean as possible. Although several of his crew caught scurvy, records claim he lost none of his men. (For more about scurvy, see the chapter "The Basics of Nutrition: Micronutrients.")

How is scurvy treated today?

Scurvy—caused mainly by a dietary deficiency of vitamin C—is relatively uncommon today. It can occur in people who are malnourished; and there are certain conditions that require more vitamin C so the person won't become deficient, such as pregnant or breastfeeding women, and sometimes infants who are breastfed.

Scurvy is usually treated by ingesting foods rich in the vitamin, such as orange juice. The symptoms improve within two days, and resolve within a week—but such treatment should be done under medical supervision.

Who was William Stark?

English physician William Stark (c. 1741– 1770) conducted one of the earliest detailed studies of what happens to a body when certain foods are consumed, but his experiments also caused his early death. Stark set out to understand how a variety of factors affect the human body—especially how a varied diet could be as healthy as a simpler strict diet— choosing to conduct all of the experiments on himself. He ate a variety of foods in several combinations. For exam-

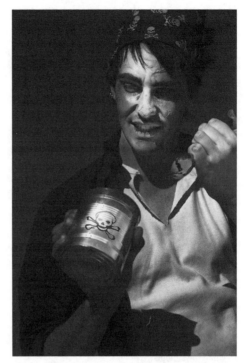

Arrrgh! Scurvy was a common ailment among sailors before the nineteenth century because they didn't have healthy diets at sea, where it was difficult to get fresh fruits and vegetables.

ple, in his first experiment, he ate bread and water, with a bit of sugar, for thirty-one days, recording his feelings, weight, how much the food weighed, the weather conditions, and even his daily bowel habits. The first diet result left him listless; in the experiments that followed, he began to gradually add certain foods, such as olive oil, veal, milk, figs, fat, and so on. But twenty-three experiments later, Stark eventually sickened on his diet and he died at the age of 29 from scurvy. His specially picked diet included little, if any, fruits and vegetables—and apparently, he had not heard of the discovery by his contemporary James Lind (1716–1794) of how a vitamin C deficiency would cause scurvy. It took almost twenty years before anyone published his meticulously recorded studies—especially what occurs in all stages when contracting scurvy.

Who was Carl von Voit?

German physiologist and dietician Carl von Voit (1831–1908) is considered by many scientists to be the father of modern dietetics. In 1865, he showed that the pathways by which food is converted were complex—noting that food is not simply burned up in the body to produce energy as previously thought, but that there are many intermediate reactions that take place instead.

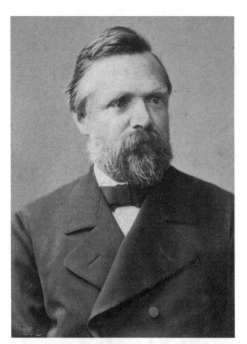

The father of modern dietetics, Carl von Voit, was a German physiologist.

Who was Henry Clapp Sherman?

In 1875, American biochemist Henry Clapp Sherman (1875–1955) was the first person to show that the ratio of calcium to phosphate in a person's diet is as important at the total amount of either mineral. He also took his investigations into the world of vitamins, especially the amounts needed in the diets of various animals.

Who was Frederick G. Hopkins?

English biochemist Frederick G. Hopkins (1861–1947; he is often called the "father of British biochemistry") was one of the first scientists to suggest that food contains ingredients essential to life—and he did not mean proteins, fats, minerals, or carbohydrates. Hopkins's publications were the first to explain the concept of vitamins, although he called these trace substances "accessory food factors"; the name "vitamin" was suggested by Casimir Funk, and finally introduced in 1912. Hopkins went on to discover a method for isolating tryptophan and understanding its structure, among other scientific discoveries; and along with Dutch bacteriologist Christiaan Eijkman (1858–1930; Eijkman originally suggested that there was an association between beriberi and the consumption of polished rice), Hopkins won the Nobel Prize in 1929.

Who was Kazimierz (or Casimir) Funk?

Kazimierz (anglicized to Casimir) Funk (1884–1967)—considered by many to be the "father of vitamin therapy"—was a Polish biochemist who presented the theory that foods contained essential chemical substances that the body needed to sustain life. Around 1911, he presented a work titled "Experiments on the Causation of Beri-Beri," based on his studies of people who ate polished rice (the pericarpium removed) and contracted the disease, and people who ate the rice polishings and did not contract the disease. (Christiaan Eijkman had already discovered the association of beriberi and polished rice in animals; Funk applied this knowledge to humans.) It was earlier thought that the endosperm of rice contained a poison, while the cortical layers, or the polishings, contained the antidote. Funk proved this wrong, concluding that there was no toxin involved (or as others thought, perhaps an infection), but the beriberi was caused by a deficiency of an essential ingredient missing in the polished rice.

Funk eventually found something referred to as a fraction B—a nitrogen-containing compound that curtailed the beriberi. He suggested that very small "trace elements" of fraction B should be called "vitamine" (a contraction of "vital amines"), with *vita* meaning "life," and *amine* meaning, loosely, a "nitrogen-containing compound essential for life." He named this first vitamin "B_1"—what we call thiamine—and presented his findings in 1912 in his paper "The Vitamines." Because the amine group is not present in all "vitamines," the word eventually became "vitamin." (We know today that a severe deficiency of the vitamin thiamine causes beriberi.)

Who was Christiaan Eijkman?

Dutch bacteriologist Christiaan Eijkman (1858–1930) was the first to discover the real cause of beriberi through studies in the tropical regions. He found that this disease, which leads to anemia, was because of a deficiency of some vital substance in rice, the major food of the region: The pericarpium (the so-called "silver skin," or covering) of the rice was removed (called polishing). This discovery eventually led to Casimir Funk's study of beriberi, polished rice, and vitamins. (For their studies on what would eventually be called vitamins, Eijkman and Frederick Hopkins [1861–1947] won the Nobel Prize in 1929.) Eijkman's studies did not stop there—he also conducted a well-known fermentation test (to see if water has been contaminated by *coli bacilli*); he researched the rate of mortality of bacteria by external factors and made a multitude of other discoveries.

Who was Albert Szent-Györgyi?

Albert Szent-Györgyi (1893–1986) was a Hungarian-American biochemist and physiologist who was, in 1928, the first person to successfully obtain a pure vitamin from a food. In his case, it was vitamin C (also called ascorbic acid) from citrus fruits. It was discovered independently of Charles Glen King (1896–1988), who claimed the same finding two weeks before.

NUTRITION IN RELIGION AND CULTURE

What is fasting?

In general, fasting most often means eliminating solid foods for a certain amount of time, and drinking only fluids such as water, tea, or juice. Or it may mean eating only raw foods for a period of time, or even restricting ingested foods to every other day. Most people usually fast for health reasons (under a doctor's care) for religious reasons or to lose weight (which most often does not work in the long term). In general, a healthy person fasting for a day or two probably won't hurt, as long as they take in enough fluids. In addition, although there has been a great deal of research examining the possibility that fasting now-and-then extends a person's lifespan, there is no conclusive evidence that this is true.

Unless under a physician's care, why can long-term fasting be unhealthy?

Although some people need to fast for various health reasons while under a doctor's care, or partake in short-term fasts (usually for religious reasons), the "trendy" idea that fasting will solve all your health problems is a myth. In fact, if you fast and even drink plenty of water, it can be harmful to your health (unless you are under a physician's care during the fast). In particular, fasting—especially for extended periods—can lower your blood pressure, cause fatigue, dizziness, and even dehydration and gallstones; fasting for even longer periods can lead to heart failure. The reason is obvious: Fasting means your body does not get enough of a variety of vitamins, minerals, and other necessary nutrients to stay healthy. In addition, for people who use fasting diets to detoxify, there really is no

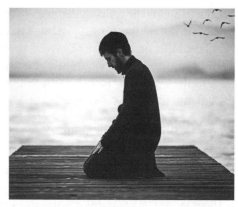

Faithful Muslims fast during the holy month of Ramadan. Fasting not only serves a religious tradition; in moderation, it can, many believe, help one's health.

evidence that such fasting will cleanse your body of impurities and toxins. In fact, those tasks are what our bodies' organs are built for—especially the removal of toxins by our liver, kidneys, colon, and even our skin (by sweating).

Can you lose weight by fasting?

No, most experts agree that if you are trying to lose weight, fasting is not a long-term solution. Most people who lose weight from fasting are merely losing water weight; in addition, your body is forced to cut into your energy stores to get the fuel it needs to accomplish your body's main tasks—so it only seems as if you're losing weight. But after the fasting is done, a person will usually go back to his or her usual diet—and rapidly gain back even more weight. As most nutritionists suggest, eating a well-balanced diet (and especially downsizing your proportions) and exercise are the best for your body—and help keep the weight down.

How are some religions connected to fasting?

For some religions, fasting was (and is) a way of cleansing the body for spiritual purposes. The following list describes a few of the religions that use fasting for religious purposes, and some general details of the fasting:

Early Christians—Early Christians believed in fasting, and Wednesday and Fridays were considered to be days of fasting (no water or food until mid-afternoon). By the Middle Ages, there was even more of an emphasis on fasting; the church ruled that on certain days, and in specific seasons and holidays (such as Lent), the faithful, especially monks and nuns, would observe fasting, sometimes for up to 24 hours. It should be noted that during longer fasting periods, such as the 40 days of Lent, fasting meant eating less food, as the Church realized such a long fast was not truly possible without health consequences. Instead, certain foods like fish, butter, meat, and eggs are forbidden on fast days.

How long can a person go without eating?

For most healthy, average adult humans, if they don't eat and are properly hydrated (drink enough water), they can last for about 30 to 40 days. There have been several historic cases of starvation—usually people starving themselves for political or religious reasons—in which the person has lived much longer; for example, in one case, a gentleman starving himself for political reasons lived for 61 days. It is thought that the result of extreme starvation is usually a heart attack or organ failure; most research indicates that death usually occurs not long after the body reaches a body mass index, or BMI, of approximately 12 or lower—if nourishment is not given. Of course, this number depends on other factors involved, including the health, sex, genetics, and size of the starving person. (For more information about Body Mass Index, or BMI, see "Nutrition and You.")

Later Christians—After the Reformation, other religions would have a much more "relaxed" attitude about fasting. The list is long: For example, Methodists have no formal rules for fasting, Quakers advocate private fasting in times of confusion or trouble, and members of the Church of Jesus Christ of Latter-Day Saints fast on the first Sunday of each month by omitting two of their three meals.

Buddhists—For most Buddhists, fasting means avoiding food during times of intense meditation.

Hindus—There is a long list of various Hindu groups who believe in fasting, but how much and when is often based on local or personal customs. Some Hindus fast certain days of the month; some have certain days of the week set aside for fasting based on personal choice or favorite deity (for example, those who follow Shiva usually fast on Mondays); and some people fast depending on the region in which they live (for example, in northern India, Tuesdays are for Lord Hanuman, and those who follow this custom are allowed to eat only fruit and drink only milk from sunrise to sunset).

Muslims—One of the more well-known fasting times for Islamic Muslims is Ramadan, a holy month (the days based on crescent moon to crescent moon) in which followers fast from dawn until sunset. They cannot eat or drink during this time, believing that they will be closer to God by abandoning bodily pleasures such as food and drink. Their fasting not only includes food and drink, but abstaining from any falsehood in speech and action—a way of developing, they hope, good behavior.

Jews—The Jewish people traditionally fast for six days out of the year, and it means completely abstaining from food and drink, including water. For example, during Yom Kippur, fasting is a means of repenting, and only those who are sick or ailing are exempt from the fasting. Another day of fasting is Tisha B'Av, in remembrance of several events (including when Babylonians destroyed the first Holy Temple in Jerusalem

2,500 years ago; and when the Romans destroyed the second Holy Temple in Jerusalem 2,000 years ago). Both of these events mean fasting from sunset to the following day's dusk.

Who were some of the first "dieticians" known?

No one really knows who the first "dietician" was—or someone who recommended certain foods for health. Some of the earliest known records of "dietary rules for health" come from the Chinese: Emperors employed Imperial dieticians as far back as the fourth century B.C.E. But perhaps some of the first dieticians were ancient humans, especially those who figured out that, for instance, one wild berry was not as good as another (and probably poisonous)!

What foods and drinks did the early Egyptians consume?

Early Egypt had one of the first cultures to embrace agriculture (thanks to the fertile Nile River basin), along with livestock breeding. Although there were regional differences—and even class differences (the rich ate well; the poor ate simply)—there were some standard foods. When it came to meats, they had plenty, and pig was one of the most common foods, as were cows and sheep, and wild game was also included, such as geese and ducks. Egyptians also ate plenty of cereal grains, such as millet; pulses, such as chickpeas and lentils; and vegetables and herbs, such as leeks, onions, garlic, and lettuces.

What did the ancient Greeks eat?

The ancient Greeks enjoyed foods from their harvests, with cereals constituting about 80 percent of the peoples' diet and total nutritional fuel. This was not because they could not grow fruits, vegetables, or meat, but because of the Greek ideology and from policies put forth by their government. They believed that they were not "barbarians" like those who hunted or picked wild berries and vegetables, but were "civilized" people who farmed as a way to control their own destiny and eating habits. Hunting to them was a sign of poverty, and not for a civilized man; meat was also thought to be eaten only by their soldiers for strength, or as a luxury, or to be used in sacrificial rituals. (Although one meat that was to their liking was fish, mainly because fish and shellfish were standard in Mediterranean cooking and very abundant.) Thus, they cultivated what they believed was "civilized" foods, including wheat bread, wine, olive oil, and some cheeses. But as a result, there was a small amount of protein in their diet, and many researchers believe that this may explain why so many ancient Greeks seemed to have health problems.

How did the ancient Greeks regard "nutrition"?

Probably one of the earliest records of nutrition was from the ancient Greeks. For example, the Greek physician Hippocrates (460–377 B.C.E.) knew the value of the moderate ingesting of foods, and the need to exercise to keep the body healthy. Greek physician and philosopher Galen (130–200; also known as Aelius Galenus or Claudius

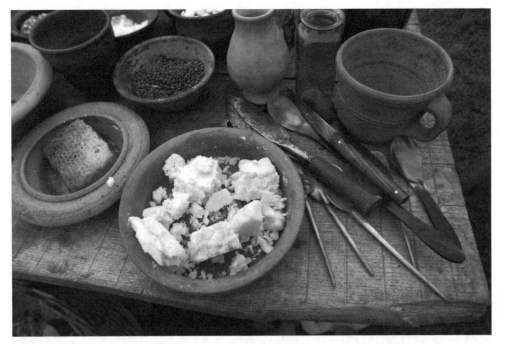

Goat cheese, beans, and a honeycomb are some examples of foods once eaten by the ancient Romans.

Galenus, better known as Galen of Pergamon) believed in Hippocrates' ideas, and added some of his own, including thoughts on the connection between diet and exercise—ideas that lasted for many centuries (both good and bad for his peoples' health).

What did people eat and drink during Roman times?

The Roman Empire lasted for centuries and there were some standard foods prevalent in the culture. For example, the richer Romans usually ate a good variety of vegetables, meats, and fish, while the poorest Romans ate more simple meals. They usually ate three meals a day, with cena (or dinner) being the main meal. Unlike most modern Western cultures, the Romans did not sit at a table to eat, but preferred to sit on couches around a low table—similar to what most of us have seen in movies depicting the Roman Empire—almost lying down to eat. As for foods, bread was a staple of their diet, as was pottage (a thick stew made from corn, millet, or wheat), to which they added spices, salt and pepper, and meats or sauces. They also liked cheese (mainly from goats) and eggs (from various birds), and sweetened things with honey since they did not know about sugar. But overall, their diet consisted mainly of vegetables, which were much easier to obtain than some other foods.

The Romans also drank mostly wine, but it was not wine as we know it today—it was very watered down. They also drank wine containing other ingredients; for example, mulsum was made of honey and wine, whereas calda (consumed only in the winter months) was made of wine, water, and special spices.

Has the ingestion of lead affected people for centuries?

Yes, the presence of lead has been known for centuries, and it's a metal that has taken its toll on countless cultures over the years—far too many to mention here. Historically, there are many reasons that people have ingested lead, including contaminated foods and/or drinking vessels containing lead, both leading to lead poisoning, or saturnism. Egyptian pharaohs used lead to glaze pottery; and the ancient Chinese used lead to make coins—both of which exposed people to lead. It was in certain recipes around the Middle Ages, as cooks put lead acetate ("sugar of lead") into foods and wine to make them sweeter. Lead poisoning has also been associated with artists, especially from the Renaissance to the nineteenth century, and is called painter's madness because of the exposure to lead in the paints the artists used. Thus, it is often theorized that famous painters with mental disorders, such as Michelangelo, Goya, van Gogh, Renoir, and others, may have been poisoned by lead.

One culture in particular was plagued by the major consumption, inadvertently, of lead: the Roman Empire. There were many reasons for this: For example, lead was part of the clay used to make Roman pottery, and when a person ate a meal off a contaminated plate or dish, he or she would also ingest the lead. The Romans even used a good amount of lead in their water pipes, and in cosmetics and coins. But the real problem came with their wine: winemakers in the Roman Empire would use nothing but the best, and to them, lead pots or lead-lined copper kettles were the best for boiling crushed grapes. This lead consumption is often noted as yet another reason for the fall of the Roman Empire, not to mention the reason why Roman Emperor Julius Caesar, who thoroughly enjoyed wine and women, fathered only one child (and his successor Caesar Augustus was sterile).

What did the ancient Roman soldiers eat?

In many movies, the ancient Roman soldiers—including the ubiquitous gladiators—are shown as heavyset and stout, and there's a good reason for this portrayal: their diet. The Romans coveted their bread and considered it a noble food (it is one of the Roman symbols). And although the general population ate some meat (but mostly vegetables), the soldiers were given a vegetarian diet, with wheat bread, along with olives, onions, figs, and oil. The reason for bulking up the soldiers had to do with the Roman way of fighting: Roman soldiers did not run into a battle, but would stay still and withstand an enemy attack. Just before battle, too, other foods were fed to the soldiers—especially garlic, which they believed would build up their physical strength (and recent studies show that they were right—garlic is one of the more healthy herbs). Some historians suggest that this somewhat inadequate diet of the Roman soldiers may have determined history—and may have been another reason for the fall of the Roman Empire.

What did people eat during Medieval times?

Historians divide the Medieval times into the High Medieval Ages and Low Medieval Ages. After the fall of the Roman Empire, the world that once was ruled by the Romans still carried on some of their food traditions. Christianity was the most influenced, with bread, wine, and oil readily in the diet, with churches and monasteries planting wheat fields and vineyards; the "barbarians," as the Romans thought of people other than themselves, never really changed their eating habits, either, and still hunted, raised animals, fished, and ate fruits, grains, and vegetables—and thus ate a good cross-section of animal protein (meat, poultry, fish, eggs, dairy), cereal grains (barley, millet, einkorn, etc.), and pulses (peas and chickpeas). In fact, many historians believe that during the High Medieval times, the people were relatively healthy, with little evidence of nutritional imbalances.

The Low Medieval Ages was a different story. An increase in population caused a higher demand on foodstuff, and in order to keep everyone fed, agriculture increase. Growing cereals was a reliable way of feeding more people; and as they ate more grains, the people ate less meat (and most of the meat they did eat came from small, thin creatures), fruits, and vegetables. Politics also came between the people and foods: There was a rise in deforestation because of the increased need for growing grains (for the "peasantry") and pasturing animals, as meat became the staple of the rich. This diet also meant that not only was there a monetary class system, but also a food-based class system, with the common people, especially in rural areas, suffering the most from malnutrition.

Do some cultures eat insects?

Yes, some cultures eat insects, and, face it, many of us have inadvertently eaten an insect or two in our lives. For Western cultures, eating insects is not a standard practice, which changed probably because when people started to grow crops and livestock, insects became "the enemy." But there are other cultures that actively seek out some insects to eat, mainly for the protein (for example, hamburger is about 18 percent protein and 18 percent fat, while a cooked grasshopper is 60 percent protein and 6 percent fat); and, as some say, because the creatures taste good.

And it's nothing new—insects have been eaten by ancient cultures throughout the centuries. For example, the Greeks and Romans dined on insects; beetle larvae fattened on flour and wine were enjoyed by Roman aristocrats, and Greek philosopher and scientist Aristotle noted that when a cicada is in its nymph phase, it is the most tasty. And

225

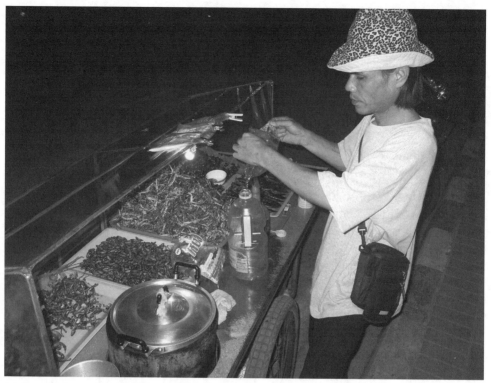

A vendor in Pattaya, Thailand, sells deep insects—a great source of protein and very little fat.

in more modern times, winged termites are collected in the spring in Ghana and are fried, roasted, or made into bread. Grubs are a New Guinea and aboriginal Australian delicacy, as are aquatic fly larvae in Japan. Some say that there may even be insect farms in our future!

NUTRITION AND CRISIS

How many Americans are affected by foodborne illnesses each year?

According to the Centers for Disease Control and Prevention (CDC), it is estimated that about 48 million Americans are affected by foodborne illnesses each year—an event the media often calls a "food outbreak." This usually results in around 128,000 hospitalizations and 3,000 deaths (especially affecting those people with already compromised immune systems). Foodborne illnesses can come from *Salmonella*, *Listeria*, and other forms of microorganisms that are in or on a certain food (for more about these illnesses, see the chapter "Nutrition and Allergies, Illnesses, and Diseases").

Contamination during a food outbreak mostly comes from either improper handling of foods (especially foods that are not fully cooked, such as pork products); a person who has an illness that is transmitted to the foods; improperly home-canned foods; or foods that contain substances that easily attract bacteria if left unrefrigerated long enough. In recent years, some food contamination has even been found in manufactured foods, sometimes discovered after the product is on the grocery shelves. Most of this contamination comes from improper handling during manufacturing or a certain contaminated ingredient from a vendor that is not detected before it is added to the product.

What were some food poisoning episodes in the past?

In the history of the United States, there have been many food poisoning events, according to *Food Safety News*. Some of the bigger outbreaks were as follows:

- In 1906, in Ithaca, New York, polluted water from a dam construction site reached public water supplies, causing a typhoid fever outbreak; 82 people died, including 29 Cornell University students.

- In 1911, in the Boston, Massachusetts, area, door-to-door delivery of raw milk caused a *Streptococcus* outbreak, in which 48 people died.

- Botulism killed 19 people in 1919, when contaminated canned ripe olives from California were distributed to three states.

- In 1922, in Portland, Oregon, door-to-door delivery of raw milk caused a *Streptococcus* outbreak, in which 22 people died.

- In one of the biggest outbreaks in U.S. history, in 1924 to 1925, contaminated oysters (exposed to polluted waters) from Long Island, New York, were distributed to many cities, including New York, Chicago, and Washington, D.C. The result was typhoid fever, in which 1,500 people became ill and 150 died.

What were some food outbreaks in the past three decades?

Food outbreaks are not just something that has happened in the past: Our modern foods have also been known to cause problems and disease. Some of the more recent severe—and not so severe—outbreaks follow, as per *Food Safety News* and the Centers for Disease Control and Prevention:

- A cheese made by a company in Los Angeles caused a *Listeria* outbreak in 1985—mostly affecting Hispanic women (many of whom were pregnant)—and 28 people died.

- In 1998, a Michigan processing plant that produced Ball Park hot dogs and Sara Lee deli meats contained *Listeria*. The meats were recalled, but still 21 people died.

- In 2002, there was an outbreak of *Listeria* from Pilgrim's Pride sliced turkey meats. People in many states were affected, and 8 died.

- In a span of time between 2008 and 2009, an outbreak of *Salmonella typhimurium* from peanut butter and paste (used as an ingredient in other foods, such as crackers) caused at least 714 illnesses in 46 states—and 9 people died.

What recent discovery may eventually be used to eliminate *Escherichia coli* bacteria in produce and meats?

In 2014, researchers at Purdue University uncovered a possible way to decrease a toxin-producing strain of *E coli* in contaminated foods (most strains of *E coli* are harmless, but some can cause severe illness). They targeted two foods that often are responsible for such illness: spinach, usually not cleaned well, and ground beef, usually undercooked. Using bacteriophages ("phages")—or viruses that attack and kill bacteria—the researchers contaminated spinach and ground beef with toxic *E coli*, then exposed the foods to three specific phages that are known to kill off *E coli*; after 24 hours, the number of *E coli* in the spinach and meats (both kept at room temperature) dropped by 99 percent or more. (Simply put, the phages penetrate the bacteria walls, injecting their own DNA into the cell; from there, it makes more phages, essentially exploding the host cell, releasing the next generation of phages.) The phages do not pose a problem to human health and can be host-specific—but time will tell how and when this study can be used to help deter some human food illnesses.

- A *Listeria* outbreak in 2011 that sickened at least 146 people in 28 states, with 36 people dying as a result, was caused by contaminated Rocky Ford cantaloupes from Colorado; the contamination was thought to have originated at the packing facility.

- In 2013, an outbreak of a parasite called *Cyclospora* was traced to a prepackaged salad mix. It sickened at least 223 people in Iowa and Nebraska, but no deaths were reported.

What was the Irish potato famine?

The Irish potato famine of 1846 to 1851 was one of the largest famines in Irish history, with an estimated one million people perishing during the famine due to malnutrition, starvation, or epidemic diseases—about an eighth of the population. The main culprit was a lethal pathogen to potato plants—the *Phytophthora infestans*. Once thought to be a fungus, it is now considered a protist, an organism that lives in humid and moist environments and spreads disease by spores. The disease spreads rapidly, and decays the leaves and stems of the plant, eventually causing the tuber to stop growing and rot. And since the Irish depended on the potato for about 60 percent of their nation's food needs at that time, the result was devastating.

But this was not the first time this protist caused problems. The disease was first noticed in the 1500s in Europe, and it has continued to show up in numerous places throughout the centuries, albeit not in as widespread and destructive a form as in nineteenth-century Ireland. Today, it is still around, and is known to farmers and gardeners as the potato "late blight."

What criteria does the United Nations use to determine a "famine"?

There are numerous reasons for a famine in a country—and it usually involves three problems: food production failure (usually from drought conditions); people's ability to access foods; and finally, how the respective government and the international donors respond politically to the famine. Overall, the United Nations has certain criteria for famines and a country's food security, all based on a five-step scale called the Integrated Food Security Phase Classification. Step five is the worst case: It means that there is a "famine/humanitarian catastrophe," and that "more than two people per 10,000 die each day, acute malnutrition rates are above 30 percent, all livestock is dead, and there is less than 2,100 kilocalories of food and 4 liters of water available per person per day."

What were (and are) some well-known famines?

Most famous famines around the world were—and are—either nature- or human-induced. Many times, people have died from starvation because of human interference—and one of world's worst was the Russian Famine of 1921–1922, which spread through the areas now called Russia, Ukraine, and Georgia. In this case, politics played a role: It was the first year that the Soviets were in power, and food shortages were caused by civil unrest and government regulations about food distribution. People scavenged for food, what food there was ended up unevenly distributed, and the unrest caused certain crops not to be sown. Add to this some major crop failures and there was even more of a food shortage. The Bolsheviks finally asked for aid from the capitalistic West—and food poured in, but not before 5 million people died from starvation or diseases such as cholera and typhus.

For a more recent example, in 2011, the African country of Somalia was experiencing a major famine, from a combination of drought (for more than two years, and that caused a loss of 50 percent of the usual harvest), war, and restrictions on aid from humanitarian groups. The famine has spread to over half of the country—a nation that has suffered from fighting and many crises since its government collapsed in 1991. To date, the famine continues—with more fighting by militant groups, little aid getting through, and many deaths caused by such diseases as measles, cholera, malaria, and typhoid.

What were some foods given soldiers during the American Civil War?

As with most wars, the foods that were available in the American Civil War had to be easy to prepare and carry, and had to feed thousands of men. There were several of these foods. For example, Northern sol-

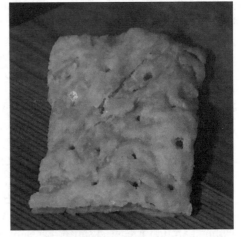

During the American Civil War, a common ration for soldiers was hardtack, a very tough-to-chew biscuit that was easy to carry and didn't easily spoil.

diers' foods included desiccated vegetables (actually the forerunner of modern dehydrated foods), ramrod bread (cornbread made by coating a ramrod with batter and baking it over an open fire), salt pork, cornmeal, coffee, and the occasional dried navy bean as a treat.

The one food eaten throughout the war was hardtack. This biscuit of unleavened flour measured about a quarter inch thick and three inches square. Both the Union and Confederate armies ate hardtack, and it was officially issued as "hard bread." But to the men who would sporadically receive about eight to ten biscuits, the food was an inedible chunk of biscuit known as "a castle for worms" and "teeth dullers." And even though hardtack was not well liked, war prisoners would often use the food as a medium of exchange, in which several biscuits would be traded for a loaf of bread or a piece of chewing tobacco.

Why did so many men die from starvation during the American Civil War?

Overall, it is estimated that 600,000 to 620,000 people died during the American Civil War—about one out of every five Americans who were alive in 1860—from a combination of battles, disease (often from malnutrition), and starvation. One reason for the malnutrition and starvation was the lack of nutritionally balanced meals in both armies. Early in the war, both the North and South had enough food, and most soldiers fared well; but as the conflict intensified, it was not uncommon for a company of soldiers to go without food for several days. (But such lack of foods also created some entrepreneurial followers: for example, sulters, or civilians licensed or permitted to operate a shop at a military post or camp, would offer foods that were not included in the special rations, operating on a cash basis, or giving credit at very high interest rates.)

The Northern armies fared better than the Southern troops, but there were certain rules to feeding soldiers. For example, in anticipation of a battle, the Union soldiers on the march would be given "three days' rations," mainly of hardtack (many diaries and letters describe that most men would eat the entire amount in a single sitting because they were so hungry). The soldiers in camp were supposed to get 22 ounces of bread or flour or a pound of hardtack daily—but this varied widely from time to time and from unit to unit. Food rations for the Confederate soldiers began to dwindle around the spring of 1862, mainly because of blockades by the North, and thus, many food supply lines were cut off. And for the rest of the war, the lack of food would affect most of the troops—becoming a major issue in almost every battle.

What Civil War battle may have been lost because of food?

The Confederate army's lack of food supplies no doubt took its historical toll, especially at Gettysburg, Pennsylvania, in July of 1863. Some historians believe that early in 1863, when Robert E. Lee's Army of Northern Virginia was growing hungry as they winter-camped around Fredericksburg, Lee sent about a quarter (two divisions) of his men to southeast Virginia to look for food supplies—a splitting of his forces that delayed his march north toward the Union line. His army was divided until the end of April of that year; but a confrontation at Chancellorsville with Major General Joseph Hooker's Union troops took a toll on Lee's troops. By the time Lee reached Gettysburg with his army, there were fewer troops—one factor thought to have caused Lee's loss at Gettysburg.

What foods did the soldiers eat during World War I?

As with most wars, soldiers had certain foods available to them in the camps and as they went into battle. For the American army, the idea of war food rations began in 1775, when the Continental Congress insisted that all soldiers receive a pound of beef, pork, or fish, bread, beer, and milk—or what was expected to feed a man for one day.

By World War I, the saying "full belly, fully ready" came into vogue. But the food guidelines had changed little from any earlier wars—so there were plenty of additional perks for the doughboys of the American Expeditionary Forces, such as potatoes, and luxuries that included butter, candy, and cigarettes. There were also mobile kitchens that would feed hot meals to soldiers, depending on weather, supplies, and, of course, enemy fire. This was also the war in which "emergency rations" were developed—a tin that kept out the pests, survived gas attacks, and offered enough food for a man for a week. It carried over 3,000 calories worth of meat, bread, coffee, and sugar to sustain a soldier if regular foods were not available.

What rations were important to soldiers in World War II?

In World War II, because of the distance from home, the military relied on mostly rations—thus, the foods had to be more nutritious. The following list describes some of the special-purpose rations that were developed:

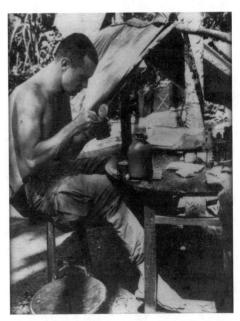

- *Field Ration D*, or the Army's emergency ration, was also a supplement to other rations. The rations included chocolate, sugar, dry milk, cacao fat, oat flour, and a flavoring—which would equal a mixture providing 600 calories a day. But it was not well received as a combat food, and was replaced by C and K rations by the end of the war.

- *Field Ration C* was mainly developed for soldiers to carry and use when cut off from the regular food supplies. It contained a ration of meat and bread components, with good, sturdy packaging. The first C rations were not well received, and they were often called a "monotonous meat diet";

A U.S. soldier in Vietnam eats C rations, including canned meat and bread.

later C rations included certain items that varied in combination, and often contained an accessory packet with cigarettes, water-purification tablets, toilet paper, matches, and chewing gum. In addition, these rations evolved throughout the war, adding essentials and more needed elements to not only better feed the men, but also to keep up morale.

- *K rations* were developed as a lightweight, easy-to-carry ration that could be used in assault and combat operations; it eventually evolved into K breakfast, lunch, and dinner rations, and was one of the most well-received combinations of food and other items by the soldiers. The list of foods and other products is long, but over the years, it was the C rations, and their continual improvements, that proved to be the most useful and nutritionally balanced for the fighting troops.

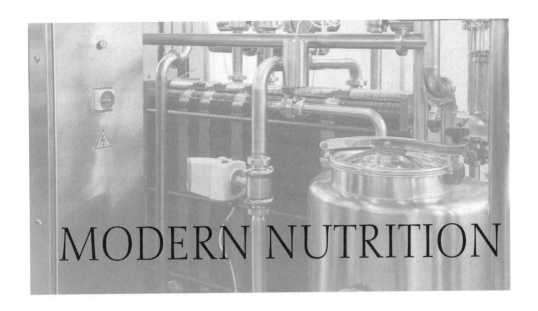

MODERN NUTRITION

What is a food system?

A food system is the process of getting our food from the source—vegetables, fruits, meat, seafood, and so forth—to our table and beyond. It includes everything that helps us feed a population, including the farms that grow and harvest the foods; those involved in processing and packaging; how the food is transported to the stores, displayed, and marketed; and even how we consume and dispose of foods. Every facet of the food system has its own processes and functions—and there are many—although each food may have a different approach. For example, how a turkey goes from growing to disposing what is not eaten is very different from growing a beet to composting the peels from the vegetable.

How has the food system affected food nutrients in the past half century?

How we process foods in the food system has changed over the last half century. In particular, when people used to grow much of their own food, there was not as much of a problem with obtaining fresh vegetables, fruits, and even some meats. But since the middle of the twentieth century, with fewer people in rural areas, a growing population (and much of it in big cities), more demands for different types of foods, and the growth of grocery stores, getting fresh foods to consumers has meant transporting foods longer distances. In turn, many of the foods that are transported for many days, even if refrigerated, often contain fewer nutrients, which is very different from the days in which most people just strolled out to their backyard gardens to pick a fresh meal.

Why did the United States eventually need an agency for food and drug safety?

Just over a hundred years ago, there was no agency to keep on eye on our foods and drugs, and no laws, regulations, or rules that would protect the consumer from potentially dangerous foods and medicines. And there were plenty of problems with the foods people consumed, including untested chemicals (mostly poisonous preservatives and dyes) in the foods. With the increase in population in cities, more food needed to be carried from distant areas, yet sanitation was primitive compared to today's standards, milk was unpasteurized (bacteriology was in its infancy), and ice was the main means of refrigeration.

Drugs were also a problem; before 1848 and the passing of the Import Drugs Act that year, the United States had become a "dumping ground" for counterfeit, contaminated, diluted, and decomposed drug materials. But it took many more decades to establish a specific agency to watch over what citizens consumed. Today, the main U.S. agency responsible for food and drug safety is the U.S. Food and Drug Administration (FDA), a part of the Public Health Service Act within the U.S. Department of Health and Human Services.

How was the FDA founded?

The steps to today's Food and Drug Administration began in 1862, when Congress created the Department of Agriculture. It was a sinuous route: The Patent Office's chemistry laboratory was transferred to the new agency, renamed the Chemistry Division, and then-President Abraham Lincoln appointed chemist Charles M. Wetherill (1825–1871) as the head; in 1890, the name was changed to the Division of Chemistry; in 1901, that division became the Bureau of Chemistry; in 1927, it became the Food, Drug, and Insecticide Administration; by 1930, it was renamed the Food and Drug Administration. But in 1940, the division was transferred from the Department of Agriculture to the Federal Security Agency; in 1953, this became the Department of Health, Education, and Welfare; and by 1979, Health and Human Services (HHS)—with the FDA as a part of the Public Health Services Act within the HHS.

Who was Peter Collier?

Peter Collier (1835–1896) was an American chemist, and the fifth head of the Department of Agriculture. He was also a major proponent of food safety—urging federal legislation to stop food alteration, and make it a crime. His proposed national food and drug law was defeated, and over the next 25 years, more than 100 food and drug laws were introduced in Congress. But it took until 1906 to enact the Pure Food and Drug Act—laws that would prohibit interstate commerce in mislabeled or altered foods, drinks, and drugs.

Who was Harvey Washington Wiley?

Harvey Washington Wiley (1844–1930) became the chief chemist of the Department of Agriculture in 1883. He specialized in the use of chemicals as food preservatives, and did intensive investigations into whether such preservatives should be used in food, and what amounts were safe for human consumption. By 1902, Wiley convinced Congress to expand the Bureau of Chemistry's food alteration studies. His idea was to determine the effects of a diet that included foods with various preservatives, using human volunteers. His famous "poison squad" studies proved that we should be concerned about preservatives, and became the impetus for new and better food and drug laws.

What was the "Pure Food Movement"?

The "Pure Food Movement" was started in the 1870s, mostly by the food trade. It was a grass-roots movement that eventually propagated the political support for the Pure Food and Drug of 1906. The Pure Food Movement began when food industry members wanted to stop the alteration of certain foods, put an end to the various rules and regulations that differed from state to state, and to control the competition from new food sources (such as oleomargarine, which threatened those who made butter).

How does the U.S. government help consumers find nutrition and health information on the Internet?

Although it is almost impossible to control what a person finds and reads on the Internet, the government does have its own sites that try to help protect consumers

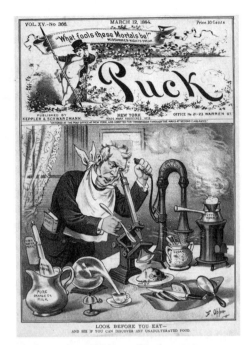

The cover of an 1882 issue of *Puck* magazine attempts to illustrate the essence of the "Pure Food Movement" by showing a scientist analyzing adulterated samples of food.

from misinformation about food, nutrition, and health. For example, the FDA regulates foods, including dietary supplements; it also monitors food product labels, claims, package inserts, and accompanying literature. At its Internet site, the FDA offers publications to help people to better evaluate health information. For instance, "Tips for the Savvy Supplement User: Making Informed Decisions and Evaluating the Information" and "FDA 101: Health Fraud Awareness" are just two of the choices.

Other government agencies are also involved in protecting consumers, including the Federal Trade Commission (FTC). This agency enforces consumer protection laws and regulates dietary supplement advertising. As part of its mission, the FTC investigates complaints about false or misleading health claims posted on the Internet; in addition, the FTC offers recommendations such as the "Operation Cure.All" page to help a person evaluate health product claims. And yet another government group, the Office of Dietary Supplements (ODS) of the National Institutes of Health, supports and distributes the results of research on dietary supplements, and provides educational material on supplements and health to the general public in the form of easy-to-understand fact sheets.

What are some recent government rulings concerning food?

In recent years, there have been several government rulings concerning foods—especially in terms of safety and nutrition. The following chronology lists some of those rulings:

- 1980: The Infant Formula Act established controls to make sure infant formulae were safe and had the proper nutritional content.
- 1990: The Nutrition Labeling and Education Act required all packaged foods to have a nutrition label, plus all of the listed health information must use the same terms as used by the U.S. Department of Health and Human Services.
- 1995: The seafood Hazard Analysis Critical Control Point (HACCP) offered regulations to ensure the safety and sanitary processing of fish and fish products (including imported seafood; for more about the fish we eat, see the chapter "Controversies with Food, Beverages, and Nutrition").
- 2010 and 2012: The Egg Safety Rule meant there were strict requirements to control the harmful bacteria *Salmonella* in eggs; the regulations went into effect for large farm egg producers in 2010, and for small farm egg producers in 2012.
- 2011: The Food Safety Modernization Act was signed into law and lets the FDA better protect public health by strengthening the food safety system, focusing more on preventing food problems instead of just reacting after the problem occurs.

Do any other governments have agencies that help maintain the quality of their respective country's foods?

Yes, there are many government agencies in various countries that deal with maintaining the quality of foods—too many to mention all of them here—including guides that outline the standards for all medicinal ingredients. For example, the guides for herbs used for medicinal purposes include the European Pharmacopoeia, British Herbal Pharmacopoeia, Japanese Pharmacopoeia, German Drug Codex, Indian Herbal Pharmacopoeia, and the United States Pharmacopeia—National Formulary.

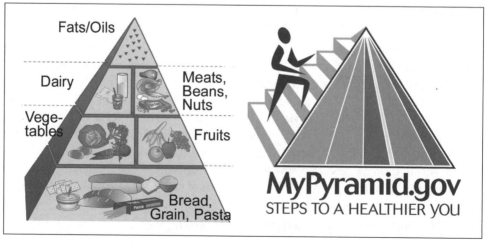

Two versions of the food pyramid that have been used by the U.S. government. At left is the older version from the early 1990s, which was replaced with the one on the right in 2005.

What was the "food guide pyramid"?

Over the years, the United States government has offered guides to Americans to help them eat better and be healthier. One of the main developments was the Food Guide Pyramid, or a way to visually show how eating a certain amount of foods from different food groups—grains, vegetables, fruits, milk and milk products, protein-rich plant and animal foods—can help a person lead a healthy life.

The Pyramid changed over the years, based on newer and up-to-date nutrition and health research. The pyramid was divided into a percent for each food group that should be consumed daily; the bigger the percent, the more you should eat of that food. But after twenty years of the government's food pyramid, it was decided that something new was needed. The first, and brief, result was the MyPyramid presented in 2005; today, the newest incarnation of the government's visual food guide is called the "Choose MyPlate" (see below).

What are the *Dietary Guidelines for Americans*?

The *Dietary Guidelines for Americans* was first released in 1980, and represent the dietary recommendations for Americans ages 2 years and older. The guidelines are not meant only to improve eating habits, but also to focus on foods and beverages that will help Americans maintain a healthy weight, promote health, and prevent many diseases that are associated with poor eating habits. The list is long, but for those who want to know more, it can be found at the USDA's website at www.DietaryGuidelines.gov. (*Note*: The *Dietary Guidelines for Americans* are different from the Dietary Reference Intakes (DRIs), or the standards for nutrient intakes in the United States, including recommendations for energy, vitamins, minerals, proteins, amino acids, carbohydrates, fats, water, and electrolytes for each sex and different stages of life. (For more about DRIs, see the chapter "Nutrition throughout Life.")

What are some ways the government helps us eat well?

The U.S. government wants to help us eat better, and therefore, there are many organizations in charge of nutrient recommendations. For example, the documents concerning DRIs are issued by the Food and Nutrition Board of the Institute of Medicine, part of the National Academy of Sciences. The Food and Nutrition Board "addresses issues of safety, quality, and adequacy of the food supply; establishes principles and guidelines of adequate dietary intake; and renders authoritative judgments on the relationships among food intake, nutrition, and health."

Here are some of more of the popular offerings from the government to help us eat well and stay healthy, all based on the DRI (the general term for a set of reference values used to plan and assess nutrient intakes of healthy people; for more about DRI, see the chapter "Nutrition throughout Life"):

Recommended Dietary Allowance (RDA) —The average daily level of nutrient intake sufficient to meet the nutrient requirements of nearly all (97 to 98 percent) healthy people.

Adequate Intake (AI) —This is established when evidence is insufficient to develop an RDA and is set at a level assumed to ensure nutritional adequacy.

Tolerable Upper Intake Level (UL) — The maximum daily intake unlikely to cause adverse health effects.

What is "Choose MyPlate"?

The "Choose MyPlate" is, to date, the latest guide by the USDA to help people eat well and maintain a healthy lifestyle; it was presented in June 2011 and is based on the government's "Dietary Guidelines for Americans." Like many other government

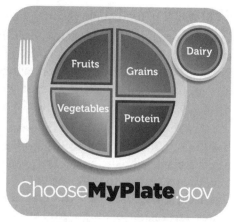

The portioned plate from choosemyplate.gov replaced the concept of the food pyramid in 2011.

programs to help people eat well, it includes a graphic of a plate divided into colors and wedges—all representing the types of foods you should eat "from your plate" each day, including grains, fruits, vegetables, protein, and a circle representing a cup outside the "plate" for dairy. The program also makes additional suggestions to go along with your "plate": how to balance calories; enjoy food but eat less; avoid larger portions; what foods to eat more often; make half the plate vegetables and fruits; switch to fat-free or low-fat milk; make half the grains you eat whole grains; determine what foods to eat less often; watch sodium intake; and drink water instead of sugary drinks.

Why do some food researchers disagree with the USDA and the "Choose MyPlate" campaign?

Not everyone is happy with the USDA's "Choose MyPlate" campaign, and as with many topics in nutrition, it is highly debated. There are many nutritionists, food experts, and sundry other specialists who believe there are major, and some minor, gaps in the government's presentation. For instance, some researchers cite that MyPlate does not address junk food, while others say that this is probably intentional, because junk food does not belong on our plates at all. Other researchers say MyPlate is too simplistic, while others say it's too complex.

And there are even organizations that have made up their own visual guidelines that are contrary to what the USDA offers. For example, because they believe there are deficiencies in the USDA's MyPlate, the Harvard School of Public Health offers the "Healthy Eating Plate." There are several changes, including differences in the beverages—specifically MyPlate displays a "dairy" circle (most people believe it represents milk), while the Harvard plate has a water glass. And of course, it comes as no surprise that there are many people who believe the Harvard version has problems—such as being too detailed and having too many food instructions for most people to easily follow.

FOOD SAFETY

What is food safety?

Food safety can mean one of two things. It can mean keeping you safe in the kitchen as you store, clean, prepare, and serve foods. It also entails what government rules and regulations—especially for the food industry—make sure the foods, beverages, and medicines you buy are safe to consume. For example, the government makes sure that food additives are safe to eat; they also have regulations in terms of the quality of the meat you eat. There are good reasons for food safety regulations and rules. According to the FDA, every year, 1 out of 6 people in the United States—about 48 million people—suffers from a foodborne illness, more than 100,000 are hospitalized, and thousands die. (For more about foodborne illnesses, see the chapter "Nutrition and Allergies, Illnesses, and Diseases.")

What are a few tips to keep you safe—food-wise—in the kitchen?

One of the main reasons for food safety in the kitchen is to stop the spread of disease. For example, keeping countertops, cutting boards, oven tops, and other food-associated areas clean is essential, as is washing and drying your hands before handling food, and keeping your towels, sponges, and cloths clean. When it comes to vegetables, it is important to wash and rinse all your vegetables before eating; there are even special non-toxic washes to clean the foods (although it is difficult to wash off the wax and some pesticides that are found on some vegetables, which is why some foods are better eaten after peeling). Even organically grown vegetables need to be cleaned well, as the soil sometimes harbors bacteria.

When it comes to meat, there are seemingly even more reasons and ways to stay safe in the kitchen. Raw meat, poultry, and fish often carry harmful bacteria, so it's essential to cook these foods thoroughly. If you cut meat on a cutting board, be sure to wash the board with hot, soapy water after each use; and wash your hands after handling raw meat. It is also thought that cooking food in stages is not the best way to make a meal—even if food is stored in the refrigerator between cooking times, the heat from the initial cooking may be just enough to allow bacteria to develop. And finally, it is best to refrigerate leftovers as soon as possible—especially meats or foods that are cooked or mixed with such ingredients as mayonnaise or eggs.

Who is in charge of recalling foods?

The U.S. Food and Drug Administration is in charge of recalling foods—especially contaminated foods that could harm the consumer. Almost weekly, the recall list at the FDA website lists yet another problem with a food or drug—usually contamination that can cause an illness outbreak—hopefully getting the offending foods off the shelf in time to keep people from becoming ill. For example, in one recent week, a spinach antipasto salad was recalled—it was thought to be contaminated with the bacteria *Listeria*. In

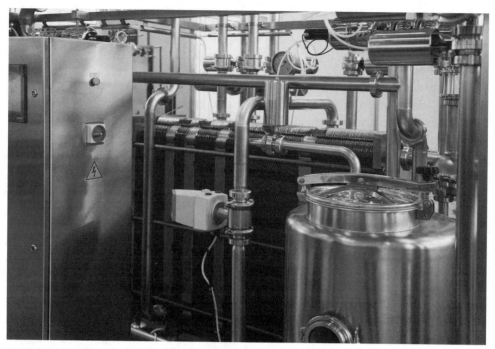

A milk pasteurization tank and pipes at a dairy factory. The process of heating milk to destroy bacteria and make it safer for consumption was developed by its namesake, Dr. Louis Pasteur.

this case (and in others that occurred), the foods are immediately taken off the grocery shelves. And to help the customer identify the offending foods (in case they purchased the item before the announcement), the FDA makes public what food brand was affected, in what states the food may be found (often the names of the grocery stores), dates the foods were sold, the "best by" dates, or the food's product numbers.

Why is pasteurization important to food safety?

Pasteurization is the process of heating liquids, such as milk or soymilk, to destroy bacteria (or sometimes other microorganisms) that can cause spoilage of foods. It is also commonly used to kill bacteria that can cause diseases in humans; for example, the bacteria known as *Salmonella* and *Streptococcus*, both common to milk and other beverages.

Who was the scientist behind pasteurization?

French chemist Louis Pasteur (1822–1895) is one of the founders of our modern study of bacteria, a field called bacteriology. Initially, Pasteur wanted to find a way to control the contamination of wine. By 1864, he developed a way to slowly heat foods and drinks—temperatures high enough to kill off most of the bacteria responsible for disease and spoilage of the foods without changing the characteristics of the foodstuff (such as curdling of milk). This was the beginning of what we call pasteurization, a well-known word we now see on food products such as milk and yogurt.

How is milk pasteurized?

Not all milk is pasteurized in the same way. One method is called low temperature holding, or LTH, in which the milk is heated to 145 degrees Fahrenheit (62.9 degrees Celsius) for about 30 minutes; another is called flash pasteurization, in which the milk is heated at higher temperatures for a shorter time (or HTST), that is, to 161 degrees Fahrenheit (71.7 degrees Celsius) for fifteen seconds. Finally, a newer method called ultra-high temperature (UHT) heats the milk to 286 degrees Fahrenheit (141 degrees Celsius) for two seconds. This may extend the shelf life of the milk, but it not only takes away much of the nutrient value of the milk (which is added "artificially" afterward), but also changes the taste of the milk—to many people, not in a good way.

What does biopreservation mean in terms of food and drug safety?

When it comes to food (and drug) safety, the term *biopreservation* means the preservation and safety of food and medicines using biological materials. For example, there is a bacterial protein that can act like a broad-spectrum antibiotic in humans. But this protein cannot be chemically created; thus, the bacteria *Lactobacillus*—which carries the protein—is used to make the protein to produce the antibiotic. All this has to be carefully monitored to make the medicine as safe for consumption as possible.

Why are food additives put in foods?

For centuries, people have added various ingredients to their foods—from flavorings and preservatives to toxins and dyes—some of them harmless, but many of them harmful. Today, there are still many additives in certain foods—and even medicines—albeit hopefully these are not as harmful as some of the old-fashioned foods and drugs (see Sidebar). Many of these additives perform useful functions; but some, although useful,

What are some of the more "scary" additives approved for use in foods?

There are some "scary" additives that are used in our foods. One of the more interesting additives is carnauba wax—which some of us know as a polish for our cars, not as belonging in our food. But if you check out the ubiquitous marshmallow treats most associated with the Easter holiday, the first ingredient is carnauba wax (used for the eyes of the "animal"). Another interesting ingredient is shellac—actually a secretion from the female lac bug in India—which, in terms of food, is called "confectioner's glaze." This additive is used to give the glossy covering to such foods as jelly beans and some other candies, and is mainly used to stop the food from drying out. From all research done on both additives, there seems to be no adverse effects—thus, they are "approved" for use in foods by the FDA.

can be harmful to those who are sensitive to that certain additive. (For more about the controversies surrounding food additives, see the chapter "Controversies with Food, Beverages, and Nutrition.")

Overall, the most common modern food additives are sugar, corn syrup, other sweeteners, and salt—all used to enhance flavor and/or prevent the food from spoiling. Still other food additives are used as preservatives, colorings, antioxidants (to prevent foods from going rancid), flavor enhancers, emulsifiers, thickeners, and stabilizers.

What are some additives added to our food to extend shelf life?

The following table lists some of the more common food additives that are used to extend the shelf life of some foods, including their functions and what foods contain such additives:

Food Additives

Additive	Function	What Foods
Nitrites and nitrates	To extend the shelf-life of a food; keep fungi and bacteria away; preserve color of meats and some dried foods	Processed meats (bacon, hot dogs, ham, luncheon meats)
BHA or BHT	To extend the shelf life of a food; keep fungi and bacteria away	Baked goods, cereals, fats, and oils—anything that can go rancid because of exposure to oxygen
Benzoic acid (and benzoates)	To extend the shelf life of a food; keep fungi and bacteria away	Soft drinks, margarine, acidic foods, some dried fruits, and beer
Sulfites	To extend the shelf life of a food; keep fungi and bacteria away	Fruit pie fillings, many dried fruits and shredded coconut, some relishes and pickles

What are emulsifiers, thickeners, and stabilizers?

Emulsifiers (to allow the suspension of one liquid in another), thickeners (to increase the thickness of a liquid), and stabilizers (to preserve the food's structure) are all food (and drug) additives, usually used to improve the consistency and texture of foods. Most sauces, soups, baked goods, frozen desserts, jams, puddings, and other such foods have some type of additive to keep the foods together or keep them creamy or smooth. They include such names as carrageenan, glycerol, gum Arabic, guar gum, pectin, lecithin, and cellulose.

What are mono- and diglycerides?

Mono- and diglycerides are considered emulsifiers—or substances that encourage liquids that would normally not combine, to combine. For example, eggs are usually called an emulsifier, but there are also many manufactured ones, including glycerides from palm, soybean, or sunflower oils, and even tallow. Most vegetable oils and animal fats

What additives often went into some "old-fashioned tonics"?

Additives, including sugar and salt, have been around for centuries, but some additives turned out to be very harmful. Some of the most harmful were the "patent medicines" that became popular by the mid-nineteenth century to early twentieth century, touted by their manufacturers or traveling salespeople to cure almost any ailment including venereal diseases, infant colic, digestive upsets, "female complaints," and cancers. But it was usually not the tonic that caused the alleged cure, but the additives—most often large doses of alcohol, morphine, opium, or cocaine were used that would make many people "feel good" (and which is why many babies who were given the tonics died).

Even though many of the tonics were called "patent medicines," there were no rules or regulations governing the concoctions. Traveling companies known as "medicine shows" would sell the tonics, which would often contain the words "Doctor" or "Professor" on the labels, such as Dr. Morse's Indian Root Pills (it supposedly "cleansed the blood"). In a show, a paid person would fake an ailment, then miraculously be cured by the "miracle" tonics. There were also a group of patent medicines promoted as liniments and ointments, which often were said to contain snake oil—which led to the phase "snake oil salesman," a term that eventually came to mean "charlatan."

have triglycerides, but the manufacturer uses certain enzymes to break the oils down into mono- and diglycerides. Overall, they help to make mixing easy, prevent separation, and even stabilize a food; they are most often found in fast-food restaurant offerings, in ice creams, baked goods, whipped toppings, puddings, certain drinks, and many more foods. Although they are "generally recognized as safe" by the FDA (they seem to pose no serious health problems), many people who try to eat a healthy balanced diet stay away from foods containing these emulsifiers.

What are some additives used as flavor enhancers?

Flavor enhancers, as the term implies, are meant to improve the flavors of a certain food. One of the most well known is monosodium glutamate (MSG), a natural flavoring that heightens your perception of taste, making the food seem as if it tastes better. Another is hydrolyzed vegetable protein, which is used in mixes and processed meats to improve the flavor of canned and processed foods. And there is even disodium guanylate, used to improve the flavors of canned meats and meat-based foods.

What are some additives used as food colorings?

There are many food coloring additives—usually to make what you eat look more appealing. Some are natural, such as beta carotene (precursor to vitamin A), and coloring from beets and carrot oils; but others are chemical compounds that have special coded listings, such as FD&C (Federal Food, Drug, and Cosmetic Act) colors, for instance, Blue #2, or Red #40. These food colors are found in almost all types of foods—from processed foods, baked goods, and cereals to frostings, jams, and even the outer skin of some fruits. (For more about controversies with food colorings, especially in the past, see the chapter "Controversies with Food, Beverages, and Nutrition.")

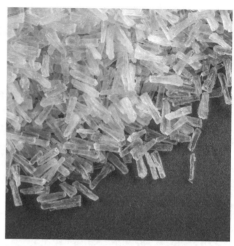

A close-up of the flavor enhancer monosodium glutamate illuminates its crystalline structure.

Are there any vitamin-based food additives?

Yes, there are several vitamins that are used as food additives—and offer some health benefits. For example, the tocopherols (vitamin E) are used in some oils and shortenings to prevent them from going rancid. Vitamin C, as ascorbic acid, and ascorbates prevent fruit juices from browning, and also stop fatty foods from becoming rancid.

Are there any additives that can affect certain organs in our bodies?

Yes, there are additives that can affect the function of various organs in our bodies. For example, the trace mineral iodine affects the thyroid; it is found naturally in food and water, but it is most familiar as an additive to table salt. The iodine turns into iodide in the body, and aids in the development and function of the thyroid gland; it is also a major part of the hormone thyroxine produced by the thyroid gland. It has a multitude of thyroid duties, including helping in energy production, and stimulating the rate of the body's metabolism. But not all additives are good for the thyroid. One such additive is a preservative called potassium bromate—a chemical that can block iodine from being absorbed by the thyroid. (For more about the thyroid gland, see the chapter "Nutrition and Allergies, Illnesses, and Diseases.)

FOOD LABELING

How does the consumer interpret certain food label claims?

Did you ever wonder about the difference between "reduced fat" and "low fat"? Or does "calorie free" on a label really mean no calories? The Food and Drug Administration has strict guidelines on how these food label terms can be used. Here are some of the most common claims seen on food packages—and there are many—and what they mean, as per the Food and Drug Administration and the American Heart Association:

Low calorie—Must have 40 calories or less per serving.

Low in saturated fat—Must have 1 gram of saturated fat or less, with not more than 15 percent of the calories from the saturated fat.

Low fat—Must contain less than 3 grams of fat per serving.

Reduced—Must contain at least 25 percent less of the specified nutrient or calories than the usual product; for example, a reduced fat mayonnaise must contain at least 25 percent less fat than regular mayonnaise.

Less—A food must contain 25 percent less of a nutrient than another certain food; for example, a pretzel can claim to contain 25 percent less fat than potato chips.

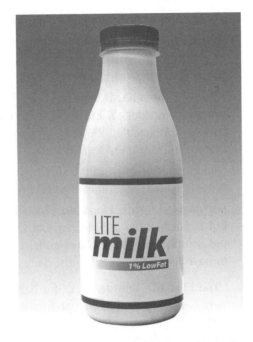

A label of "lite" can only be placed on this bottle of milk if it has no more than half the fat or two-thirds the total calories of regular whole milk.

Good source of—Must provide at least 10 to 19 percent of the Daily Value of a particular vitamin or nutrient per serving; for example, to be a good source of calcium, the food must contain 10 to 19 percent of the daily value for calcium.

Light (or lite)—A food must have one third fewer calories or half the fat of another certain food, or the sodium in a low-fat, low-calorie food must be reduced by 50 percent; for example, light mayonnaise must contain at least 50 percent less fat than regular mayonnaise.

Calorie free—Must contain less than five calories per serving.

Fat free/sugar free—Must have less ½ gram of fat/sugar per serving.

High in—Provides 20 percent or more of the Daily Value of a specified nutrient per half a serving.

High fiber—Must contain 5 or more grams of fiber per serving.

Good source of fiber—Must contain 2.5 to 4.9 grams of fiber per serving.

Lean meat—Must contain less than 10 grams of total fat, 4.5 grams of saturated fat or less, and less than 95 milligrams of cholesterol per serving.

Extra lean—Must have less than 5 grams of fat, 2 grams of saturated fat, and 95 milligrams of cholesterol.

245

High protein—Must contain 20 percent (or more) of the daily value for protein.

Natural flavoring—The FDA standard states that foods with this label must be extracts from nonsynthetic foods, such as essential oils, spices, and so on; its function in the food is flavoring, not nutrition.

Fresh—Although this term has been misused over the years, it originally meant unprocessed, uncooked, and unfrozen foods (with washing and coating [usually wax] of fruits and vegetables allowed). Fresh-frozen is also included, or food that is quickly frozen, and is usually seen in association with fresh fish.

Good source—This means a serving must contain between 10 and 19 percent of the recommended daily value of a certain nutrient, such as vitamin A or D.

Fortified—A fortified food must have 10 percent or more of a daily value per serving, but it can be used only to represent vitamins, protein, minerals, dietary fiber, and potassium; for example, most milk in the United States is fortified, thus one cup has to have about 30 percent of the daily value for vitamin D.

The FDA also sets standards for health-related claims on food labels to help consumers identify foods that are rich in nutrients and may help to reduce their risk for certain diseases. For example, the manufacturers can make health claims that highlight the link between calcium and osteoporosis, heart disease and fat, or even high blood pressure and sodium.

How is a food's cholesterol listed on labels?

Cholesterol has its own label rules and regulations. Cholesterol-free means the food has to have less than 2 milligrams of cholesterol and 2 grams or less of saturated fat per serving. Low cholesterol means the food has to have 20 or fewer milligrams of cholesterol and 2 grams or less of saturated fat. And finally, reduced cholesterol means the food has to have at least 25 percent less cholesterol than the regular product, and two grams or less of saturated fat.

How is sodium often listed on food labels?

Because sodium in our diet has been linked to several health concerns, in particular heart disease, there are several ways that the consumer can determine just how much sodium is in a specific food based on the label. The terms include: *Low sodium,* or the food must contain 140 milligrams or less of sodium per serving; *very low sodium,* or the food must have 35 milligrams or less of sodium; *reduced or less sodium,* or the food must have at least 25 percent less sodium than the regular product; and, *sodium free or no sodium,* in which the food must have less than 5 milligrams of sodium and no sodium chloride in the ingredients.

How have "gluten-free" product labels changed?

People who have celiac disease or those who have a hard time digesting gluten (the starch and proteins found in certain grassy grains like wheat, barley, and rye) need to pay attention to each food's nutrition label. If not, the result may be mild to extreme gastrointestinal distress. This has been tricky in the past, as there were often traces of gluten in a label marked "gluten-free." But in 2013, the FDA finally set a standard on the labeling of "gluten-free" products—with the agency setting a gluten limit of 20 parts per million in such foods. This is good news because the number of people who have been diagnosed with celiac disease (or are thought to be gluten-intolerant) has dramatically increased in the past decade.

How do some labels "trick" consumers?

Even though it is estimated that close to 50 percent of consumers read food labels before buying, sometimes those labels can be misleading. Here are some of the more common confusing labels:

Low fat—Many people on a diet look for the low-fat label. And this may mean that, as per regulations, the product has 3 grams of fat or less. But oftentimes, when one ingredient is missing, food manufacturers often add something to make up for it—and in the case of "less" or "low fat," it usually means more sugar, sodium, and calories that can cause weight gain.

Low sugar versus reduced sugar—Many people want less sugar in their diet, but be aware of two phrases: "reduced sugar" means that the product has 25 percent less sugar than the regular version; but "low sugar" has no standard definition.

Sugar free—This means that the food has to have less than half a gram of sugar per serving, but if you check out the "serving size," it may be very small. For example, a serving size can range from a tablespoon to a cup! In addition, sugar-free products may cause gastrointestinal problems in people, especially those sensitive to other sugar substitutes, such as sorbitol. (For more about sugar substitutes, see the chapter "The Basics of Nutrition: Macronutrients and Non-nutrients.")

Gluten free—Most products that say gluten-free are usually just that—but they may have refined starches or extra sugar to compensate for the lack of gluten, thus adding unwanted calories to the diet.

Whole grain versus multigrain—This is another trick that food producers use, especially for breads and baked goods. A 100 percent whole-grain food has to be labeled as such; and if the product has a "whole grain" stamp that is black and gold, it follows all the requirements from the Whole Grains Council. But the term *multigrain* is not as explicit—and usually just means the product contains many grains, and probably not all of them whole grains, but milled or refined.

Antibiotic free/No antibiotic residues—These two listings are actually something to ignore—after all, the USDA does not authorize such claims on any foods. Since no one really approves or has a specific measurement of such claims, these two terms should mean nothing to consumers.

Made with organic ingredients—Many people now look for the "organic" label on their food, especially if they are concerned about the amount of pesticides, herbicides, and insecticides—not to mention the possible genetically modified organisms (GMOs)—in their foods. But the terms are not the same: *Organic* means at least 95 percent of the product's ingredients are truly organic; *Made with organic ingredients* means at least 70 percent of the ingredients are organic. (See below for more about organic foods.)

Does the term *fat-free* on a label mean no calories?

No, this is one of the myths propagated by advertisers' use of the word "free"; just because the food claims to have no fat, there can still be calories, usually in the form of carbohydrates. In fact, a food product container may state it is fat free, but still contain added flours, salt, starch, or sugar. This improves the flavor of the fat-free food, but also can add many calories, and you gain more weight. And although fat free (and zero fat means the same thing), there is one "trick" that manufacturers don't seem to mention—the kind of fat. In addition, even though a product claims to have 0 grams of, for example, trans fat, it may really have up to half a gram of the fat per serving. As always, the best way to truly see if the food has a great deal of calories is to check the label.

Why is there a problem with the term *serving size* on labels?

Sometimes nutrition labels are tricky to read—and make you think you're eating less when you're truly eating more. Usually, under "Nutrition Facts," you can find out the number of calories in the food you eat by noting the "serving size" and "servings per container"; below this is usually listed the amount of calories per serving. Thus, if the serving size is one cup, with one serving per container, and the number of calories is 200, then you know if you eat one cup of the food, you will consume 200 calories.

But sometimes the label will be misleading—or misread—and if you don't pay careful attention to the labeling you may eat more calories than you want or need. For example, a serving size may be "1 cup," the servings per container "4," with calories per serving being "200." If you're not careful, you may think the entire contents contain only 200 calories—but in reality, the entire container has 800 calories (4 times 200).

Why will food labels change in the near future?

A great deal has changed since the Food and Drug Administration sent out guidelines for nutrition labels in 1993—especially with the American diet. The FDA label's serving size standards were based on the Reference Amounts Customarily Consumed (or RACCs)—numbers based on consumption in the late 1970 and 1980s. But Americans eat more now—as evident in the increase in heart diseases and obesity—and instead of a third of an English muffin (the "serving size"), a person eats the entire muffin (which means more calories consumed). Now the FDA wants to emphasize this difference in serving size, and give more realistic numbers; it also wants the food manufacturers to be more realistic, and if most people eat the entire muffin, label the package as "one serving," not several. These changes will help consumers not only to make better decisions about how much they truly want to eat, but also to make healthier choices.

What are examples of common and future food labels?

Most food labels have to include certain nutritional information. The figure at right shows a common food label.

What are the "traffic light" food labels?

Although just catching on in the United States, the voluntary use of "traffic light" food labels by the food industry has already been introduced into Europe in the past few years. These food labels use traffic light colors to help people see, at a glance, a food's level of fat, saturated fat, sugar, and salt—especially foods that are highly processed. (The main reason for such labels is the rise in obesity and heart disease.) In general, red means "enjoy once in a while," (for example, it usually indicates that the fat in the food exceeds 100 grams, and/or saturated fat exceeds 100 grams); amber means "you can probably eat this food most of the time"; and green means "this is a healthy food to eat often."

But not everyone is happy with the traffic light system—and there has been a recent call for some changes in the labels. For instance, people who like to eat a healthy Mediterranean diet, and especially those who sell olive oil (thought to, in moderation, be a healthy food because of

Nutrition Facts	
Serving Size 5 oz. (144g)	
Servings Per Container 4	
Amount Per Serving	
Calories 310 **Calories** from Fat 100	
	% Daily Value*
Total Fat 15g	**21%**
Saturated Fat 2.6g	**17%**
Trans Fat 1g	
Cholesterol 118mg	**39%**
Sodium 560mg	**28%**
Total Carbohydrate 12g	**4%**
Dietary Fiber 1g	**4%**
Sugars 1g	
Protein 24g	
Vitamin A 1% • **Vitamin C** 2%	
Calcium 2% • **Iron** 5%	

*Percent Daily Values are based on a 2,000 calorie diet. Your daily values may be higher or lower depending on your calorie needs:

		Calories	2,000	2,500
Total Fat	Less Than		65g	80g
Saturated Fat	Less Than		20g	25g
Cholesterol	Less Than		300mg	300mg
Sodium	Less Than		2,400mg	2,400mg
Total Carbohydrate			300g	375g
Dietary Fiber			25g	30g

Calories per gram:
Fat 9 • Carbohydrate 4 • Protein 4

Food labels like this one are required on foods sold in the United States; they show the calories, ingredients, and nutritional values contained in each serving.

its low saturated fat and higher good fat contents), would be "given two red lights" when it comes to fat and saturated fat—because olive oil is 100 percent fat, with 14 grams of saturated fat per 100 grams!

Are consumers affected by the color of a label when purchasing various foods?

In a recent study from Cornell University, researchers found that consumers are truly affected by colors on labels when purchasing foods. The researchers asked 93 university students to imagine they saw a candy bar in the grocery checkout lane—and that they were hungry. When shown a candy bar with a green or red label, and asked which was healthier, the green "won"—even though both had the same number of calories. Still another group was asked to compare a white- versus green-labeled bar, and once again, the green was chosen as the healthiest. The next time you're in the grocery store, you may want to remember this experiment—and if you pick up a food with a green label, it's more important to check the nutrient label than to trust your "green" instincts!

Is there a difference between a serving and a portion?

Yes, there is a difference between a serving and a portion. A serving is part of the U.S. Food and Drug Administration (FDA) nutrition label that appear on most packaged foods. The serving size is mentioned, along with how many calories per serving, total fat, cholesterol, sodium, total carbohydrates, protein, and any relevant vitamins and minerals. A portion is how much food you decide to eat at one time, from eating at a restaurant or at home. In many cases, our food portions do not match the serving size, because many people eat a larger portion than what is considered a serving size—which is one of the possible reasons for a person's weight gain.

Are there differences between infant and adult food labels?

Yes, there are definite differences between infant and adult food labels. For example, the most obvious difference has to do with serving size—an infant's serving size dif-

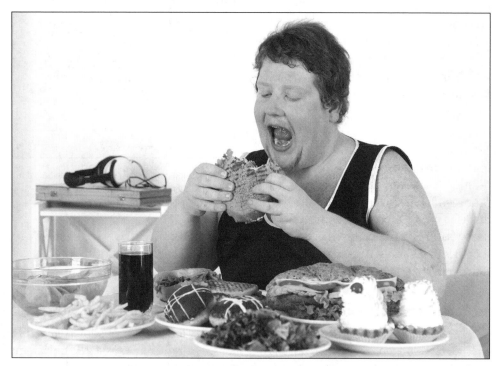

One reason why many Americans are overweight is that they eat portions that are much larger than recommended serving sizes.

fers greatly from an adult's serving size because adults need more food to survive. Another difference is that the total fat content on infant food labels does not list calories from fat, saturated fat, or cholesterol as on adult labels; this is because babies under two years old need fat in their diet, whereas most adults want that information in order to control the amount of fats they eat each day (to help control weight, in particular). And finally, the daily value percentages for protein, vitamins, and minerals are usually listed on the labels for infants and children under 4 years old; but the daily values for fat, cholesterol, sodium, potassium, carbohydrates, and fiber are not listed—mainly because the FDA has not determined the daily amounts of these nutrients for children under 4 years old.

How are some meats labeled in terms of quality?

Not all cuts of meat are top quality, and thus, many governments have a grading system so consumers can understand the quality of the meat they buy. For example, beef is often graded on how much marbling the meat contains (for more about marbling, see the chapter "Food Chemistry and Nutrition"). From superior to least quality, the meat is most often labeled: prime, AAA, AA, and A. In order to have a higher grade, too, the meat has to be inspected by the respective government agency; for example, in the United States, it is the U.S. Department of Agriculture. But not all meat is inspected—mainly because of a lack of inspectors.

How are some meats labeled in terms of where the animal is raised?

There is a growing concern about where certain cuts of meat come from—and especially where the animal was raised. For example, beef has certain labels indicating where the cattle are raised, such as "grass-fed" (cattle raised exclusively on forage); "grain-fed" (cattle raised mostly on forage, but at the end of their lives, to fatten them up, fed grains in a feedlot); "antibiotic-free" (no antibiotics given to the cattle or in their feed); or "organic" (mostly indicative of cattle raised without any added hormones [such as growth hormones], antibiotics, or pesticides, herbicides, or chemicals in their food or where they graze; this classification can vary widely depending on the type of meat.

What does the word "natural" mean on a label?

"Natural" is one of the most baffling words found on a product label. Although in most peoples' minds, "natural" is thought of as something positive in a food, there is truly no formal definition, especially when applied to products that don't contain eggs or meat. In fact, sugar, bark, and beans are all "natural" when you think about it—but if it's on a label, people will more likely pick up a product (and the sugar, bark, and beans can be contaminated with pesticides—and still be "natural"). Thus, consumer advocates warn shoppers not to put too much trust in the "natural" label—and even the terms *simple* and *wholesome* need to be ignored. Your best bet is reading the contents on the nutrition label to see if the food is truly nutritious to eat.

Are there various "certifications" when it comes to organic foods?

Yes, there are many organizations that certify organic foods. The following list describes some of those groups to date (and as the demand for organic food continues to grow, the list of certifying agencies will no doubt also grow):

USDA Organic/USDA Process Verified—This is considered the best, or gold standard, in organic labeling. It is overseen by the government's National Organic Program, which deals with all organic crops, livestock, and agricultural products; these products, in turn, must meet the standards of the USDA. But the label doesn't mean the product is completely organic—the USDA organic seal means that the product has 95 percent or more organic content. This also means that there have been no synthetic fertilizers or sewage sludge applied on the soil, and no irradiation or genetic engineering has been used.

Non-GMO Project Verified—This means that there are no genetically modified organisms (or GMOs; for more about GMOs, see below and the chapter "Controversies in Food and Nutrition") in the plants or animals that are eaten as foodstuff. This project is attempting to preserve the non-GMO food supplies, and is one of the only independent verification groups in North America that deals with GMO avoidance.

Certified Naturally Grown—For smaller farmers, direct market farmers, and beekeepers, one of the best ways to comply with the USDA's requirements is to join the CNG—a nonprofit group that offers a similar certification. Those who are certified do not use synthetic herbicides, pesticides, fertilizers, antibiotics, hormones, or genetically modified organisms. Even though the certification follows the USDA's standards, the farmers cannot call their products organic under this label.

American Grassfed—This is a certification by the American Grassfed Association that promotes the grassfed industry. The standard requirements include that the animals eat only grass and forage from weaning to harvest; that the animals have not been raised in confinement; and that the animals have never been fed growth hormones or antibiotics. (Interestingly enough, the USDA grassfed standards allow the use of such substances in grassfed animals.)

Fair Trade Certified—Fair Trade Certified products include such foods as coffee, tea, herbs, cocoa, fresh produce, sugar, beans, and grains, and the term is usually associated with imports from various countries. The label is usually used on products for which the growers paid their workers a fair wage; and although the foods are usually not certified organic, Fair Trade tries to promote such practices.

When it comes to eggs, is "cage-free" the same as "free-range"?

No, if a hen is cage-free, it is not the same as a hen that is free-range, but it's a way that many egg producers tend to label eggs to entice the public to buy the product. Cage-free means only that the hens were kept not in a cage; in reality, many of these hens are tightly crowded together in a large barn. Free-range means the hens probably did go outside whenever they wanted, but with their food and water usually inside a barn, no one really knows how much time the animal spends outside or inside.

What are genetically modified organisms (GMOs)?

Genetically modified organisms—or GMOs—are those organisms (plants, animals, and other organisms, such as bacteria) in which the codes or organization of the genetic material within the organisms have been changed. This is usually carried out in a laboratory using special techniques that manipulate the DNA of the organisms. The resulting plants, animals, and bacteria (so far) that result from these genetic techniques do not occur in nature. Many of our foods and meats are now labeled with the international symbol for genetically modified foods. (For details and the controversies surrounding GMOs, see the chapter "Controversies with Food, Beverages, and Nutrition.")

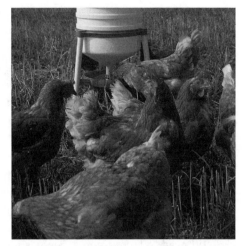

When chicken is labeled "free-range" it means that the birds were allowed to roam outside a barn or cage when they wished to.

NUTRITION, FOOD, AND THE FUTURE

What is the Svalbard Vault?

The Svalbard Global Seed Vault is an underground facility found in Svalbard, Norway. It is located about a half mile from the Longyearbyen Airport, and is part of an ocean archipelago only 621.4 miles (1,000 kilometers) from the North Pole, at about 426.5 feet (130 meters) above sea level. This facility, with its claimed "endless lifetime," is meant to hold plant seeds that represent the genetic diversity of the world's food crops; overall, it can store 4.5 million different seed samples. It has three separate underground chambers, all with a constant interior temperature of –0.4 degrees Fahrenheit (–18 degrees Celsius); because it is located deep in a mountain, if there is a loss of power, the local permafrost would help hold the temperatures low enough for the seeds. Specifically, the vault is meant to contain duplicates of the world's seed collections, in case of war, natural disasters, or simply a lack of resources to grow certain crops. In addition, with the loss of biodiversity on the Earth today, along with global climate change and new plant diseases, the hope is that this vault can essentially "jumpstart" certain lost crops and reestablish them where needed.

Is it more expensive to eat a healthy diet?

In most high-income countries, it is more expensive to eat a healthy diet than an "unhealthy" one (processed foods, meats, and refined grains). In 2013, the Harvard School of Public Health released data that noted, over the course of a year, a diet of fruits, vegetables, fish, and nuts would increase costs for one person by about $550 per year (this is based on 2013 U.S. dollars—and did not include such parameters as droughts or floods in major agricultural regions). Even though the researchers suggested new policies and production changes to increase the availability (and to lower the price) of healthy foods, they also pointed out that compared to the economic costs of diet-related diseases, this increase in the costs for a healthy diet are much, much less.

How much is organic farming predicted to grow in the next 25 years?

According to estimates by many (optimistic) researchers, organic farming will probably grow tenfold in the next two and a half decades. This is because of a new generation of farmers—and consumers—who are not only demanding more control over the foods they eat, but who want to stop agricultural industries' effects on the environment. Major obstacles still need to be overcome, such as more government policies to help small organic farmers, and better access to land and resources.

But not everything is "perfect" in the organic world, and there are other obstacles brought about by the nature of organic farming. For example, rules and regulations regarding organic farming differ between states—and also between countries; some intense organic growing methods put stress on water resources; runoff from the farms can still cause local problems with water supplies; and raising animals for meat or milk often uses up a great deal of land for grazing.

What is global climate change, or as it is more commonly called, "global warming"?

Global climate change (with the unfortunate common label of "global warming") is caused by the rising temperatures around the planet. This is thought to be caused mainly by rising carbon dioxide and other greenhouse gas concentrations; some of the greenhouse gases are natural, but the majority of scientists believe most of the gases are human-made from the burning of fossil fuels and industrial activities.

And some signs of global climate change might already be seen in recent extreme weather events, such as the prolonged droughts in California; more heat waves, such as the heat wave and resulting drought in 2012 in the "American Corn Belt" (central United States); extreme cold, as in the record-breaking cold from polar air masses that covered the northeast during the winter of 2013 to 2014; and heat, as in the excessive heat waves in Europe in the summers of 2003 and 2013.

Does food production emit greenhouse gases that contribute to global climate change?

Yes, how humans produce food can be a significant emitter of greenhouse gases. It also causes some environmental concerns, too, such as using up land for grazing cattle, or cutting down forests for growing crops. Overall, according to the Grantham Research

Institute on Climate Change and the Environment, agriculture alone contributes about 15 percent of all greenhouse gas emissions in the world, which is similar to what transportation adds. If everything about how we produce food is taken into account—such as taking over land or other environmental factors—the percent of emissions may be closer to 30 percent. This means that to feed more than 7 billion people—and more in the future—and to lower carbon emissions, future food production will, like humans, have to change and adapt to a warming global environment.

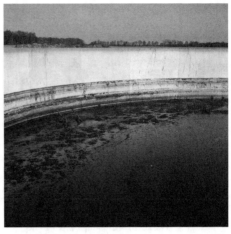

Manure pits like this one have become a smelly side effect of large factory farms. They also emit a lot of methane gas that contributes to global warming.

Do scientists believe that global climate change will affect the world's food chains and/or food webs?

Yes, some scientists believe that future global climate change will definitely affect the world's food chains and food webs, although it may affect pockets of change all over the world, not the entire planet at once. Some debate that even small local changes in certain organisms will create a domino effect, causing food chain and food web changes all over the planet. Either way, increases in sea surface and air temperatures, and changes to ocean circulation resulting from warmer temperatures, will no doubt be a challenge to certain ecosystems—and thus food chains and food webs—around the Earth.

For example, in one recent study, ecologists estimated that as the global temperatures increase, populations of herbivores—important to the human food supply chain—will decrease. In particular, they believe if small organisms in the oceans called zooplankton decrease in numbers with warmer temperatures, there will be less food for fish, and less seafood for humans. Another study in the Arctic showed that the melting and subsequent decline in ice, along with warmer temperatures, has changed vegetation and organisms along and on the Arctic coasts—and thus changed the local marine and land-based (terrestrial) food chains. In particular, they found that larger plankton (small organisms in the upper part of the ocean waters) thrive, replacing the smaller but more nutrient-dense plankton—which may eventually change the marine food web in the region. The loss of ice has also caused many marine animals to change their migration paths, and has opened up new pathways for other marine animals. (For more about food chains and food webs, see the chapter "Nutrition though the Centuries.")

How will global climate change affect our overall food system?

Time will tell how much global climate change will affect our food supplies, but most scientists believe that the location where certain foods will be grown and harvested will definitely change. To date, there is some evidence that climate change has affected the quality and quantity of foods, but it is a small amount when compared to the overall production of food supplies around the world. And so far, there are some reports of small changes—for example, a recent study found that worldwide production of maize and wheat would have been about 5 percent higher in the past few years if it had not been for the effects of climate change.

According to the Union of Concerned Scientists, there are some climate-related threats that will affect our global food systems; for instance, climate change could easily disrupt and destabilize the world's food supplies. They cite a reduction in the yield of some crops because of high temperatures and/or drought-related stress; more water would be needed to irrigate crops, especially in long-term drought areas—water that may not be available; good growing areas may shift north because of warmer temperatures, but the soils (and especially nutrients) in the north may not be conducive to growing certain major crops; and there may be an increase in pests, insect and otherwise, because of warming, which can cause major crop damage.

Will global climate change be bad for all crops?

No, not all changes in the climate will be detrimental to all crops. According to a recent report by the Intergovernmental Panel on Climate Change (IPCC), a rise in global temperatures will also help increase production of some food crops—such as rice, soybean, and wheat—depending on where they are grown. Note that this does not take into account an increase in pests (especially those organisms that affect vegetation), floods, droughts, wildfires, or extreme weather events. The biggest challenge will be not only changes in what grows where, but how and if humans can adapt to such changes.

How many people will have to be fed by 2050?

There are several educated guesses as to the number of people who will live on Earth by the year 2050. By 2015, there will be about 7.5 billion people on the planet. By the year 2050, some experts predict that the population will reach about 12 billion on the planet; according to other researchers, such as the Pew Research Center, a more reasonable number is be closer to 9 billion, as the world's population levels off and even declines, mainly because falling birth rates. Either way, there will be plenty of mouths to feed, and therefore many experts wonder if we will have enough food. As of 2014, there was an estimated 1 billion people undernourished around the world. But it's not only the number of people—there are a few more factors that need to be added to the mix. Will we have enough good land to grow food? Will rising sea levels mean less land to grow foods, but more people demanding food? Will we be able to provide enough food in regions where it is needed, such as those areas with long-term drought conditions? Will transportation of foods around the planet—which means more greenhouse gases in the atmosphere—increase the effects of global climate change? And how we will use our land in the future for food production?

For example, as more countries become wealthier, they usually demand more food. In particular, there is usually more of a disproportionate desire for meat in wealthier countries than in poorer countries. Growing cattle and other animals for meat requires much more land and water resources per calorie consumed—mainly because of the need for grasslands to feed cattle and other "consumable" animals. All these questions and many more—including the necessity of modifying our growing practices for grains, legumes, and other plant-based foods because of changes in our climate—are the challenges humans will face in the future.

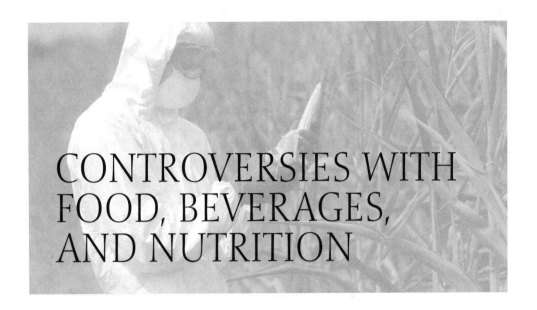

CONTROVERSIES WITH FOOD, BEVERAGES, AND NUTRITION

PROBLEMS WITH ADDITIVES AND DRUGS IN FOOD

What additives have been banned in the past decade?

There have been many food additives that have been banned in the United States and other countries. For example, dye Red #2 is banned in the United States; it is not banned in Canada. Another dye, Red #40, is used in the U.S. to replace the Red #2, and is also used in Canada, but it is banned in much of Europe (Austria, Belgium, Denmark, France, Germany, Norway, Sweden, and Switzerland). The banned-not-banned problem can create a dilemma for those who eat imported foods from all over—and may have an adverse reaction because they are not aware that a particular dye is in the food. (For more about food additives, see the chapter "Modern Nutrition.")

What is BPA and why has it become a concern?

BPA (Bisphenol A) is a plastic additive that is found in some plastic water bottles, and in the inner coating of many food cans . Research has connected this chemical—which mimics the hormone estrogen—with several types of cancer; for example, one recent study showed that a male fetus exposed to the chemical could have an increased risk for prostate cancer later in life. Because of the problems with BPA, many manufacturers are now selling their products without BPA; for the consumer, the best way to stay away from BPA is to avoid the containers that have the chemical—or to look for products that advertise they are "BPA-free."

Is there a controversy concerning farmed fish versus wild-caught fish?

Yes, there is definitely a controversy with farmed fish versus wild-caught fish: Fish farming has always been thought of as the solution to overfishing, but it's not been as suc-

> **Is there a link between childhood obesity and the plastic additive BPA?**
>
> Yes, according to a recent study by the New York University School of Medicine, the plastic additive BPA may be partially to blame for some children's obesity. In particular, the researchers found that children exposed to the most BPA had the highest rates of obesity, even after correcting for several factors, such as how long the children sat and watched television and the average number of calories consumed per day.

cessful as hoped. For example, fish farms are inherently inefficient, having to feed their fish a great deal of other fish; to compare, it takes about 12 pounds of grain to produce a pound of beef, whereas it takes about 70 wild-caught feeder fish to produce one salmon on a fish farm. In addition, many fish farms, in order to keep fish disease in check, will give their fish foods with antibiotics that can eventually reach the consumer's plate; many fish farms raise the fish in a confined area and allow the fish wastes and water to flow unchecked into the ocean, and nearby creeks, streams, and rivers; and for fish that are genetically modified, some can escape into the wild (with many researchers wondering about the consequences in terms of interbreeding or food competition with wild populations).

Thus, most research tends to emphasize the more environmentally sound and better health value of wild-caught fish, with a caveat: The fish should be caught using sustainable practices. But there is another controversy that is much harder to mitigate—or even slow down: Not all people agree with such health and environmentally sound practices, especially those in countries that do not adhere to the practice of sustainability.

What are "indirect" or "accidental" additives?

Some research refers to "indirect additives," or those additives in our food over which we have little or no control. For example, mercury in fish is thought of as an indirect additive (see below); and, much to many people's dismay, sometimes pieces of insects can be in foods such as grains or rice (it's inevitable in some foods, especially those foods grown outside). And in a way, there are also antibiotics in some meats—mainly from the medicines given to cattle, pigs, and other livestock to fight disease—that eventually find their way into our foods.

What types of toxic chemicals are often found in the food chain?

There are numerous toxic chemicals—from the agriculture and manufacturing industries, along with pollution from factories, cars, and other sources—that enter our food chain. A short, but well-known, list includes the heavy metal mercury; PCB (polychlorinated biphenyl), a synthetic, organic chemical compound; mirex (a chlorinated hydrocarbon that has been banned, but was once used as an insecticide); and dioxin (a

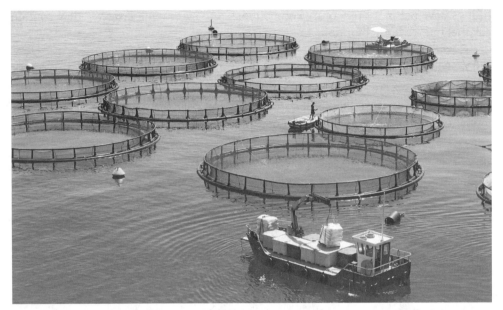

Fish farms were once thought of as an environmentally friendly solution to catching fish in the wild, but they cause concentrated pollution (fish waste) and require a lot of antibiotics to keep the fish healthy.

group of toxic chemical compounds, many of them resulting from incineration, backyard trash burning, and some industrial processes).

Why is there mercury in our food chain—especially in fish?

The majority of this heavy metal in our environment comes from coal-burning electrical plants, some industrial waste, and pesticides. In the case of burning coal, particles enter the atmosphere and eventually make their way (mostly through precipitation) into the oceans, lakes, and rivers; mercury from industrial facilities and pesticides are usually flushed into waterways as waste-water or runoff. Once in the water, the mercury becomes more toxic, as it is converted into methyl mercury by natural bacteria living in the water systems. Fish absorb the methyl mercury through their skin or ingest algae that eat the bacteria, and the heavy metal settles into fishes' fatty layers. Mercury is not like some toxic substances—it does not dissipate, nor is it eliminated from a fish's body after it is absorbed by the fatty tissues. And the amount of mercury in a fish is directly proportional to the size of the fish. Thus, when we catch, fillet, and eat a fish, we are eating that fat—and the methyl mercury it contains.

The eating of fish is not the only way in which we are exposed to this heavy metal—we can either inhale or ingest it. For example, industrial workers are often exposed to the mercury-containing products they manufacture, which can cause major problems if it is an extreme exposure. But there are also some minute amounts we are exposed to each day. For example, some cosmetics contain mercury compounds to kill bacteria; some dental fillings may contain mercury (older fillings may contain mercury; the newer fillings have better, nonmercury compounds); and even some laxatives may contain calomel (mercurous chloride).

What seafoods are thought to have the most amount of mercury?

Probably most sea creatures have some mercury in their bodies, but there are some fish that seem to have more than others. The following chart lists some levels of mercury found in common seafood (from the Food and Drug Administration):

Seafoods with Mercury

Seafood Type	Approximate Mean Amount of Mercury (in parts per million)
Catfish	0.07 ppm
Halibut	0.20 ppm
Lobster	0.30 ppm
Scallop	0.05 ppm
Swordfish	1.00 ppm
Tuna (canned; light)	0.20 ppm
(canned; white)	0.30 ppm
(fresh/frozen)	0.30 ppm

What is the accepted level of mercury that a person can consume?

It is thought that mercury can be harmful to humans when foods containing the heavy metal are ingested in large quantities. For example, many fish products, and even fresh fish, contain mercury. The accepted amount of mercury in our foods, set by the government's Food and Drug Administration, is 0.25 parts per million (and there are special age and sex considerations concerning the amount of mercury ingested; see below). From the chart above, some fish definitely exceed that amount. Overall, it is thought that the average intake of mercury by most people from food is about 0.5 milligrams per day—and toxic symptoms usually are thought to develop when a person ingests around 100 milligrams of mercurous chloride per day.

Are there special FDA warnings about the intake of mercury based on age and/or sex?

Yes, there are suggestions made by the Food and Drug Administration about consumption of foods containing mercury depending on your sex and age. For example, children's intake of foods possibly con-

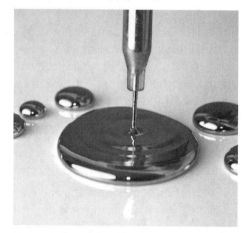

Mercury is the only metallic element that is a liquid at room temperature. It therefore can easily leach into the environment to contaminate rivers, lakes, and oceans.

taining mercury should be monitored, as the metal has been shown to affect a child's developing brain. Plus, it is estimated that about ten percent of the mercury ingested accumulates in the brain—which not only depletes the brain's tissues of zinc, but can also cause nerve and genetic defects.

For women of childbearing age or who are already pregnant, fish that have the higher levels (in parts per million) of mercury, such as swordfish, should be avoided, and the woman should also limit her intake of any type of fish to 12 ounces (340 grams) per week. The reason for these recommendations is based on research, most of which shows that exposure to mercury—even at lower levels—can affect a fetus, especially in terms of neurological and behavioral problems after birth (studies have shown such children are slower to develop and learn). In addition, if a pregnant woman eats fish from certain areas, she should be aware of any government warnings (many times this is listed in brochures or handouts when purchasing a fishing license, or on the Department of Environmental Conservation [DEC] or FDA websites) concerning the consumption of fish from that particular river or stream. For example, according to the New York State Department of Health, women under 50 years of age (or who are pregnant) and children under ten years old, should not eat any fish from almost all of the lakes, rivers, and tributaries in the St. Lawrence Valley region of New York. (To find out about this region, link to the Internet website at www.health. ny.gov/fish, or write in your own state's health department in a search engine.)

What is irradiation of food?

Irradiation is often used to extend the shelf life of various foods; this method exposes the food to x-rays or other forms of radiation, killing off the harmful molds, insects, and bacteria that lead to food decay and spoilage. Fruits are irradiated to keep them fresh longer; vegetables are irradiated to extend the shelf life for such foods as potatoes and onions (so they won't sprout as fast); and meats and seafood are irradiated to kill off harmful bacteria. Foods that are irradiated—either from the United States or other counties—must carry the international symbol.

What are some effects on foods from irradiation?

Overall, some research indicates that irradiation of foods preserves more of the nutrients in fruits, vegetables, and meats, especially niacin, thiamine, and some B-complex vitamins, than do other methods of sterilization. But contrarily, irradiation can also destroy vitamins A, E, and K—or

If you see this symbol on a package it means the food has been preserved using radiation.

the fat-soluble vitamins. In addition, the effects on the food depend on the type of irradiation: there is radiation that merely passes through the food; other types of irradiation use much higher doses to destroy bacteria, and when used on certain meats, the flesh can darken, and fish can become spongy and soft.

Why is irradiation so controversial?

The process of irradiation is extremely controversial. Some environmental, consumer, and health groups object to the idea, because they believe that radiation may create harmful "mutants" in terms of foods. For example, when meats are irradiated, the animal fats create compounds called 2-alkylcyclobutanones, which can break strands of DNA, creating possible conditions such as the growth of cancers in humans. But others disagree, stating that the overall health benefits—not to mention the increase in the availability of foods, because irradiation stops most spoilage—outweigh the possible health risks from potentially harmful "mutant" compounds.

GENETIC MANIPULATION AND FOOD

How long have humans been "genetically modifying" organisms, including foods?

GMOs, or genetically modified organisms, are those organisms in which there is a change in the code or organization of the genetic material. Today, this is done by using techniques in the laboratory, manipulating the DNA of various organisms, including foods and meats. But in a way, the term can also apply to what humans have done for centuries—but not in a laboratory: examples include modifying crops and other edible plants by cross-pollination, crossing various breeds of domesticated animals to obtain a certain characteristic, and even using bacteria to develop various medicines.

What do the abbreviations GMO, GE, and GM stand for in terms of food?

Most of us have seen these abbreviations before—especially in terms of the foods we now buy from the grocery stores. GMO stands for "genetically modified organisms," or organisms with DNA that is genetically modified by specific genetic engineering laboratory techniques, such as gene splitting, and not by natural or traditional crossbreeding methods. GE means "genetically engineered," and is often used in reference to crops. For example, GE seeds were introduced commercially in 1996 are now used in many countries around the world—especially in places that grow corn, soybeans, and cotton. In particular, the main purposes behind GE crops are to withstand the direct application of chemical herbicides or to produce engineered toxins within the plant that kill certain insect pests. GM stands for "genetic modification," and usually refers to food, as in GM foods, which are produced from GMOs.

How was "Flavr Savr tomato" connected to the movement against genetically modified organisms?

The Flavr Savr tomato, also known as CGN-89564-2, was genetically developed in response to consumer complaints that tomatoes were either too rotten to eat when they arrived at the store or too green. Growers had found that they could treat green tomatoes in the warehouse with ethylene, a gas that causes the tomato skin to turn red—but the tomato itself stayed hard.

Genetic engineering of the tomato came in the late 1980s, when researchers discovered that the enzyme polygalactouronase (PG) could control rotting in tomatoes. They reversed the DNA sequence of PG, resulting in tomatoes that turned red on the vine and yet the tomatoes' skins remained tough enough to withstand the mechanical pickers. However, before the Flavr Savr tomato was introduced to the market in the mid-1990s, the company disclosed to the public that the tomato was bioengineered—thus causing a public protest that led to the worldwide movement against genetically modified organisms (GMOs).

What is the difference between a hybrid and a GMO plant?

There is definitely a difference between a hybrid plant and a GMO plant—two very different plants that often cause confusion. For example, when talking about fruits, a hybrid fruit is merely a product of crossbreeding between two similar plants of a related species. This process has been around for centuries—and actually occurs naturally all over the world without humans intervening. When a farmer produces a hybrid fruit, it means that two parent fruit trees are cross-pollinated to create a hybrid fruit tree. This is usually done to take the best-desired qualities of the parent plants and replicate them in the plant's offspring.

On the other hand, genetically modified organisms (GMOs) are done on a much smaller scale—and are the result of combining the DNA molecules from different sources to alter the genes of a plant. This bioengineering is purely human-driven—and results in, for example, a fruit that has some specific characteristic, such as a resistance to a certain insect or to climate elements, such as droughts.

How widespread is the global use of GMO crops?

As of 2002, more than 120 million acres (40 million hectares) of fertile farmland were planted with GMO crops. This in-

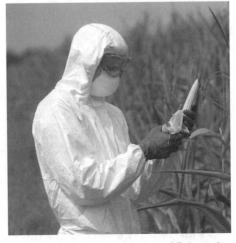

A crop inspector wears protective gear while inspecting GMO foods. Images like this one have caused many people to suspect that GMO foods are unsafe.

cludes mostly four countries: the United States, with 68 percent of the total acreage, Argentina with 22 percent, Canada with 6 percent, and China with 3 percent. And the numbers have increased in the past decade—by 2012, GMO crops grew on over 420 million acres of land in 28 countries worldwide, a record high according to the International Service for the Acquisition of Agri-biotech Applications (ISAAA), an industry trade group. This means that the land devoted to genetically modified crops has increased 100 times since farmers first started growing the crops commercially in 1996. The ISAAA found that these countries have planted and replanted GMO crop seeds on a total of about 3.7 billion acres, or an area 50 percent larger than all of the United States. And to date, the numbers continue to increase.

But not everyone agrees—and there is a total of over 64 countries around the world, including Australia, Japan, and all of the countries in the European Union, that are concerned about the possible health problems with GMO foods. Thus, they have significant restrictions, labeling laws, or outright bans on the production of GMOs—mostly because these foods still have not been proven to be safe.

How widespread is the use of GMO crops in U.S. foods?

The list of GMO crops in U.S. food products seems to grow every year. According to the United States Department of Agriculture, to date, it is estimated that around 93 percent of soy, 93 percent of cotton, and 86 percent of corn grown in the United States have GMOs; and there are also GM varieties of sugar beets, squash, and Hawaiian papaya. It is also estimated that over 90 percent of the canola grown in the U.S. contains products that are genetically modified. And according to estimates, about 75 to 80 percent of processed foods found in the average United States and Canadian grocery stores have GMOs, which are found in such ingredients as corn oil, soy meal, sugar, and corn syrup.

At this time, most of these GM products are required to be labeled as genetically engineered, although there are still some products that don't have to be labeled—but the

What was once called "Frankenfood"?

"Frankenfood" was first used as a term to describe any food that was genetically modified or that contained genetically modified organisms (GMOs). It was the invention of several environmental and health advocacy groups—all of whom wanted to stop the genetic modification of foods for many reasons. They believed that the gene pool of "natural" plants could be altered permanently if exposed to pollen from genetically altered plants; that natural pollinators, such as bees and butterflies, would disappear; and that there would be genetic contamination of seeds from GM plants. There was (and continues to be) a fear that people and animals that consume GM food might have allergic reactions to altered protein—or could develop health problems later.

rules are rapidly changing. Thus, if you are concerned about GMOs, look for the "non-GMO" label on the products you buy.

What are the biggest problems with GMOs?

One of the biggest problems with GMOs is that there is no proof whether they are safe or not, or that they will (or can) cause health problems, not only in humans, but in various species of plants and other animals. In fact, an independent study by Biofortified of GMOs in 2010—a study not funded by the industry—found that there was "no scientific evidence associating GMOs with higher risks for the environment or for food and feed safety than conventional plants and organisms." This was followed by similar comments from the World Health Organization, and the National Academy of Sciences, among others.

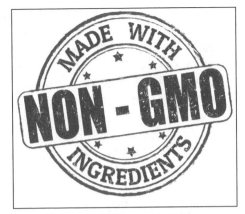

This label clearly indicates that a food item has not been genetically modified.

Another problem involves GMO versus organic crops: There is concern from farmers who use organic methods of growing their crops, because the organic plants can be crossbred with GMO-grown plants. It is not done on purpose, but it mostly occurs through natural means called drift, as the winds, pollinating bees, and birds do not discriminate between both types of plants. In many instances, the organic farmer can reduce the amount of contamination by growing crops a certain distance from GMO crops or use a wide buffer zone between the plants; or organic farmers can plant their seeds earlier than farmers who grow GM crops, so that the plants flower at different times.

Why do many people *like* GMOs?

Reasons in favor of GMOs are obvious: Genetically modified plants, in many cases, can mean an increase in yield, a decrease in disease, and even less of a need for pesticides. And for a third world country or even smaller farms that may have problems with plant disease, droughts, or even insect infestations, such stronger and more resilient plants will feed many more people. In addition, many researchers have been able to produce foods that are more nutritious, such as corn with increased protein, or even rapeseed that can make the resulting canola oil contain more of the healthy unsaturated fatty acids.

MAJOR CONTROVERSIES WITH FOODS

Why is there concern over foods labeled "organic" in terms of consumer perception?

Contrary to what many consumers believe, not all foods labeled "organic" are as healthy (and nonfat) as they may think. In fact, a recent study conducted at Cornell University showed that consumers really believe the organic label means the food is better for health and/or is lower in fat—an example of the "halo effect." In psychology, this is used to describe perceptions: If a person perceives one trait of an object, it can influence the other traits of the object. This idea agrees with some research that shows that if a fast-food eatery claims to serve "healthier" foods, people tend to consume more calories when they eat at that establishment. In the Cornell study, organic-labeled foods benefit from what the researchers called the "health halo," with many consumers buying the product because of the organic label. But not all organic foods are created equal, and the organic label may actually cause consumers to overeat a certain food that can also be higher in fat and calories than the same nonorganic foods.

Does organic milk have more helpful fatty acids than nonorganic milk?

For people who like milk, some research indicates that there are advantages to drinking organic milk over conventional milk. In particular, a recent study found that organic milk may help lessen the risk factors for cardiovascular disease because it is more balanced in both omega-3 and omega-6 fatty acids. The researchers believe that, because organic milk is from dairy cows that eat natural grasses—instead of the usual fare of the corn-based diet (high in omega-6) offered to "nonorganic" cows—organic milk is healthier. This, of course, is debated by many other researchers, especially those who believe that any cow—or animal-based—milk is not healthy for humans. (For more

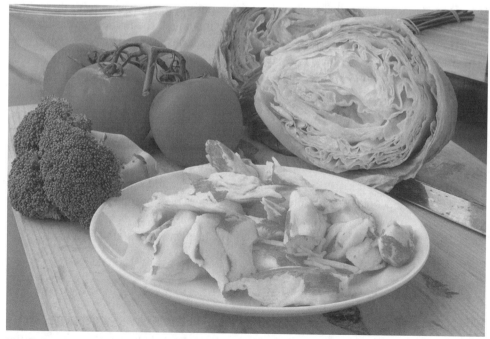

This imitation crabmeat has the texture, flavor, and color of crabmeat but is made from processed white fish such as pollock. It is cheaper than real crab and is low in fat but can have a lot of salt.

about omega-3 and omega-6 fatty acids, see the chapter "The Basics of Nutrition: Macronutrients and Non-nutrients.")

Are simulated (fake) foods nutritious?

Like most foods that are processed, there can be some nutrional benefits, but in most cases, simulated (fake) foods can be high in sugar, fats, sodium, gums, artificial flavors, dyes, and so on. For example, imitation crabmeat is a cheaper "crab," and to most people, tastes the same as real crab. It is made with a ground-up fish (surimi); from there, the producer adds fillers, flavoring (sometimes including sugars and salt), and color to the product to mimic the taste, texture, and color of real crab. In this case, most fake crabmeat is low in fat and calories, but can be extremely high in sodium; most fake crabmeat can contain up to 800 milligrams of sodium or more in a three-ounce serving, and the daily recommendation for sodium is 1,500 to 2,300 milligrams per day.

Other examples include fake cheeses, most of which contain fillers, oils, and emulsifiers (called "processed cheese" by most producers); frozen dairy desserts that have to contain a minimum of 10 percent milk fat, but are also high in corn syrup, gums (like guar gum), whey, and even fake, dehydrated potato flakes that also come with preservatives, emulsifiers, artificial flavorings, and trans fats. In other words, it's best to read the label—or eat real foods that aren't processed if you want the best nutritional value!

Why do some people say cutting back on meat is "good for the environment"?

Just over a decade ago, a trend called "meatless Mondays" began, asking Americans to go without meat one day a week. To date, the trend continues and grows—mainly because there is more and more evidence that eating less meat and more fruits and vegetables helps most people stave off diseases and illness. In fact, it is estimated that a person can cut saturated fat intake by 15 percent just by cutting out meat for one day a week.

But it's not just for our health—many researchers say such a cut is good for the environment, too. For example, growing animals for meat takes an enormous amount of water and grassland. In fact, it is estimated that if all Americans avoided meat and cheese just one day a week for one year, it would be comparable to taking 7.6 million cars off the road.

Do humans produce sodium nitrites?

Yes, although sodium nitrites and nitrates have long been thought to be harmful when eaten in excess—sodium nitrate is used to cure and preserve such processed foods as hot dogs, which converts it to sodium nitrite—our bodies do the same thing. When we ingest natural sodium nitrate from fruits, vegetables, and grains, our digestive processes naturally convert it to sodium nitrite.

Is there arsenic in rice?

Arsenic occurs naturally in our environment; it is a chemical element found in the soil and in rock in many parts of the world. This element is also used in manufacturing, especially in treating wood, and in pesticides, although in many countries, its use has become greatly restricted. Because it has been used in industry and agriculture, it has also become a contaminant—especially in water supplies. Thus, because rice is a very water-intensive crop to grow, arsenic has been detected in many rice products.

In 2012, the FDA came out with a study that examined more than 1,300 samples of rice grain (from white to basmati), rice products (pastas, cereals, etc.), and beverages (beer, rice wine, etc.) to determine the amount of arsenic present, and if there was a cause for concern. Overall, the arsenic ranged from 2.6 to 7.2 micrograms per serving of rice (instant rice was at the low end, while brown rice was at the high end), and 0.1 to 6.6 micrograms of arsenic per serving in the rice products. Accordingly, they determined these levels were not high enough to cause any immediate or short-term health effects.

Why are foods that contain phytoestrogens—mainly soy products—so controversial?

The connection between phytoestrogens and humans—especially people who eat soy products—has long been a highly debated subject. For example, there are those researchers who feel that phytoestrogens may lower testosterone levels in men, and also create problems for those women whose breast tissue is sensitive to estrogen, and so can't defend against certain breast cancer cells—often referred to as estrogen- or hormone-sensitive breast cancers.

Other research indicates that phytoestrogens only weakly mimic the body's natural estrogen, and thus, problems with eating foods that contain phytoestrogens for most people is really not an issue. To date, there is no conclusion and the debates go on, with both camps continuing to do research to support their claims. (For more about phytoestrogens, see the chapter "The Basics of Nutrition: Macronutrients and Non-nutrients"; for more about soy products, see the chapter "Nutrition in Eating and Drinking Choices.")

Why are soy products often called health food?

The connections between eating soy products began when researchers noticed that Asian people who ate soy products as a dietary staple seemed to suffer fewer symptoms of certain diseases. For example, many Asian women who regularly eat soy experience fewer menopausal symptoms; there also appears to be some cardiovascular benefits from eating soy for both males and females.

But many researchers have questioned the soy-health connection—mainly because there is a big difference in the foods Asian and American people eat. In particular, most of the soy sold in the United States is very different from the soy eaten in Asia. Americans eat mostly processed tofu and soy products, including some that have little nutritional value, such as soy chips and ice cream (often referred to as "health-junk-food"); whereas most of the soy eaten in Asia is naturally fermented, such as tempeh, miso, and soy sauce (fermented the "old fashioned" way; for more about this process, see the chapter "Food Preservation and Nutrition"), which retains many of the soy products' valuable nutrients.

Why are soy products in general so controversial?

Besides the phytoestrogens found in soy, these products also contain other controversial elements—especially the nonfermented ones. For example, some studies point to a natural toxin (some call it an antinutrient) in soy—specifically one that inhibits enzymes needed for protein digestion; the controversy is that the same inhibitors are believed by some researchers to have some anticancer benefits. Another study points to a substance that is found in soybeans called haemagglutinin that causes red blood cells to clump; other substances called goitrogens suppress thyroid function. Most nutritionists therefore recommend eating a moderate amount of tofu and other such soy products (nonfermented); but for the best health benefits, choose the fermented soy products, such as tempeh and miso, or even the less processed, high-protein, green soybeans called edamame (usually found as a salted snack, but can be found as frozen [plain] soybeans).

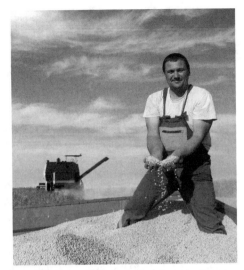

Soy crops have proliferated throughout the United States because soy has so many uses, but some concerns have been raised about natural toxins in the bean.

Why is there a controversy with gluten intolerance?

So far, there is no true reliable test for gluten intolerance, and most of the claims of gluten sensitivity are based on subjective results. This means that many times after a person eats foods containing gluten, he or she notes feelings of bloating or foggy thinking, and then self-diagnose gluten intolerance. One study even estimates that two-thirds of the people who think they are gluten-intolerant are actually not; and many experts note that self-diagnoses is often based on reading about scientific studies in the popular media—research that has few participants and/or no control groups. Other research also indicates that gluten may not even be the problem—but that specific sugars called fructans found in wheat products may be responsible for the symptoms. (For more about gluten intolerance, see the chapter "Nutrition in Allergies, Illnesses, and Diseases.")

Why are omega-3s and omega-6s so controversial in terms of health?

There has been a great deal of debate in the health literature about the benefits—and possible harmful effects—from omega-3s and omega-6s, and the research studies and

271

Do some people think that beans are bad?

Besides the usual reason that some people stay away from beans (flatulence), there are others who believe that beans are bad for one main reason: the amount of lectins, or substances that originally evolved in beans and grains to fight off insect predators. It is know that a portion of the lectin can bind with our body's tissues and create certain problems—especially for genetically susceptible people with autoimmune diseases. (For more about this controversy, see "Appendix 3: Comparing Diets," under "Paleo Diet").

But since the average person is usually not in the genetically susceptible category, most nutritionists advocate eating beans—especially for people who eat a vegetarian diet, or for those people who want to try eating more meatless meals. Most beans not only cost less, but they can help protect you from diabetes, heart attacks, strokes, and even help you to lose weight. Most are filled with antioxidants (such as black beans, lentils, and red kidney beans), and may help prevent LDL cholesterol (the "bad" one) from oxidizing (oxidation of LDL cholesterol is thought to trigger artery-clogging plaque that can lead to heart attacks and stroke). People who eat beans can usually lose weight—mainly because the fiber-like compounds called resistant starch, along with the beans' proteins, may help a person feel full faster (so you eat less) and burn more fat.

their conclusions are often confusing. The following lists only a few of the findings to date (for more about omega-3 and omega-6 fatty acids, see the chapter "The Basics of Nutrition: Macronutrients and Non-nutrients"):

- Some researchers believe it is actually the amounts of both fatty acids that cause health problems—in particular, the Western diet seems to contain too few omega-3s (of any kind) and too many omega-6s (which is high in calories). This imbalance has two major reasons: Most people who eat a Western diet consume too many calorie-rich omega-6s, found in many fast- and processed foods; and second, omega-3 and omega-6 fatty acids compete for the same conversion enzymes in the body, and because of this, researchers believe the quantity of omega-6 in the diet directly affects the conversion of omega-3's alpha-linolenic acid (ALA, found in plant foods) to the long-chain omega-3's eicosapentaenoic acid (EPA) and docosahexaenoic acid (DHA)—both of which protect us from many diseases.

- On the other hand, there are experts who don't believe the ratio of omega-3s to omega-6s is significant, while other researchers believe that the actual health benefits of omega-6s—the fatty acid many say to cut back on in our diets—are being ignored.

- There is also research that says our omega-6 choices are suspect. For example, some omega-6s come from highly refined and processed vegetables oils, such as soybean and corn oils, which removes the "real" omega-6 benefits. In addition, this refinement actually takes away the antioxidants that were once in the oil—making them virtually worthless in terms of health benefits.

- Another study showed that extremely high doses of omega-3's pose health risks such as impairing the body's immune system response to fighting infection, or can increase the effects of inflammatory conditions such as IBD (irritable bowel disease; although it was noted that the researchers pointed to mega-doses of omega-3, which is not what the average person would consume.

- Recent studies show that healthy elderly people taking omega-3 supplements did no better on thinking and verbal skills tests than those taking a placebo. But researchers also admit that omega-3 fats may still help the brain and the heart somehow, but tests need to be done for a longer time.

- Still another study points to the possible connection between the rise in inflammatory diseases and illnesses—such as obesity and metabolic syndrome—and the increase in omega-6 fatty acid consumption. This is because omega-6 is called "pro-inflammatory," while omega-3 is considered to be neutral.

- Overall, more research needs to be done, but for now, most nutritionists recommend moderate consumption of foods containing omega-3s, along with a balance of (or much fewer) foods containing omega-6s.

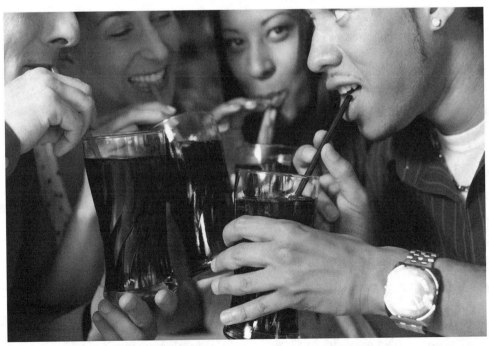

High-fructose corn syrup, which is sometimes fingered for rising rates of diabetes in America, is found in most regular sodas.

Why is the role of carbohydrates in the human diet so highly debated?

The role of carbohydrates in our diet is a hotly debated subject—with issues ranging from eating low to no carbohydrates to eating a seemingly excessive amount. The reason is clear: Many popular diets, especially a low-carbohydrate diet, propose that the only way to lose weight is to eliminate carbohydrates. And because of such "trend" diets, for many people, the word "carbohydrate" has taken on an inherently bad meaning. But there seems to be more of a case for the other side: Carbohydrates are fuel for the brain, nervous system, muscles, and various organs; in fact, they are more high-quality fuels than fats and proteins—mainly because it takes little for the body to break them down and release their energy. Thus, the body metabolizes these simple carbohydrates (sugar) and starches into glucose (blood sugar), which becomes the body's primary fuel sources—as long as they are eaten in moderation.

Fiber, another form of carbohydrate, has the most major health benefits. For example, whole grains are important for reducing the risk for colon cancer and keeping the body's digestive tract in good working order. Many long-term studies have shown that a diet with the most whole grains and cereal fibers—especially nutrient-rich grains and fibers that are less milled or processed—can provide protection from diabetes, certain cancers, and heart disease. (For more about carbohydrates, see the chapter "The Basics of Nutrition: Macronutrients and Non-nutrients.")

How much sugar is too much?

Sugar consumption—no matter what the type—is yet another one of those hotly debated subjects when it comes to nutrition and our health. One study conducted by the Food and Nutrition Board, Institute of Medicine of the National Academies concluded that there is no scientific evidence that any level of sugars increases the risk for dental cavities, changes in behavior, cancer, obesity, and high cholesterol. This was, of course,

Why is high-fructose corn syrup so controversial?

High-fructose corn syrup is formed by changing the simple sugar glucose into another simple sugar called fructose. The combination of the two sugars is cheap to produce, and acts as a preservative to extend the shelf life of many sweets and baked goods. Unfortunately, cheap as it is to make, it is high in calories and low in nutrition; and because it is in so many beverages and processed foods, it is also linked to obesity. But not everyone agrees; for example, the Mayo Clinic notes that there is "insufficient evidence to say that high-fructose corn syrup is less healthy than any other type of sweetener." But it does add that any added sugar, not just high-fructose corn syrup, can contribute many unnecessary calories that are linked to health problems such as weight gain, type 2 diabetes, and metabolic syndrome—all of which increase your risk for heart disease, too.

countered by the World Health Organization (WHO) and the Food and Agriculture Organization of the United Nations (FAO); they stated that sugar leads to obesity, especially when it replaces other more nutritious foods in the diet, and that sugar definitely does cause dental problems. More recent studies seem to agree. For most people, the intake of sugar affects us on an individual basis. What is a good intake for one person may lead to obesity in another—and thus, the debate continues. (For more about natural sugars, see "The Basics of Nutrition: Macronutrients and Non-nutrients"; and for more about obesity, see "Nutrition and Allergies, Illnesses, and Diseases.")

Why is sugar so controversial when it comes to our modern foods?

Various types of sugars have been used for centuries—for example, refined sugar has been widely available since the 1500s—usually to flavor or to preserve certain foods. But in the past half century, the use of sugars for flavoring in various food products has increased, mainly because sugar from sugar cane, beets, and corn is very cheap to produce. This is also why many health-care professionals believe obesity is on the rise—especially in Western and industrialized countries. In general, most doctors and nutritionists suggest that the average adult (excluding those people with such diseases as diabetes) make sugars be less than 10 percent of their daily calories (according to the World Health Organization)—a great deal less than most of us consume.

And there is a good reason: Although many of us think we're cutting back on sugar, recent research has shown that the food industry is hiding more and more sugar in certain foods we eat. For example—and keep in mind that a teaspoon of sugar is equal to about 4 grams—if you drink a Starbucks® caramel Frappuccino® with skim milk, and whipped cream, you are consuming 44.4 grams of sugar per serving (serving size is "tall," or small; this is equal to about 11 teaspoons of sugar); Ragu® tomato and basil pasta sauce has 13.8 grams of sugar per serving (a 200-gram serving size; equal to about 3 teaspoons of sugar); Heinz® tomato ketchup has 4 grams of sugar per serving (serving size of 15 milliliters; equal to about 1 teaspoon of sugar). Even some nonfat yogurts, with flavoring, have the equivalent of 5 teaspoons of sugar.

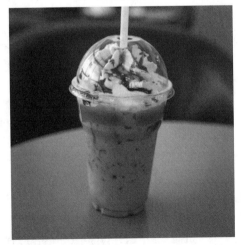

Why are artificial sweeteners so controversial?

Artificial sweeteners are added to many foods, providing a sweet taste without the calories. But there are concerns—especially for people who consume large quantities of the artificial sweeteners, or have allergies or severe reactions after ingest-

Sugary coffee drinks popular at coffee stores and fast food chains are incredibly high in sugar and fat calories.

ing certain sweeteners. For example, the artificial sweetener aspartame often gives susceptible people a headache about 10 to 20 minutes after it is consumed; even more of a concern is, although rare, the triggering of seizures in epileptics who ingest aspartame. (For more about artificial sweeteners, see the chapter "The Basics of Nutrition: Macronutrients and Non-nutrients.")

PROBLEMS WITH BEVERAGES

What are some major concerns surrounding cow's milk?

There are several major concerns surrounding the consumption of cow's milk (for more about milk, see the chapter "Nutrition in Eating and Drinking Choices"). One concern is that cows are injected with recombinant bovine growth hormone, or rBGH (for more about rBGH, see below), along with the antibiotics, steroids, and pesticides included in their feed. Another (highly debated) concern comes from how much milk we consume—with some researchers saying that the recommended three to four servings of dairy per day is too much; while others say that milk is a good source of protein, is usually fortified with necessary vitamin D, and is thought to be a beneficial source of calcium for strong bones and teeth—not to mention it may lower the risk for high blood pressure and colon cancer.

Still another concern about drinking milk is that many people are lactose intolerant—they do not have enough of the enzyme in their digestive tracts to break down the milk sugar (lactose). Many people are unaware they have such an intolerance—but to those who are lactose intolerant and know it, drinking most milk or milk products is not even an option. (For more about lactose intolerance, see the chapter "Nutrition and Allergies, Illnesses, and Diseases.")

What is the controversy surrounding bovine growth hormone, or rBGH?

The recombinant bovine growth hormone (rBGH), or recombinant bovine somatotropin (rBST), is a genetically engineered hormone—one of the earliest applications of genetic engineering that made its way into our foods. It was initially developed to increase the milk production of lactating cows; when injected into the cows, the rBGH resulted in a 20 percent increase in milk production—thus, farmers were able to avoid fluctuations in the amount of milk produced by their cows. Although this was good news to the farmer, the controversy over the genetically engineered hormone grew. Consumers became concerned because the hormone can be detected in the milk we drink, and no one knows the effects of such a hormone on the human body, especially infants who drink the milk. (In fact, the FDA recently stated that there is apparently no significant difference between rBGH and non-rBGH milk, and no test so far can distinguish between either milks—but this is highly debated.)

Other people were concerned about the cows that are given rBGH, because the animals would then produce more milk than they normally would, making many of them more susceptible to diseases. And there was yet another problem—if a cow became ill, it was fed antibiotics, and there was a concern that those medicines were passed on to the humans who consumed the milk (see below). Still another claim is that the hormone stimulates another hormone called insulin-like growth factor-1, or IGF-1—which promotes cell division, and is, in this instance, possibly an impetus for cancer growth in humans who consume the rBGH milk.

What is the controversy over antibiotics in our milk and meats?

Most people associate antibiotics with an infection in their system, usually prescribed by doctors. But antibiotics are also given to many animals to prevent infection—and some of those animals are consumed by people, or the animals' milk is ingested. Thus, the controversy: Just how much of the antibiotics from the consumed animals do we ingest—and what are the consequences to humans if we do ingest these antibiotics?

Antibiotics were first given to healthy animals—a "subtherapeutic" dose—which caused the animal to grow faster and fatter. But there were concerns, especially that humans were ingesting unnecessary antibiotics. Several health-care organizations became concerned about overdosing humans with the drugs; but to date, most research has found that there is no direct effect on people who eat such meat. But the real problem started later, as researchers realized that the bacteria the antibiotics fought against were becoming more resistant to the drugs. Ingesting antibiotics from animals, along with the overprescribing of these drugs to humans, has caused (and continues to cause) antibiotics to become less and less effective against fighting off many human infections and diseases. And this, in turn, has caused many food manufacturers to ban the use of antibiotics, subtherapeutic or not.

What are some controversies over fast foods?

There have been many controversies over fast foods, or those foods sold at restaurants that serve your meal more rapidly than a "regular" restaurant. According to the Harvard Medical School, fast food, and even restaurant food, is often heavy on fat and sugar; if eaten in excess, such foods can lead to potential weight gain and the development of some chronic diseases, such as obesity, heart disease, and diabetes for adults.

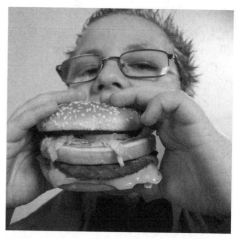

Modern American children too frequently dine on fast foods because parents find themselves too busy to fix dinner at home. The trend is another factor blamed for obesity in young people.

But much of the controversies with fast foods have to do with the effects of such foods on children. For example, in 2013, a study found that there may be a good reason why obesity has become a concern for teenagers and children: Many children and teens consume more calories in fast food and other restaurants than they do at home. For younger children, that can mean about 160 extra calories daily, and for teens, as many as 310 calories a day. In yet another study, 500,000 kids from 31 countries in two age groups were surveyed, representing ages 6 to 7 and ages 13 to 14. In both groups, the children who ate fast food three times a week or more had increased risks of asthma, rhinitis, and eczema; for example, there was as much as a 39 percent increase in severe asthma risk for teens and 27 percent for younger children (in this case, many of the health issues cleared up when the children and teens ate more fruits and vegetables per day).

What are the top ten sources of calories in the United States diet?

According to the USDA Center for Nutrition Policy and Promotion's Dietary Guidelines Advisory Committee—a panel of nutrition experts that help develop the federal nutrition standards—people in the United States don't always consume what the dietary guidelines recommend. Instead of concentrating on a daily diet that contains plenty of vegetables, legumes, fruits, and whole grains, many Americans reach for foods filled with refined grains, sugar, fat, and calories. The following (source: Report of the 2010 Dietary Guidelines Advisory Committee) lists ten of the top sources of calories for most Americans—both food and beverages:

1. Grain-based deserts, such as cakes, donuts, cookies, crisps, and granola bars
2. Yeast breads
3. Chicken and dishes that contain chicken mixed with other foods
4. Soda and energy and sports drinks
5. Pizza

6. Alcoholic beverages

7. Pasta dishes

8. Mexican mixed dishes

9. Beef and dishes that contain beef mixed with other foods

10. Dairy desserts

What are some controversies with the so-called "energy drinks"?

Energy drinks are beverages that boast that they boost your energy levels, improve your mental performance, and even aid in weight loss. They are high in caffeine, sugars (varying in the types of sweeteners), and herbal compounds (presented as supplements). And because they claim to be dietary supplements, the FDA does not regulate the safety of the ingredients, meaning the manufacturers are responsible—which is the first major controversy with "energy drinks."

Another controversy stems from the ingredients in the drinks, and their effects on our system. For example, the Society for Cardiovascular Angiography and Interventions notes that, in adults, the high amount of caffeine in energy drinks can alter a person's activities and mood, and can even become addictive; a dose of caffeine can cause heart palpitations, and increase blood pressure and heart rate; and can also be toxic—even fatal—at higher concentrations. This also leads to the next controversy, the consumption of energy drinks by children and adolescents, with most health-care professionals saying children and teens should not drink such beverages.

WATER CONTROVERSIES

Is our drinking water safe?

One of the major debates in the past few decades has been the safety of our drinking water. In general, the United States has some of the world's safest and most reliable water supplies (of course, this depends on where you live in the country). But as more contaminants enter our water supplies, and an increase in population raises the demand for more water, some of that "pure" water will carry waterborne illnesses, heavy metal contamination, and toxic runoff from farms, industry, and even nuclear power plants. (For more about water and our health, see the chapter "The Basics of Nutrition: Macronutrients and Non-nutrients.")

How much arsenic is allowed in our drinking water?

According to the Environmental Protection Agency (EPA), arsenic is a semi-metal element in the periodic table that is odorless and tasteless. It enters our drinking water supplies from natural deposits in the earth, or from agricultural and industrial practices.   There is a set arsenic standard for drinking water, 0.010 parts per million (or 10 parts per billion) to protect consumers served by public water systems from the effects of long-term, chronic exposure to arsenic. This water standard was put into effect in 2006, with all water systems around the country complying to protect the U.S. water supplies.

What are some harmful contaminants found in drinking water?

The following chart lists some of the major contaminants that often affect our drinking water supplies:

Contaminants in Drinking Water

Contaminant	Source and Possible Health Consequences
Chlorine	Chlorine is added to our drinking water to destroy some disease-causing bacteria. But it can combine with other organic components to form some harmful byproducts, including trihalomethanes, which are linked to an increased risk for certain cancers (especially bladder and colon cancers).
Lead	Lead is mostly a problem in water that travels through holding tanks and pipes in your home; this toxic heavy metal can build up over time, damaging organs and blood cells; hot water tends to hold more lead than cold water.
Arsenic	Usually from agriculture or industrial processes, and includes runoff from those activities; noncancer effects can include thickening and discoloration of the skin, stomach pain, nausea, vomiting; diarrhea; numbness in hands and feet; partial paralysis; and blindness; it has been linked to cancer of the bladder, lungs, skin, kidney, nasal passages, liver, and prostate.
Parasites	There are a multitude of parasites, including bacteria, viruses, protists, or other microorganisms; parasites in water can cause many gastrointestinal diseases. For example, if the parasite *Giardia lamblia* gets into the water supply via sewage or animal waste, and even if a small amount is ingested, it can cause diarrhea, dehydration, and vomiting.

Is a home filter system necessary?

One of the major debates in the past few decades has been the safety of our drinking water—and that includes whether to filter our water or not. Most drinking water, depending on where you live, is safe, especially in the United States. But if you have a question, experts suggest you contact your local public health agency and ask for information on contaminant levels in your drinking water. For people who have wells, there are county extensions and state agencies that can help you, usually for a nominal fee, to check out your water for contaminants. If you believe your water might be contaminated—or you just want it to taste better—you can buy a water filtration system for the home. Just make sure you chose a filter system that can effectively remove any specific contaminants. One of the best sites to check is the NSF International in Ann Arbor, Michigan (www.nsf.org, under "Consumer Resources"), a nonprofit agency that works closely

with the U.S. and Canadian governments to set water standards for many areas—including the use of water filter systems. (For more about water, see the chapter "Nutrition in Eating and Drinking Choices.")

Why is the addition of fluoride to our potable water supplies so controversial?

The addition of fluoride to our water supplies—especially in cities and towns (but not usually in rural areas where wells are used) is called fluoridation—and has been controversial for over 50 years. The initial addition of fluoride in the water was done to combat dental cavities: adding such minute amounts was thought to help fight against tooth decay, with some studies showing that there could be fewer cavities in places with fluoride than places without fluoride. The amounts are very minute— one part fluoride for every 1 million parts of water (or 1 ppm, parts per million; it is known that 2 parts per million is toxic) is all that is needed to reduce cavities by up to 40 percent.

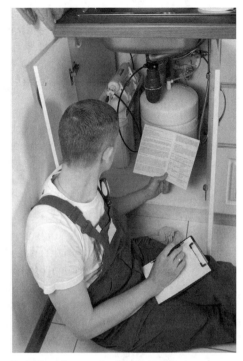

Installing a home water filtering system is one way to ease concerns about drinking tap water, but federal water guidelines—especially for city water— help ensure that water supplies are safe.

Although the scientific consensus is that water fluoridation is absolutely safe and extremely effective, there is still controversy, especially regarding the effects of the fluoride on the public health. And even though over twenty different countries have fluoridation and there have been hundreds of studies, there are still people who point to children, saying that the effects on youngsters are greater than adults. But so far, there have been few studies that can actually prove that there is a connection between any disease or illness and fluoride in the water.

MAJOR PROBLEMS WITH NUTRIENTS

What is the biggest problem that needs to be researched when it comes to nutrients and food?

The biggest question with nutrients and food is obvious: Just how many nutrients are truly in the foods—especially fruits and vegetables—we eat? One problem is that there are very few research studies that combine findings regarding all the nutrients, food, and the various conditions that foods are exposed to—from fresh from the fields to your mouth. For example, a great deal of research has been done on the vitamin C content of various vegetables under certain storage conditions, but little has been done on the availability or loss of vitamin B in stored vegetables over time.

Why is geography a problem when it comes to fresh fruits, vegetables, and their nutrient values?

A big problem with fresh fruits and vegetables and their respective nutrients deals with geography—in other words, where the produce is grown and where you live. There is a great demand for certain fruits and vegetables, especially for people who live in the north during the colder, non-vegetable-producing winter months. And some research has shown that some fruits and vegetables transported longer distances to the market often have fewer healthy nutrients.

For example, if a vegetable such as spinach is being transported from California to New York, and is kept at a warmer temperature in a shipping truck for a few days, by the time a person buys the vegetable from the store, cooks it, or just chops it up for a salad, most of the nutrients may be gone. Not all vegetables suffer this fate, but many of them do. Research also shows that even if the food is kept at temperatures closer to that of a refrigerator (around 39 to 40 degrees Fahrenheit [3.9 to 4.4 degrees Celsius]), it will still lose some nutrients as it travels across country to your plate.

How much of the food in the United States is imported?

To date, it is thought that almost a quarter of the average American's foods are imported. For example, many of the processed foods usually have at least one ingredient from China; fruits and vegetables often come from South America or Mexico; seafood, and many canned or frozen fruits and vegetables often come from Asian counties, such as China, Thailand, and Vietnam. The reason for this move from growing our own foods to imports is obvious: Many food companies cut costs by using foods and ingredients from emerging countries such as China where labor is cheap.

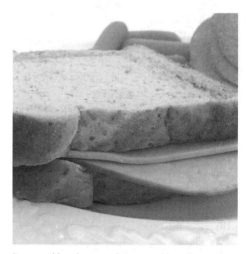

Why are processed foods such a concern to our nutrition?

Although many processed foods are fortified with vitamins, minerals, and other nutrients, a diet that consists of all processed foods is a concern to many nutritionists. In particular, the "replacement nutrients" are in the food artificially—and, in many

Processed lunch meat, cheeses, and breads may be a problem because the nutrients are added artificially, rather than naturally occuring. Such nutrients are not as easily absorbed by the body.

cases, these nutrients are not as easily absorbed into our systems as the natural nutrients found in fresh meats, fruits, and vegetables.

But your consumption of processed foods can be balanced. According to the Academy of Nutrition and Dietetics, "processed" foods can mean anything you process in your own food processor to packaged frozen pizza. And although some processed foods are not too bad for you (such as canned beans, vegetables, etc.), the Academy cautions against consuming too many of the heavier processed foods. In particular, it warns consumers who do buy processed foods to be aware of what is listed on the food label, and especially how much—such as sugars (added as a sweetener to everything from ice cream to pasta sauce, but also for such things as browning breads), fats (for flavor and to make the food last longer on the shelf), and sodium (for almost all foods, for enhanced flavor and as a preservative). Too much of any of these ingredients can add on the weight that can eventually lead to certain chronic diseases.

PROBLEMS WITH SUPPLEMENTS

What is an ORAC score?

ORAC stands for Oxygen Radical Absorbance Capacity—or an analysis used to measure the total antioxidant power of certain foods and chemicals. Some researchers claim that the higher the ORAC score, the more the antioxidant potential of the fruit, vegetable, or chemical. For example, the following chart gives some ORAC scores for various fruits and vegetables (measured for 3.5 ounces [100 milliliters] of food):

Sample ORAC Scores

Fruit or Vegetable	ORAC Score
Prunes	5,770
Raisins	2,830
Blueberries	2,400
Strawberries	1,540
Raspberries	1,220
Oranges	750
Kale	1,770
Spinach	1,260
Brussels sprouts	980
Broccoli	890

Why are ORAC scores so controversial?

There is a great deal of controversy surrounding ORAC scores. According to a 2010 report by the U.S. Department of Agriculture's Nutrient Data Laboratory, there is mounting evidence that "the values indicating antioxidant capacity have no relevance to the effects of specific bioactive compounds, including polyphenols, on human health." The main concern of the USDA is that ORAC scores are misused by food and dietary supplement companies to promote their products—and through advertising and erroneous statements, people believe such claims.

There are many reasons for questioning the validity of ORAC scores. For example, no one really agrees on how to measure antioxidant capacity in foods—in fact, there is no single method that measures the "total antioxidant activity" in any food. In addition, there are a number of compounds that are thought to have a role in preventing or helping improve the effects of certain diseases, but too much is still unknown about the body's associated metabolic pathways to determine their connection to antioxidants and human health. And still yet another reason is that most of the ORAC studies are carried out in test tubes in a laboratory, with little "human evidence" that higher ORAC scores truly prevent disease.

Is it really necessary to take vitamin and mineral supplements?

Although many people do need to take vitamin and mineral supplements to augment their nutritional needs—especially if they have certain diseases or illnesses—the number of people who take such supplements, and don't really need them, alarms many doctors and researchers. Many people who are "too busy to eat well" and/or believe they are deficient in micronutrients, believe the imbalance can be offset through vitamin and mineral supplements—instead of taking the time to eat a balanced diet rich in nutrients. And most of the time, it is done without asking the advice of their doctor.

Thus, taking supplements will continue to be a debated subject, mainly because of advertisements that convince people they can cure something "just by taking a pill." In addition, many people follow supplement trends (especially by unsubstantiated information on the Internet)—and some of those "health promises" may actually be harmful to their health. Almost all health experts agree that micronutrients obtained from foods are always better, as foods contain other compounds that your body needs—most of which are absent in pill formulations.

How many people are on supplements in the United States?

It is estimated that in the United States, about half of adults regularly take dietary supplements—and less than one quarter of those people take the supplements based on their doctor's recommendation. The most common supplement taken is multivitamins; the second most consumed is calcium, followed by omega-3 fatty acids. Supplement purchases rank among the most expensive items that consumers buy. In fact, worldwide sales to date are over $70 billion per year.

What is the best way to obtain micronutrients?

Although this is still a hotly debated subject, almost all research indicates that micronutrients obtained from food are always better than those from pills. Most nutrition experts also argue that people need only the recommended daily allowance, or RDA—in other words, the amount of vitamins and minerals we get from eating a well-balanced, routine diet.

Should vegetarians take vitamin supplements?

The answer to this question depends on the person—especially what he or she decides to eat or has any health issues that need special supplements. If you eat eggs and dairy products (a lacto-ovo vegetarian), along with fermented soybean products, many doctors say that there is no reason to take vitamin supplements (as long as you eat enough and your diet is balanced). If you are strictly a vegan, some doctors recommend taking B_{12} supplements. But, overall, if you're a healthy vegetarian or vegan and eat a balanced diet of nutrient-rich foods, you won't need to take supplements.

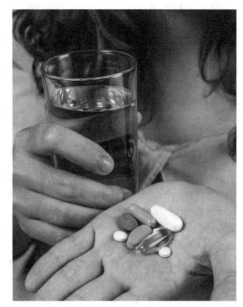

It's always best to get vitamins from natural foods. Vitamin pills might help, but taking too many vitamins is a waste because your body can absorb only so much.

If you take vitamin supplements and then stop, does that lead to a vitamin deficiency?

No, if you take vitamin supplements and then stop, your body does not have an increased demand for the vitamins. In fact, any excess of certain vitamins, such as vitamins A and C, is excreted in the urine. If you stop taking supplements, the body takes in those vitamins naturally—from the foods you ingest—which is actually better for you in the long run than taking supplements.

What have studies revealed about taking certain supplements?

There are many—albeit controversial—studies that deal with health problems in people who take certain nutritional supplements. For example, in 1996, *The New England Journal of Medicine* published a study of 18,000 people who were at an increased risk for lung cancer, mainly because of smoking or being exposed to asbestos. All the participants received a combination of vitamin A and beta carotene, or a placebo (a pill with "nothing" in it); the study was stopped when researchers found that, for those who took the vitamins, the risk for death from lung cancer was about 46 percent higher. An even more recent example was in *The Journal of the American Medical Association* in 2011: it tied vitamin E supplements to an increased risk for prostate cancer in men.

What is the connection between large doses of supplements, antioxidants, and free radicals?

Many researchers believe that the connection between taking supplements and the advent of some disease in people (who take large doses of supplements) has to do with antioxidants (for more about antioxidants, see the chapter "The Basics of Nutrition: Macronutrients and Non-nutrients"). In general, when the body converts food to energy in our cell's organelles called mitochondria, the process needs oxygen (called oxidation). When this occurs, it also produces what are called free radicals that can damage DNA, the lining of arteries, and even the cells' membranes. In fact, free radicals are the reason why we age—and often why we have a propensity toward cancers and heart disease; on the positive side, we also need some free radicals to kill off bacteria and eliminate cancer cells.

There are people who take large doses of supplements thinking that those vitamins will make them healthier and able to fight off free radicals better than good foods—but this does not happen. In fact, researchers have shown that people who take large doses of supplements actually upset the balance of "good and bad" free radicals, weakening the immune system enough so harmful invaders are not killed off, in what researchers call the "antioxidant paradox." Thus, if you're a healthy person, and you eat a balanced cross-section of nutrient-rich foods, not only will your body produce free-radical-fighting antioxidants, but the good food you eat also carries antioxidants to combat free radicals—and keep them both in balance.

If large doses of vitamins can increase the risk for some diseases, why doesn't the U.S. government control vitamin supplements?

The U.S. government, in particular the Food and Drug Administration, does not regulate the sale of megavitamins that are often offered in magazines, newspapers, and on the Internet. The reason goes back to the late 1970s, when the FDA, concerned that people were consuming larger quantities of vitamins, announced a plan to regulate supplements that contained more than 150 percent of the recommended daily allowance (RDA). Because the vitamin industry would have to show that megavitamins were safe before they were sold to the public, they lobbied to prevent the FDA from such regulations. Even though supporters of the bill showed that taking large quantities of vitamins was not natural—and little was known at that time of the health risks—the bill was defeated. Thus, since that time, megavitamins are still sold without regulation, much to the concern of many physicians, health researchers, and nutritionists.

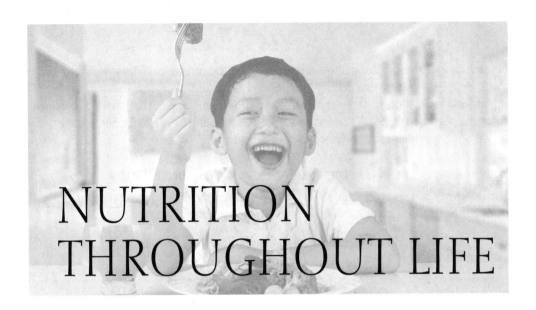

NUTRITION THROUGHOUT LIFE

GENERAL NUTRITION

What are some general nutritional requirements for all humans?

This is one of the most difficult questions to answer—mainly because every human is unique in terms of physical and chemical makeup. That being said, there are some "average" nutrients everyone should be aware of, and whether you ingest them should be between you and your health-care provider. A comprehensive list of just how much of each nutrient you should be getting for your age and sex can be found at the website sponsored by the government's Office of Dietary Supplements at http://ods.od.nih.gov.

What are the various government centers that watch our foods?

There are several watchdog agencies that keep track of the safety of our foods. For example, the Center for Food Safety and Applied Nutrition, known as CFSAN, is one of six product-oriented centers (with some nationwide field forces) that carry out some of the tasks of the Food and Drug Administration (FDA). Overall, the FDA is a scientific regulatory agency responsible for the safety of the nation's domestically produced and imported foods, cosmetics, drugs, biologics, medical devices, and radiological products.

How does the government help us eat healthier?

It may seem confusing (and it often is a bit difficult to follow), but the government uses several ways to convey to us what it thinks are the best amounts and the most nutritious foods to eat, depending on age, sex, and health. For example, the recommended intakes of nutrients vary by age and sex and are known as Recommended Dietary Allowances (RDAs) and Adequate Intakes (AIs); and one value for each nutrient, known as the Daily Value (DV), is selected for the labels of dietary supplements and foods. A DV is often, but not always, similar to a person's RDA or AI for that nutrient. DVs were developed by the FDA to help consumers determine the level of various nutrients in a standard serving of food in relation to their approximate requirement for it. The label actually provides the percent DV (%DV) so that you can see how much (or what percentage) of a serving of a specific product contributes to reaching the DV.

What is an example of a Recommended Dietary Allowance (RDA)?

The following table is an example of an RDA (Recommended Dietary Allowance) for iron from the National Institutes of Health website, from birth to adult:

Recommended Dietary Allowances (RDAs) for Iron

Age	Male	Female
Birth to 6 months	0.27 mg*	0.27 mg*
7–12 months	11 mg	11 mg
1–3 years	7 mg	7 mg
4–8 years	10 mg	10 mg
9–13 years	8 mg	8 mg
14–18 years	11 mg	15 mg
19–50 years	8 mg	18 mg
> 51 years	8 mg	8 mg

*Adequate Intake (AI)

What is an example of a Daily Value?

There are many examples of a Daily Value on the government site. The following chart gives an example of a Daily Value based on a caloric intake of 2,000 calories for adults and children older than four years old:

Daily Value Examples

Food Component	Daily Value
Total Fat	65 grams (g)
Saturated Fat	20 g
Cholesterol	300 milligrams (mg)
Sodium	2,400 mg
Potassium	3,500 mg
Total Carbohydrate	300 g
Dietary Fiber	25 g
Protein	50 g
Vitamin A	5,000 International Units (IU)
Vitamin C	60 mg
Calcium	1,000 mg
Iron	18 mg
Vitamin D	400 IU
Vitamin E	30 IU

Daily Value Examples

Food Component	Daily Value
Vitamin K	80 micrograms µg
Thiamin	1.5 mg
Riboflavin	1.7 mg
Niacin	20 mg
Vitamin B$_6$	2 mg
Folate	400 µg
Vitamin B$_{12}$	6 µg
Biotin	300 µg
Pantothenic acid	10 mg
Phosphorus	1,000 mg
Iodine	150 µg
Magnesium	400 mg
Zinc	15 mg
Selenium	70 µg
Copper	2 mg
Manganese	2 mg
Chromium	120 µg
Molybdenum	75 µg
Chloride	3,400 mg

The nutrients in the table above are listed in the order in which they are required to appear on a label.

What is a Dietary Reference Intake?

The Dietary Reference Intake (DRI) is the standard for nutrient intakes in the United States, including recommendations for energy, vitamins, minerals, proteins, amino acids, carbohydrates, fats, water, and electrolytes for each sex and different stages of life. The list of the various dietary reference intakes depending on age and sex is long, and can be found at http://iom.edu/Activities/Nutrition/SummaryDRIs.

How do you choose a vitamin and mineral supplement?

There are many ways to choose a vitamin and mineral supplement, if you and your doctor decide you need to take them. Your health-care provider may help you choose the right supplement, or he or she may recommend a nutritionist who can guide you. And there are general charts suggesting amounts of supplements a person can take if necessary; for example, the USDA offers the Daily Reference Intake (DRI) charts, based on the vitamin and mineral, and a person's stage of life, found at the site http://fnic.nal.usda.gov/ dietary-guidance/dietary-reference-intakes/dri-tables.

Can you ingest too many vitamins and minerals?

Yes, you can ingest too many vitamins or minerals; but if you're concerned about your nutrient intake, there is a way to tell safe upper limits of certain vitamins and minerals (and, of course, always check with your doctor before taking any vitamin and mineral supplements).

In particular, there is a list of Tolerable Upper Intake Levels (ULs), first established in 1997 by the United States Institute of Medicine (IOM). This list shows, according to the IOM, "the highest level of daily nutrient intake likely to pose no risk for adverse health effects for almost all individuals in the general population." Because of this claim, many other countries use this data to educate the general population about ULs.

Which vitamins does a woman need more than a man?

An adult woman should consume certain vitamins more than an adult man—and vice versa—and there are too many to mention here. But there are some common ones; for example, according to the Institute of Medicine, men and women have the same basic requirements for calcium and vitamins D, E, and B_{12}, and women who are pregnant or nursing need extra amounts of these (and other) vitamins and minerals. Men need a little more vitamin C than women (90 milligrams for men each day versus 75 milligrams for women); and premenopausal women need more iron (18 mg for women versus 8 mg for men). For postmenopausal women, the iron quota is the same as for men—8 milligrams for both.

What is malabsorption?

Malabsorption is when the body fails to completely absorb nutrients—predominantly certain sugars, fats, proteins, or vitamins from food—in the gastrointestinal tract, leading to many health complications. It can be caused by a huge list of mild to severe problems, with estimates of two hundred causes or more—from interference by medications to genetic predisposition. Researchers divide malabsorption into selective (such as the inability to process lactose [milk sugar] in milk, or lactose intolerance); partial (such as an inherited disorder that causes a problem with absorption of fats or fat-soluble vitamins); or total (as with celiac disease). Some causes can also be from a specific disorder; for example, iron-deficiency anemia is the inability to absorb iron in the small intestines—and can be caused by celiac disease, of malabsorption.

What are some "nutrient-dense" foods?

There are many nutrient-dense foods that can be eaten to help a person meet his or her daily requirements for good nutrition. They include fruits, vegetables, whole grains, low-fat dairy products, seafood, eggs, low-fat meat and poultry, and beans. More detailed information about the types of nutrient-dense foods is listed in the *Dietary Guidelines for Americans* (see Sidebar).

What is the National Nutrient Database?

The National Nutrient Database is managed by the USDA, and presents the nutrient information for over 8,000 foods. You can search by food item or group to find the nutrient information for your particular food items. This Internet website can be found at http:// ndb.nal.usda.gov/.

What are the *Dietary Guidelines for Americans*?

The *Dietary Guidelines for Americans* was first released in 1980, and is considered to be the main federal nutrition policy for the United States. The DGAs are jointly issued and updated every five years by the Department of Agriculture (USDA) and the Department of Health and Human Services. According to the USDA, the guidelines "provide authoritative advice about consuming fewer calories, making informed food choices, and being physically active to attain and maintain a healthy weight, reduce risk for chronic disease, and promote overall health."

The *Dietary Guidelines for Americans* listings are different from the Dietary Reference Intakes—which are the standards for nutrient intakes in the United States, including recommendations for energy, vitamins, minerals, proteins, amino acids, carbohydrates, fats, water, and electrolytes for each sex and different stages of life (see above). The DGA recommendations are for ages 2 and over, including those who have an increased risk for a chronic disease. The guidelines encourage people to eat better, focus on nutrient-dense foods and beverages that help them maintain their health and weight, and as an incentive, suggest that such a lifestyle will help prevent most major diseases—especially those diseases associated with poor nutrition habits. The list can be found through the USDA's Center for Nutrition Policy and Promotion at www.cnpp.usda.gov or the USDA's www.DietaryGuidelines.gov. The guidelines listed on the Internet were published in 2010 (the seventh edition since 1980); the latest guidelines, the eighth edition, are to be published in late 2015.

What are some numbers to pay attention to for better nutrition?

There are plenty of numbers to pay attention to if you want to consume the best nutrients. For example, there are lists of the certain nutrients available in specific vegetables. One good example is the list of vegetables with beta carotene, the precursor to vitamin A: A cup of sweet potatoes has 11 milligrams of beta carotene, a half cup of pumpkin has 1.8 milligrams, a cup of carrots has 4.4 milligrams, a half cup of asparagus has 2.5 milligrams, and a half cup of kale has 1.5 milligrams. An example of proteins includes: A half a cup of tofu has 10 grams of protein, a half cup of lentils has 9 grams, a half cup of black, kidney, or lima beans has 6 to 7 grams, and one medium artichoke has 10 grams. For a listing of some foods and their nutrient and non-nutrient numbers, go to the government site: http://ndb.nal.usda.gov/ (the USDA's Nutrient Database).

What is an example in the *Dietary Guidelines for Americans*?

There are many recommendations in the Dietary Guidelines for Americans. The chart on the following page is from the 2010 edition: the "estimated calorie needs per day by age, gender, and physical activity level."

		Physical Activity Level[b]		
Gender	Age (years)	Sedentary	Moderately Active	Active
Child (female and male)	2–3	1,000–1,200[c]	1,000–1,400[c]	1,000–1,400[c]
Female[d]	4–8	1,200–1,400	1,400–1,600	1,400–1,800
	9–13	1,400–1,600	1,600–2,000	1,800–2,200
	14–18	1,800	2,000	2,400
	19–30	1,800–2,000	2,000–2,200	2,400
	31–50	1,800	2,000	2,200
	51+	1,600	1,800	2,000–2,200
Male	4–8	1,200–1,400	1,400–1,600	1,600–2,000
	9–13	1,600–2,000	1,800–2,200	2,000–2,600
	14–18	2,000–2,400	2,400–2,800	2,800–3,200
	19–30	2,400–2,600	2,600–2,800	3,000
	31–50	2,200–2,400	2,400–2,600	2,800–3,000
	51+	2,000–2,200	2,200–2,400	2,400–2,800

Estimated amounts of calories needed to maintain calorie balance for various gender and age groups at three different levels of physical activity. The estimates are rounded to the nearest 200 calories. An individual's calorie needs may be higher or lower than these average estimates.

a. Based on Estimated Energy Requirements (EER) equations, using reference heights (average) and reference weights (healthy) for each age/gender group. For children and adolescents, reference height and weight vary. For adults, the reference man is 5 feet 10 inches tall and weighs 154 pounds. The reference woman is 5 feet 4 inches tall and weighs 126 pounds. EER equations are from the Institute of Medicine. Dietary Reference Intakes for Energy, Carbohydrate, Fiber, Fat, Fatty Acids, Cholesterol, Protein, and Amino Acids. Washington (DC): The National Academies Press; 2002.
b. Sedentary means a lifestyle that includes only the light physical activity associated with typical day-to-day life. Moderately active means a lifestyle that includes physical activity equivalent to walking about 1.5 to 3 miles per day at 3 to 4 miles per hour, in addition to the light physical activity associated with typical day-to-day life. Active means a lifestyle that includes physical activity equivalent to walking more than 3 miles per day at 3 to 4 miles per hour, in addition to the light physical activity associated with typical day-to-day life.
c. The calorie ranges shown are to accommodate needs of different ages within the group. For children and adolescents, more calories are needed at older ages. For adults, fewer calories are needed at older ages.
d. Estimates for females do not include women who are pregnant or breastfeeding.

These dietary guidelines—based on sex, age, and physical activity—come from the U.S. government site www.health.gov.

How much water does a person need to drink per day—depending on your stage of life?

As we age, there are differences in water consumption needs—although not everyone agrees on the exact amount. The following list gives some general guidelines (and remember, many of these water requirements are highly debated):

Infants—Most infants—especially from birth to 6 months—don't need to have extra water because hydrating liquids come from breast milk or formula.

Young children—Most young children need to drink enough water because they are more active and growing; most say enough water to keep their urine a pale yellow (not dark).

Pregnant women—When a woman is pregnant, she needs more water for the amniotic fluid, the expanded blood volume of having a child, and meeting the needs of the fetus. In fact, if you're pregnant, your blood volume increases by 40 percent—and more water also means you *and* the baby are hydrated. Thus, many experts recommend anywhere from 8 to 10 cups per day—and some say even more.

Nursing women—After the child is born, a nursing woman needs to increase her water intake to produce milk—which is about 87 percent water. Some doctors recommend drinking an extra glass of water before each nursing.

Average adult male—This is where the debates really appear—but for the most part, research shows that men need about 6 to 8 cups of water a day.

Average adult female—Again, this is debated, but for the most part, women need a bit more water than males—about 7 to 9 cups of water a day.

Elderly—This is truly debated, mainly because most elderly people take certain medications or can have various health problems that call for different daily water requirements. For example, people who are on a diuretic medicine are often told to drink more water because the medication causes them to urinate more frequently—and lose water. But overall, it is often recommended that an older person, if possible, drink about 6 to 8 cups of water daily.

NUTRITION FOR PREGNANT AND LACTATING WOMEN AND INFANTS

How does the government help food manufacturers know what nutrients are needed for, say, pregnant and lactating women, and infants?

There are many guidelines offered by the U.S. government (and other countries) that give food manufacturers an idea of what nutrients people need at various stages of life. For example, the following chart is from January 2013, called "Guidance for Industry: A Food Labeling Guide (15. Appendix G: Daily Values for Infants, Children Less Than 4 Years of Age, and Pregnant and Lactating Women)," published through the Food and Drug Administration (this is only one example—there are many more in government guideline databases):

Recommended Nutrients for Young Children and Pregnant and Lactating Women

Vitamin or Mineral	Infants	Less Than 4 Years	Pregnant and Lactating Women	Units of Measure
Vitamin A	1,500	2,500	8,000	IU*
Vitamin C	35	40	60	mg
Calcium	600	800	1,300	mg
Iron	15	10	18	mg
Vitamin D	400	400	400	IU
Vitamin E	5	10	30	IU
Thiamin	0.5	0.7	1.7	mg

Recommended Nutrients for Young Children and Pregnant and Lactating Women

Vitamin or Mineral	Infants	Less Than 4 Years	Pregnant and Lactating Women	Units of Measure
Riboflavin	0.6	0.8	2.0	mg
Niacin	8	9	20	mg
Vitamin B_6	0.4	0.7	2.5	mg
Folate	100	200	800	mcg
Vitamin B_{12}	2	3	8	mcg
Biotin	50	150	300	mcg
Pantothenic acid	3	5	10	mg
Phosphorus	500	800	1,300	mg
Iodine	45	70	150	mcg
Magnesium	70	200	450	mg
Zinc	5	8	15	mg
Copper	0.6	1.0	2.0	mg

*The abbreviation "IU" is used for International Units, "mg" for milligrams, and "mcg" for micrograms. The abbreviation "µg" may also be used for micrograms. Also, the agency has modified the units of measure for four nutrients. Calcium and phosphorus values are expressed in mg and biotin and folate values in mcg.

Is it true that, when pregnant, a woman is eating for two?

Yes, it is true that women are "eating for two" when pregnant, but that does not mean doubling your intake of foods. According to research from the University of Washington, it is recommended that women increase their caloric intake by about 100 calories in the first trimester, and about 300 calories in the second and third trimesters. In terms of foods, this is not much: For the first trimester, it is about the amount of an extra snack, such as a few walnuts; for the second and third trimesters, it is about an extra bowl of cereal a day. And some sources also mention checking with your doctor or health-care professional about adding extra vitamins to your diet, either as supplements or eating more nutrient-dense foods.

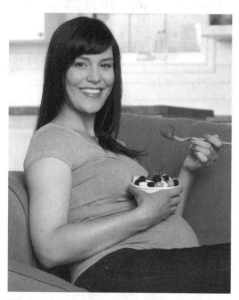

The U.S. government has developed guidelines specific to what pregnant women should eat compared to those who are not pregnant.

What is the concern about caffeine and pregnant women?

One controversial question for women has always been the consumption of caffeine while pregnant. Some studies say that drinking one or two cups of coffee a day may be associated with a very small increased risk for miscarriage, while other studies suggest that drinking large amounts of caffeine daily while you are pregnant will increase the risk for a miscarriage or a low-weight-birth child—even a premature delivery. But as with all such studies, the consumption of caffeine by pregnant women remains controversial. (For more about caffeine, see the chapter "Nutrition in Eating and Drinking Choices.")

What is lactation?

After a child is born, the mother secrets milk from her mammary glands, a process called lactation. The actual preparation for lactation begins in early pregnancy, when the hormones estrogen and progesterone cause the storage of "maternal energy," mainly in the form of fat. After the baby is born, the woman goes through changes in her ductless glandular system—allowing the secretion of milk that contains nutrients and important antibodies for the child.

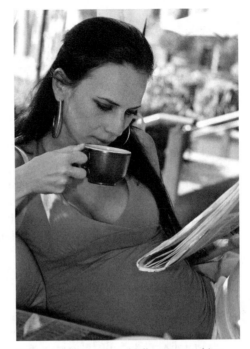

Drinking large amounts of caffeine is something pregnant women should avoid because it could increase the risk for having a miscarriage

Why is breast milk so nutritious for a baby?

A woman's breast milk is extremely important for her baby's nutrition. The milk has an amazing constant composition: in most mothers, it is almost a "perfect food" (although it is usually low in vitamin D and fluoride). The nutrition of the breast milk is directly related to the nutrition of the mother; in particular, if the nursing mother has poor nutrition, it is often the amount of milk rather than the quality that suffers. Some studies also indicate that a baby who is breastfed has a lower incidence of diabetes in later years (although, realistically, it also depends on lifestyle).

Why is the first breast milk from the mother good for a newborn baby?

Human milk has often been compared to blood—a living fluid that constantly changes composition so as to meet the needs of the baby, from birth to about a year old. The first milk produced is called "colostrum," a thick, yellowish fluid in a woman's breast late in her pregnancy and in the first days after the child is born (postpartum). During the first days after the child is born, this colostrum, although small in amount, is nutritionally valuable to the child, allowing a newborn to get off to a healthy start. This is because the child has not yet developed any immunity to germs, and the intestinal tract has never had food. One of the benefits of colostrum is that it includes the immunity-building immunoglobulin, also known as "secretory IgA," which coats the baby's digestive system and prevents germs from getting through.

How does breast milk change as a baby grows?

A mother's first milk, or colostrum (see above), lasts for just a few days after a child is born. After that, the hormone levels change in the mother, and she starts to make more plentiful amounts of milk. This is called "mature milk," and consists of plenty of fats, proteins, lactose, vitamins, minerals, and water for the growing baby.

Why does a baby push food out with his or her tongue as it eats?

We've all seen babies—usually between the age of 6 months to a year when they start ingesting more solid foods—eating mashed carrots, potatoes, or other foods. The baby seems to push the food out with their tongue, with food going in and out as the tongue moves back and forth. This is not because they want to frustrate their parents—it is because the baby is learning how to perfect the swallowing reflex—and without this ability, the baby would not be able to take in food.

Why do most nutritionists suggest that babies drink milk from their mothers—not from other mammals?

The milk from a human mother's breast is filled with all sorts of necessary nutrients needed for the baby's healthy growth. This is thought to be true for all mammals' milk, not just humans. But the proportions of the milk's ingredients—fats, proteins, lactose, vitamins, minerals, and water—differ from mammal to mammal, along with the types of fats and proteins. Because of this difference, most nutritionists believe other mammals' milk—for example, a cow-milk-based formula—is inferior in nutritional offerings for human babies. In other words, they advocate human breast milk because it is made for humans!

Why do most nutritionists suggest that human babies drink milk from their mothers, and not artificial milk?

Nutritionists have long known that artificial milk, or formula, is not as nutritious as human breast milk, although the quality has improved in the past few decades. Most of the formulae offered for babies have a basic recipe of fats, proteins, carbohydrates, vitamins, minerals, and water; the biggest

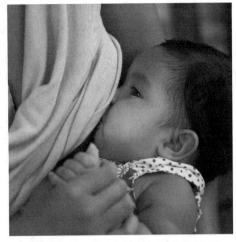

Breastfeeding is better than feeding an infant with formula for two reasons: mother's milk is the most suited for infants and the physical contact is emotionally healthier.

difference is the sources of these ingredients, from cows or from soy or some other base. In most of the formulae, the base (for example, cow's milk) contains most of the nutrients necessary, but in the wrong proportion; the manufacturers of the formulas then add ingredients until the artificial milk approximates human milk as closely as possible.

But for those who cannot breastfeed (or choose not to for some other reason), many times it becomes necessary to feed the baby formula. Choosing a formula isn't always easy, and many times the nutritional content listed on the label is difficult to interpret. The best way to approach finding the most nutritious formula is to compare proteins, fats, and carbohydrates. Also keep in mind certain vitamins and minerals babies need; for example, most babies from 6 to 12 months old have daily iron and calcium requirements that increase quickly (check with your child's doctor for amounts). And don't be surprised by the amount of saturated fatty acids in an infant formula—babies under the age of two years need fats to meet their energy needs, and to supply raw material for their cell membranes. In fact, most infant formulas contain 30 to 50 percent saturated fatty acids—about the same as human breast milk.

What is the concern about caffeine and lactating women?

When it comes to caffeine, there is a slight concern about women who breastfeed. Most experts recommend if you want to have, for example, coffee while breastfeeding, to drink it in moderation—about 16 ounces of brewed coffee per day (it's estimated that about 1 percent of it ends up in your milk). But try drinking it three hours before breastfeeding; this is because the caffeine in your breast milk peaks about an hour after you consume caffeine. Although the caffeine can be transferred to the breastfeeding baby, most experts believe it usually causes no problem (of course, this depends on the baby). But many nursing mothers who want to be on the safe side usually give up their caffeine intake until the baby is weaned.

What is a "follow-up" formula?

A follow-up formula is associated with artificial baby milk—and is meant to be a bridge between formula and regular cow's milk, usually for the infant older than six months. Most nutritionists suggest that you don't feed your baby cow's milk until after the age of one year—and some people suggest, because children often develop, or already have, lactose intolerance, not to give them cow's milk at all (for more about lactose intolerance, see the chapter "Nutrition and Allergies, Illnesses, and Diseases").

Why do infants need fats to help their brains?

According to most research, infants need fats, especially to help brain development and performance. In the first two years of life, an infant needs fats in order to help the rapid growth of their brains; an infant's brain triples in size by the first birthday, when the brain uses 60 percent of the total energy consumed, and the brain itself is around 60 percent fat. This is why around 50 percent of an infant's daily calories come from fat in their first year (when they are breastfed), and why around 50 percent of the calories in a mother's milk come from fats.

But it's not only the amount of fat, it's the type. Infants' brains grow faster than their bodies. And because humans have such highly developed brains, human milk is low in saturated fats and high in brain-building fats, such as the omega-3 fatty acid known as DHA. In fact, DHA is the primary structural component of brain tissue; some research also seems to indicate that many infants who have low amounts of DHA in their diet also often have reduced brain development.

If infants drink breast milk or formula, do they also need water?

According to the American Academy of Pediatrics, from birth to about 6 months, if an infant is breastfeeding or drinking formula, he or she usually doesn't need any extra water (but consult your pediatrician, especially if the baby is vomiting or has diarrhea, as such conditions can dehydrate the child). This is because most mother's milk or a formula has enough water for the growing baby. Too much water can flush the sodium and electrolytes from the baby's kidneys; it can also fill the baby and replace needed calories, bringing on malnutrition. From six months to a year—when babies are often transitioning from a liquid diet to a solid food diet—they can drink around two to four ounces of water a day; but this is not really essential, especially if they are still breastfeeding or ingesting formula (and if you do give them water, it should be given gradually during the day).

NUTRITION FOR CHILDREN, TEENS, AND YOUNG ADULTS

What are some healthy beverages for a preschooler?

According to the American Academy of Pediatrics, a preschooler can consume many drinks—more than when they were babies. But they recommend that preschoolers should not have more than 2 to 3 cups of milk per day; by age two, you can introduce the child to reduced fat milk, which is a much better "habit" than drinking whole milk! Soft drinks are not really what a child should drink (too many sugars and additives), but pediatricians do recommend 100 percent fruit drinks. But buyers beware: Make sure the label reads 100 percent fruit *juice*, not fruit *drink*, which often contains little, if any, fruit juice; it's also best to dilute the juice with two or even three parts water, especially for very young children. And if they don't like the fruit juice, try to encourage them to eat whole fruits (which are better for them) instead.

Why should you eat healthy in early childhood?

One big reason to eat healthy in your early childhood has to do with your health in later years. For example, according to several recent studies, the clogging of a person's arteries with fatty tissues (atherosclerosis) can start in childhood, especially in those children who eat too many sweets, salty foods, and fatty meats. Overall, it takes about 20 to 30 years or more for the vessels to become clogged enough to show symptoms. And since the clogging of the arteries is directly related to heart disease, and even fatal heart attacks, eating healthy early in childhood seems like a good prescription

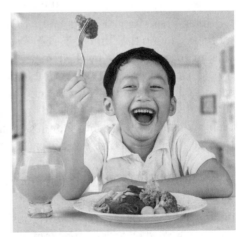

Eating healthy foods early in childhood will help establish good eating habits throughout one's lifetime.

299

for a lifetime! There is a long list of other diseases that can catch up with a person who eats poorly in childhood and on through middle age (such as heart disease or type 2 diabetes), which is why there are so many government programs that target elementary, middle, and high schools, emphasizing to young people the need to eat well.

Is there any connection between heredity and nutrient absorption?

Yes, there seem to be some connections between our genes and the ability to absorb nutrients. For example, one of the most well-known conditions that have a genetic component is gluten intolerance, mainly celiac disease, which often runs in families. This is a condition in which the immune system is abnormally sensitive to gluten, a protein found in wheat, rye, and barley; it is also considered an autoimmune disorder, in which the immune system malfunctions, attacking the body's own tissues and organs.

Recent studies have also shown that celiac disease is commonly, but not exclusively connected to type O blood (people with other blood types can also be gluten intolerant). And even though it is estimated that about 33 percent of the Western population has type O blood, no one really knows how many of these people will become or are truly gluten intolerant. (For more about gluten intolerance and celiac disease, see the chapter "Nutrition and Allergies, Illnesses, and Diseases.")

Does sugar make a child hyperactive?

It depends on what research you examine—but according to the National Institute of Mental Health, although the idea that refined sugar causes ADHD (Attention Deficit Hyperactivity Disorder) or makes symptoms worse is popular, there is definitely a need for more research. The studies that have been done so far have shown some interesting results: for example, in one study, children were given foods containing either sugar or a sugar substitute every other day; those who ingested sugar showed no different behavior or learning problems from those who received the sugar substitute.

In another study, it appeared that the results were more subjective—based on the mothers', not on the children's, responses. All the children in the study (who were considered sugar-sensitive by their mothers) were given the sugar substitute aspartame (brand name NutraSweet), but half the mothers were told their children received refined sugar, and the other half NutraSweet. The mothers who thought their children ingested sugar rated their offspring as being more hyperactive than the other children, and were even more critical of their children's behavior—in comparison with the mothers who thought their children received aspartame.

How can you help your child eat more nutritious meals?

Besides the obvious—cooking nutrient-rich meals—there are ways to help your child understand that eating more nutritiously is easier than they think. Children are not only bombarded by advertising from all directions, but many of their peers also influence what they choose to eat. But you can help them eat better in several ways—and the following are only a few hints: Try cooking more meals at home (especially getting your child involved in cooking the meals, and even making their own bagged lunch for school—so you can show them how to cook a healthy meal that uses less salt, fats, or sugar); get them involved in the actual growing of food (if you have the room, have a small garden out back or even some containers filled with easy-to-grow plants such as lettuce, Swiss chard, or beet greens, so they can "pick their own dinner"); let your kids help you with the grocery shopping, and use it as a learning experience (let them pick out the "vegetable or fruit of the week," or explain to them why it's more fun to eat an orange than a bag of greasy potato chips!); keep a variety of healthy snacks around the house (including fruits, vegetables, and healthy beverages); and keep an eye on their portion sizes so they don't gain unhealthy weight (don't insist they clean their plates— that could lead to not wanting to eat at all—and don't use food as a reward or bribe).

Do growing brains have nutritional needs?

Yes, the growing brains of young people have nutritional needs, as do the brains of adults. Overall, like ever other system in the body, the brain needs good food in order to work better; in fact, no matter what age, the brain uses 20 to 25 percent of the total energy we consume, so the more (and better) you feed the brain, the better it works. If you want to help your brain—and especially your children's brains—offer such foods as asparagus, avocados, bananas, brown rice, broccoli, cheese, chicken, eggs, flaxseed oil, legumes, milk, oatmeal, peanut butter, peas, lettuce, potatoes, salmon, spinach, wheat germ, yogurt, and soybeans to eat—in other words, foods that boost the body and brain. And beware of the "brain drainer" foods, such as artificial food coloring and sweeteners, colas, corn syrup, frostings (and most junk food sugars), white bread, hydrogenated fats, and high-sugar drinks.

How can diet help alleviate the symptoms of PMS (premenstrual syndrome) in young women?

There are many ways in which a woman can help alleviate PMS symptoms—especially bloating, cramping, fatigue, and mood fluctuations. The following list offers some di-

---

What are some of the best "sugars" to serve growing children?

If you want to serve your family some "sweets," the best sugars for the brain (excluding children and adults on special diets) are fruit sugars and complex carbohydrates, or what used to be called starches (they include chickpeas, lentils, oatmeal, soy, sweet potatoes, whole-grain pastas and cereals, and whole grains, such as whole wheat and brown rice). This is because starches and fruit sugars (fructose) do not cause the roller-coaster mood swings that refined sugars do. Complex carbohydrates also have long molecules—thus, the intestines take a longer time to break them down into the simple sugars the body can use. Simple sugars go into your system, giving a peak of energy followed by a sudden drop—not good for you or your children.

etary suggestions that may help you get through the week before and during your "period" (as per the National Institutes of Health):

- Drink plenty of fluids (water or juice, not soft drinks, alcohol, or other beverages with caffeine) to help reduce bloating, fluid retention, and other symptoms. (Some research also indicates that eating omega-3 fatty acids helps with cramps; if possible, try eating more fish or taking fish oil or flaxseed oil supplements.)

- Eat frequent, small meals. Leave no more than 3 hours between snacks, and avoid overeating.

- Eat a balanced diet with extra whole grains, vegetables, and fruit, and less or no salt and refined sugar (sugar can worsen mood swings, while salt worsens water retention and bloating).

- Your health-care provider may recommend that you take nutritional supplements. Vitamin B_6, calcium, and magnesium are commonly used. Tryptophan, which is found in dairy products, may also be helpful.

- Some research shows that cutting out dairy helps relieve some symptoms.

Do females' diets—and nutrients—change because of menstruation?

Yes, there are some dietary and nutrient changes that occur during a female's menstrual cycle. This is mainly caused by the fluctuation in hormones that cause her energy levels to fluctuate, too; for example, during the premenstrual phase, the energy intakes are higher,

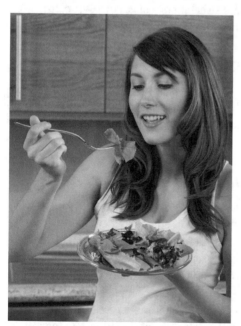

Eating foods high in iron, such as spinach, is a good idea for women who are menstruating, which results in a lot of minerals being lost.

so some women have food cravings as their period approaches. Women also may experience fluid retention before their periods, because some hormones help to hold salt in the body; thus, many health-care professionals recommend slowing down on your salt intake before your period. A major nutrient change during your period comes from the loss of iron, the mineral that helps the blood carry oxygen throughout your body; it is estimated that when a woman is menstruating, she can lose about 1 milligram of iron a day. This can be counteracted by eating iron-rich foods, including lean red meats, lentils, spinach, almonds, and iron-fortified cereals.

How much iron should women ingest throughout life?

According to the government guidelines, women of childbearing age have an RDA of 15 milligrams of iron per day—with the need for iron almost doubling when a woman becomes pregnant, to about 27 milligrams. Women over 51 years of age do not need as much iron—around 10 milligrams per day (unless there is an illness that calls for more or less)—because they are no longer losing blood (and therefore iron) from menstruation.

Deficiencies can be for a multitude of reasons, such as iron loss through the menstrual cycle, a low dietary intake of iron, frequent dieting, and a low intake of vitamin C. If you do have a deficiency of iron, it can cause several symptoms, such as fatigue and weakness; a deficiency can also lead to iron-deficiency anemia. Finally, if you take both an iron and calcium supplement, take them separately at different times of the day for better absorption of each.

What are some nutritional needs of young men?

Not every young man thinks about nutrition. Because their lives seem filled with busy schedules, bad eating habits, such as too much fast food and snacks, and skipping meals become part of their routine. Some also drink heavily, and all of these dietary habits can cause weight gain or lack of energy. According to many experts, certain nutrients are essential when young. These include calcium, at least 1,000 milligrams per day, to keep bones and teeth healthy; vitamin D to not only help absorb calcium, but to give strength to bones and teeth as well as helping nerves, muscles, and the immune system to function properly; and minerals. The mineral zinc, for example, helps the immune system, along with being necessary for wound healing; it improves the senses of taste and smell, and helps with protein and DNA synthesis. Males aged 9 to 13 years need 8 milligrams of zinc daily; those aged 14 to 18 years need 11 milligrams daily. And overall, the energy requirements for men aged 19 to 30 are between 2,400 and 3,000 calories per day, depending on activity level and overall health.

NUTRITION IN ADULTHOOD AND BEYOND

What diet-related diseases affect men more than women in adulthood?

According to the American Heart Association, at least 83.6 million Americans are living with some form of cardiovascular disease (including high blood pressure) or the aftereffects of a stroke; and according to the American Cancer Society, about 8.2 million Americans alive today have a history of cancer. These statistics include both males and females, young and old.

But as we age, there are several diseases that affect adult men more than adult women; in fact, some research shows that men may have the highest rates of diet-related diseases. (But there is one caveat: There have not been as many health studies on women as there have been on men, so many of these statistics will probably change over time as more women participate in health studies.) The following list describes some of the "more male than female" diseases, primarily in the United States:

- Men have approximately 1.5 times the death rate from total cardiovascular diseases as women.
- According to the American Cancer Society, men have an almost 23 percent chance of dying from cancers, while in women, it is around 19 percent.
- Men have more of a risk for dying from lung cancer than women—1 in 15 men versus 1 in 20 women.
- Men have a risk for dying from colon and rectal cancer a bit more than women—1 in 48 men versus 1 in 53 women.

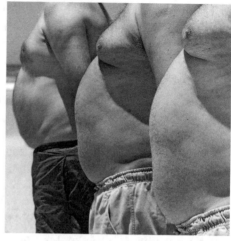

Obesity rates in the United States have risen to 35 percent in adults over the age of twenty, contributing to disease and higher medical costs.

How much has obesity increased for everyone in recent years?

According to the Centers for Disease Control and Prevention (CDC), obesity has risen over the past decade. The latest statistics for the United States show that 35 percent of adults over the age of 20 are obese, as are 18.4 percent of adolescents between 12 and 19 years old. And for those who do carry too much weight, their health is in jeopardy—obesity is related to heart disease, stroke, type 2 diabetes, and certain cancers; these people are also more prone to inflammation, hypertension, and other chronic disorders. The estimated annual medical cost of obesity in the United States in 2008 was $147 billion—and it continues to grow.

How can diet help with premenopausal symptoms in women?

About ten years before a woman reaches menopause—the average age is about 51 years old for "the change"—her reproductive system prepares for a change in its production of hormones that were available in her childbearing years. These "perimenopausal" (premenopausal) years can create different symptoms in women, such as hot flashes or weight gain. Diet can relieve many of those symptoms, and can help a female through her body's transition. For example, a female needs to boost her calcium intake (and to help with absorption, vitamin D and magnesium); this will help support bone health and prevent osteoporosis. If she is experiencing hot flashes, limiting wine, sugar, white flour products, and coffee—along with eating one or two tablespoons of ground flaxseed (rich in lignans that stabilize hormone levels) a day—can help reduce the discomfort of feeling like she is in a sauna—when there is no sauna around!

What foods can cause osteoporosis in women?

According to the National Osteoporosis Foundation, there are many nutritious foods women can eat to slow down or even lower the risk for osteoporosis due to age. There

Is obesity in later life often connected to a person's early life?

Yes, one recent study indicated early obesity can be connected to obesity later in life. The researchers looked at the body mass index (BMI) of males when they were 25 years old and if they became obese later in life. They discovered that males who were obese by that young age have a much higher risk—almost 25 percent—for being severely obese after the age of 35. But when a male had a normal weight at age 25, the chance of being severely obese after age 35 was only 1.1 percent.

But it wasn't just men who had a problem. The researchers also studied women, and found that the chance for obesity at age 35—if they were obese at 25 years of age—was even higher, at about 46.9 percent. When a female had a normal weight at age 25, her chances of being severely obese after age 35 was only 4.8 percent. But the researchers also noted that if a person lost weight at any stage of life—especially by eating a well-balanced, nutritional diet—he or she could reduce the risk for cardiovascular and metabolic disease no matter what he or she weighed when young.

are some foods and drinks to watch, too—most of which interfere with calcium absorption: proteins (too much can cause a woman to lose calcium); phytates (they interfere with calcium absorption and are found in such foods as beans—but don't quit eating nutrient- and fiber-rich beans, as you can reduce phytates by soaking the beans in water for several hours before cooking); and too much salt and too much alcohol (too much of either can cause problems with calcium absorption).

How does menopause in women change their nutritional needs?

A menopausal woman does have different nutritional needs than when she was of childbearing or premenopausal age. For example, according to the American Academy of Orthopaedic Surgeons, premenopausal women should consume about 1,000 mg of calcium daily; after menopause, they should consume 1,200 mg of calcium per day (see below). Vitamin D is also important for calcium absorption and bone formation—and in one study, women with postmenopausal osteoporosis who took vitamin D for three years significantly reduced their risk for spinal fractures. But there are disagreements as to what amount of this vitamin is healthy, as too much vitamin D can cause kidney stones, constipation, or abdominal pain, especially in women with kidney problems.

The nutritional guidelines recommended by the National Research Council of the National Institutes of Health include the following for menopausal women:

- Choose foods low in fat, saturated fat, and cholesterol; a menopausal woman's fat intake should be less than 30 percent of her daily calorie intake.

- Eat fruits, vegetables, and whole grains (including cereals), especially those high in vitamin C and beta carotene.

- Consume 20 to 30 grams of fiber daily (which is recommended for all ages, too, not just menopausal women).

- Get plenty of calcium to support bone health. This is important because women are at a greater risk than men for developing osteoporosis. Dairy products are high in calcium, but they often have too much animal fat and protein that can accelerate bone loss (and cause weight gain if eaten in excess)—thus, it's best to get calcium from plants, such as kale, broccoli, beans, and collard greens.

- Avoid foods and drinks with refined or processed sugars (too many empty calories and they can cause weight gain).

- Avoid salt-cured and smoked foods such as sausages, smoked fish, ham, bacon, bologna, and hot dogs. These foods are high in sodium, which can lead to high blood pressure, a serious risk for aging women.

- Don't eat too much animal-based protein; in fact, ignore most diets that recommend low-carbohydrates and/or high-protein. These diets are not good for older women, because eating too much protein over time can lead to calcium loss, and thus, a decrease in bone density that leads to osteoporosis.

- And of course, along with eating well, exercise!

What types of fats should older men and women eat for better health?

The best fats you can eat to help your brain to function when older (and also to help your moods and to maintain a healthy weight) are called healthy fats. This does not mean stocking your cupboard with all types of fats, but rather that it is advisable to choose "good" fats such as the mono- and polyunsaturated fats found in olive and canola oils, olives, nuts, fish, some peanut butters, and avocados. Ignore the "bad" fats, such as trans and saturated fats, that can increase your risk for diseases, including heart attacks and strokes.

Can an older person's sense of taste and smell affect their eating habits?

Yes, it is thought that the sense of smell, in particular, is most accurate between the ages of 30 and 60 years old. After age 60, the ability to smell declines—and along with that, taste. Not only does a person lose their sense of smell, they lose their ability to discriminate between smells. Research has shown that more than 75 percent of people over the age of 80 years show evidence of

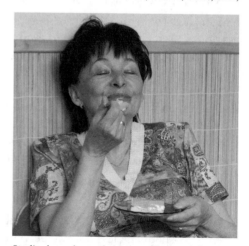

Studies have shown that many older people have a less acute sense of smell, which can affect their enjoyment of food.

What foods may be better to eat fermented rather than unfermented, especially for older people?

There are some foods that are thought to be better eaten after rather than before fermentation. Some of the most controversial are soybean products: There are some nutritionists who believe that older people who eat a great deal of tofu—or soybean curd—may have more of a risk to develop dementia or memory loss as they age. The researchers believe that the phytoestrogens in the soy may be harmful to older brains, and recommend that older people who like tofu eat more of the soy product called tempeh (a soy product that is fermented with *Rhizopus oligosporus*, a fungus used as a starter culture; tempeh resembles chunks of soybeans pressed together in a thin rectangular cake). They believe that the fermentation process increases the amount of folate (also called folic acid, folacin, and B$_9$), a water-soluble vitamin that protects your brain. (For more about fermentation, see the chapter "Food Preservation and Nutrition.")

major olfactory impairment, and that olfaction declines considerably after the seventh decade. (For more about smell and taste, see the chapter "Nutrition in Eating and Drinking Choices.")

The reasons seem to be many, and vary with each person; but overall, it often has to do with the normal aging process, drug use, infections (especially upper respiratory), changes in the mouth (such as dentures or tooth loss), and even the reduction of saliva. Thus, because smell and taste are so intertwined with our perception of foods and eating habits, a large proportion of elderly people who lose their smell don't eat well—and become nutrient deficient.

Do the foods you eat affect your sleep patterns when you're older?

According to the National Sleep Foundation, everyone's sleep patterns change as they get older as part of the normal aging process. As we age, it becomes harder to fall asleep—and stay asleep compared to when we were younger. But it's not only the normal progression of life—sleep patterns can change when we're older because of the foods we eat or beverages we drink. For example, eating too much or too little can disrupt sleep; in particular, too much food can cause discomfort in your digestive tract that keeps you awake. And if you eat too much fat with a meal before you sleep, or for a bedtime snack, it can give you indigestion and heartburn, which keeps you awake.

Does nutrition affects diseases we may encounter as we age?

Yes, nutrition plays an important part in helping develop—or stopping—certain diseases that are often associated with aging. For example, older people have a more difficult time with the absorption of calcium, and less calcium in the system can often lead to osteoporosis (the gradual loss of bone structure). Another ailment that is affected by nutrition is arthritis; some foods such as processed or fried foods, cause more inflammation in our bodies, while foods, such as fresh vegetables and fruits, along with nuts and teas, can reduce the inflammation that can affect a person's arthritic joints.

And of course, there are other challenges that seniors have when it comes to nutrition, especially trying to take in enough nutrients to stay healthy. This can be for a multitude of reasons, including a loss of appetite (from medications or illness), problems with chewing and swallowing (difficulty with dentures or lack of teeth), and a need to reduce the intake of fats and sugars that are associated with certain chronic conditions (sugars and fats provide energy, but also add weight that can lead to diseases). (For more about some of these diseases, see the chapter "Nutrition and Allergies, Illnesses, and Diseases.")

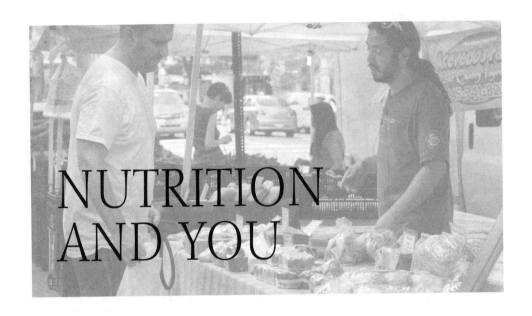

NUTRITION AND YOU

YOUR NUTRITION, HEALTH, AND NUMBERS

What is your body mass index, or BMI?

One of the first people to realize the connection between your body mass, weight, and height was Adolphe Quételet (1796–1874), who created the index in 1830. Body mass index (BMI), as the name implies is a statistical way of measuring your body's mass—based on body weight and height of a person. Most doctors use BMI to determine how you are weight-wise for your age, gender, and size. According to the Centers for Disease Control and Prevention, in general, for an adult female (males have a bit higher BMI numbers), if you have a BMI less than 18.5, you are considered underweight; 18.5 to 24.9 means normal weight; 25.0 to 29.9 means overweight; and over 30.0 is considered obese. (For more about BMI, see the chapter "Nutrition throughout the Centuries.")

Why do some doctors consider your BMI to be important to your overall health?

According to the Centers for Disease Control and Prevention, people with very low or high BMIs tend to have the greatest health risks—but remember that your BMI is only one factor in your overall health. For example, if your BMI falls into the normal weight category, you still may have a higher risk for health problems, especially if you smoke, don't participate in regular exercise, don't eat nutrient-rich foods, and/or eat an excess of foods that contain fats and sugars. But there is good news: If your BMI is in the overweight category, you can lower your overall health risk if you exercise regularly; have blood pressure, blood sugar, and cholesterol levels in the "normal" range; and eat a healthy diet.

How do you determine your BMI?

To determine your BMI, take your weight in pounds and your height in inches. Then multiply your weight times 703, and divide that number by your height squared (or

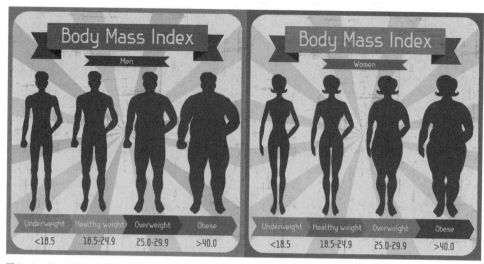

This visual provides an idea of how the Body Mass Index relates to body shapes in men and women.

height times height). For example, if you are 5 feet 4 inches tall (or 64 inches tall) and weigh 133 pounds, the calculation would be as follows: 133 x 703 = 93,449; 64 inches squared = 4,096; divide 93,449/4,096 = 22.83—thus, your BMI is in the normal range.

For more about BMI ranges—in metric and standard measurements—see the chart below:

Calculating Your BMI

Measurement Units	Formula and Calculation
Kilograms and meters (or centimeters)	Formula: weight (kg) / [height (m)]^2

With the metric system, the formula for BMI is weight in kilograms divided by height in meters squared. Since height is commonly measured in centimeters, divide height in centimeters by 100 to obtain height in meters. Example: Weight = 68 kg, Height = 165 cm (1.65 m); Calculation: $68 \div (1.65)^2 = 24.98$

| Pounds and inches | Formula: weight (lb) / [height (in)]$^2 \times 703$ |

Calculate BMI by dividing weight in pounds (lb) by height in inches (in) squared and multiplying by a conversion factor of 703. Example: Weight = 150 lbs, Height = 5'5" (65"); Calculation: $[150 \div (65)^2] \times 703 = 24.96$

What is viewed as overweight, underweight, and normal?

The major way that most health-care professionals determine whether a person is underweight, normal, overweight, or obese is through what is called the body mass index (BMI). As the name implies, BMI is a statistical way of measuring your body's mass—based on your body weight and height. Most doctors use BMI to determine how you are weight-wise for your age, sex, and size. According to the National Institutes of Health, the following chart gives the average range for people who are overweight to obese, based on a person's BMI:

BMI of Adults Age 20 and Older

BMI	Classification
18.5 to 24.9	Normal weight
25 to 29.9	Overweight
30 +	Obesity
40 +	Extreme obesity

What is an example of a person's BMI at a certain height and weight?

Depending on your height, which is usually considered to be a constant, you can determine what weight range will send you into another BMI category. For example, here are the weight ranges, the corresponding BMI ranges, and the weight status categories for a person with a sample height of 5 feet, 9 inches:

Sample BMI Range

Height	Weight Range	BMI	Weight Status
5'9"	124 lbs or less	Below 18.5	Underweight
	125 lbs to 168 lbs	18.5 to 24.9	Normal
	169 lbs to 202 lbs	25.0 to 29.9	Overweight
	203 lbs or more	30 or higher	Obese

How are BMI numbers interpreted—especially for obesity?

As seen in the chart above, the categories of BMI weight status are as follows: underweight (BMI of <18.5), normal weight (BMI of 18.5 to 24.9), overweight (BMI of 25 to 29.9), and obese (BMI equal to or greater than 30). And according to the National Heart, Lung, and Blood Institute, obesity is further divided into three grades: Grade 1 obesity is defined as a BMI of 30 to less than 35; grade 2 obesity, a BMI of 35 to less than 40; and grade 3 obesity, a BMI of 40 or greater.

Is BMI calculated for children, teens, and adults in the same way?

No, the calculations are different. For adults 20 years old and older, the BMI interpretation is same for both sexes; but for children and teens, it is both age- and sex-specific. While BMI calculations for children and teens use the same formula as adults, the criteria used to define obesity and overweight are different for young people because of two major factors—the body fat differences between boys and girls, and the variations in body fat at different ages.

Why are body mass index readings different for children?

The body mass index readings differ for children, especially because growth is faster or slower, depending on the child, so it's difficult to tell if they are definitely overweight. To determine if a child is overweight or obese, the government publishes a listing of statistics based on data collected; thus, the BMI charts for children and adolescents ages 2 to 19 are based on a comparison of height and weight to other children of the same sex and age. The following chart gives the listing; you can find a children's BMI calculator at the Centers for Disease Control and Prevention at http://apps.nccd.cdc.gov/dnpabmi/Calculator.aspx:

BMI of Children and Adolescents Ages 2–19

BMI	Classification
At or above the 85th percentile	Overweight or obese
At or above the 95th percentile	Obese

Is a low or high BMI number cause for concern?

Yes, many health-care professionals and nutritionists are concerned when a person has a very low or high BMI number. In studies done over the past decade, it has been shown that lower BMI numbers can be a cause for concern, as a person becomes underweight; higher BMI numbers means a person is usually overweight or obese—and for most, that means they carry a risk for many diseases over time. In one major study by the American Cancer Society, the data showed that as the body mass index increased, the risk for death increased (based on the optimum body mass indices of between 23.5 and 24.9 for men and 22.0 and 23.4 for women). Men and women with body mass indexes of 40.0 or higher increased their risk for death by 250 percent and 200 percent, respectively; in contrast, underweight men and women, with body mass indexes of 18.5 or lower, increased the risk by 26 percent and 36 percent, respectively.

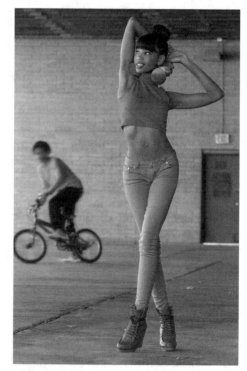

Fashion models can reflect an unrealistic expectation of what our bodies should look like. Computer programs can add to the perception that super-thin bodies are beautiful.

Why should older people keep track of their BMI?

Although a recent study in *The American Journal of Clinical Nutrition* showed that, for older populations, being overweight was not found to be associated with an increased risk for mortality, the researchers did find that there is an increased risk for those at the lower end of the recommended BMI range and that mortality actually increased for older people with BMIs under 23, which is why the average,

What BMI numbers have been reported in fashion models?

According to a study done in 2011, it is estimated that 20 to 40 percent of fashion models suffer from some type of eating disorder—so much so that some groups are urging the fashion industry to ban the use of size "0" models. This is because size 0 usually corresponds to someone who has a body mass index (BMI) below 18.5 (a BMI between 18.5 and 24.9 is considered to be at a healthy weight).

healthy older person—meaning those 65 years old or older—should try not to lose too much weight. Of course, it's not only a lower BMI that older people should be aware of: the much higher numbers are also a concern, as is true for all ages (see above).

How reliable is BMI as a health indicator?

For several reasons, not everyone thinks that the BMI is a person's best indicator of health. For example, although the connection between the BMI number and the fatness of a person is fairly strong, the numbers all vary by sex, race, and age; for instance, at the same BMI, older people (on the average) tend to have more body fat than younger adults, and highly trained athletes may also have a high BMI, but it is because of more muscle than body fat.

Another objection is that the BMI is only one factor related to risk for certain diseases. Thus, some organizations look at other factors to understand a person's likelihood of developing overweight- or obesity-related diseases. For example, the National Heart, Lung, and Blood Institute guidelines recommend looking at two other factors: a person's waist circumference (because abdominal fat is often a predictor of risk for obesity-related diseases) and whether a person is at risk for diseases associated with obesity (for example, if they have high blood pressure or are physically inactive).

What is blood pressure, and what is hypertension?

Your blood pressure is actually the force of blood pushing against the walls of all your blood vessels throughout the body, from capillaries to arteries. As the heart pumps (beats), it sends your blood into the arteries, and on through veins and capillaries throughout your body; when we take our pulse, or even feel our blood pulsing through our neck, we are actually feeling the blood being pushed through arteries. But if you have high blood pressure (also called hypertension), the pressure in the arteries is high (also said to be above the normal range)—making your blood pressure reading high.

Does salt affect your blood pressure?

Most health-care professionals agree that, for most people, ingesting too much salt can cause the body to develop high blood pressure over time. In fact, when you eat too much salt, it causes your body to hold extra water in order to eliminate the salt from your system. For some people (but not for all) this causes extra pressure in the blood vessels—causing a rise in blood pressure. The additional water also puts stress on the blood vessels and heart—and when your pressure increases, this creates even more stress on your vessels and heart.

What is the recommended daily maximum of salt?

The majority of Americans eat too much salt, which is often associated with hypertension and promotes fluid retention. Thus, several organizations, including the American Heart Association and the USDA, recommend that people ingest only a certain amount of salt each day. The government recommends, for a healthy adult under 51 years of age, a maximum of 2,300 milligrams daily; for an adult 51 years or older, African-Americans, or for someone who has diabetes or chronic kidney disease, the number is lower, at about 1,500 milligrams daily. In addition, the American Heart Association suggests that people with high blood pressure, or a tendency toward developing high blood pressure, should eat foods lower in fat, salt, and calories—and that they also take in no more than 1,500 milligrams of sodium per day (a teaspoon of salt is about 2,400 milligrams of sodium). (For more about salts, see the chapter "The Basics of Nutrition: Micronutrients.")

Are there any Internet sites to help calculate a person's daily macronutrient needs?

Yes, there are plenty of Internet websites that help you to calculate your daily macronutrient—carbohydrates, fats, and protein—needs, but there are too many to mention here. The best sites include the government sites, for example, the Dietary Reference Intakes from the Institute of Medicine's Healthy Macronutrient Distribution at http://www.iom.edu/~/media/Files/Activity%20Files/Nutrition/DRIs/DRI_Macronutrients.pdf (for more about Dietary Reference Intakes, see the chapter "Nutrition throughout Life"). Other sites are also available, and usually reflect the government guidelines. For example, there is a site that concentrates on daily macronutrient needs called "The MacroNutrient Calculator" at http://macronutrientcalculator.com. Another site is "Active" (mostly for athletes) at https://www.active.com/fitness/calculators/nutrition that has a calculator for nutritional needs (again, the macronutrients: carbohydrates, fats, and proteins), and is based on National Institutes of Health's Institute of Medicine's Healthy Macronutrient Distribution.

YOU AND SUPPLEMENTS

Why don't most people get enough nutrients?

According to the USDA, there are many reasons why certain people don't get enough of the essential nutrients through the food they eat. And the list is long: For example, many people skip meals, and do not make up the nutrients they lack in other daily meals; many people do not consume many fruits, vegetables, or whole grains, which are all important for nutrients and fiber requirements; people on a low-calorie diet may not get enough nutrients unless their foods are nutrient-dense; many vegetarians, because they may not consume dairy products, do not get enough calcium in their diet, and this also often applies to people who do not eat dairy products because of lactose intolerance; people who have had weight-loss surgery and have changes in their intestinal tract that often makes it harder for their bodies to absorb vitamins and minerals from foods; pregnant women who are unaware of their increased nutritional needs, such as for more folic acid, iron, and calcium; and people who do not realize that nutritional needs change at different stages of life, such as women after menopause needing more calcium and vitamin D.

Who really needs a daily supplement?

There are seemingly a billion varieties of supplements touted for a wide range of effects by the media, including those promising anything from preventing heart disease, cancer, and stroke to delaying the progression of dementia and Alzheimer's. And although research has linked certain vitamins, minerals, and other compounds to health-promoting activity in our cells, there is a lack of clinical evidence to prove that taking supplements has any long-term benefits. Thus, overall, most researchers agree that if you eat a healthy diet of nutrient-rich foods, there should be no reason to take supplements.

That being said, there are some conditions in which a person needs to supplement his or her diet with vitamins and/or nutrients; for example, during an illness or if a person is malnourished, and oftentimes, the elderly need more vitamins and minerals. But the biggest obstacle to stopping the unnecessary ingestion of supplements seems to be money—it is estimated that the worldwide supplement business takes in close to $70 billion or more each year. (For more about the controversies surrounding vitamin and mineral supplements, see the chapter "Controversies with Food, Beverages, and Nutrition.")

Is there a worldwide standard listing of nutrient dosages?

No, there is no worldwide standard that lists dosages for such nutrients as vitamins, minerals, and even non-nutrients such as flavonoids. In fact, many of the nutrients touted on vitamin and mineral pill containers have no standard either—which is why it's so difficult for the general public to determine if the hype they read in the popular media is accurate or not!

How are nutrient supplements often measured?

The measurement of supplements is not always straightforward. In general, vitamin and mineral supplements are generally measured using international units (IU), usually the most common way to measure a recommended dose of a vitamin or mineral, with each pill containing relatively the same dosage of IUs. Another measurement is RAEs, which stands for retinol activity equivalents, and is a way to measure the amount of vitamin A from retinols (obtaining vitamin A from meats, as opposed to vitamin A from beta carotene, or through plants). The standard measurement is 1 RAE = 1 microgram (mcg) retinol or 12 mcg beta carotene. And finally, some vitamins are measured using mcg, or micrograms.

Overall, these measurements can often become rather confusing, especially if a vitamin has several different forms. For example, vitamin A has additional units: the amount of vitamin A may be listed in IUs, or in Retinol Equivalents (REs), in which 1 RE is equal to 3.3 IU of the retinol form of vitamin A and 10 IU of beta carotene; 1 RE is also equal to 1 microgram (mcg) of retinol or 6 mcg of beta carotene!

What does RDA mean in terms of vitamins and minerals?

RDA stands for the Recommended Dietary Allowances and is used to recommend the optimum dosage of each vitamin or mineral per day. The RDAs are set to "meet the known needs of all healthy people," and are governed by the Institute of Medicine (one of the U.S. National Academies). For example, the RDA for vitamin E, for adult males and females over 19 years of age, is 15 milligrams. There is also something called the daily adequate intakes (AIs), which are used rather than RDAs when the scientific evidence is insufficient to estimate an average requirement. (For information about the controversies surrounding supplements, see the chapter "Controversies with Food, Beverages, and Nutrition.")

NUTRITION AND FOOD MYTHS ... OR NOT

Is MSG (monosodium glutamate) bad for you?

Monosodium glutamate (MSG) has long been a flavor enhancer, and is produced by growing a special type of bacteria on sugar (or molasses and corn); it is also found naturally in dried seaweed. It is often found in Chinese foods, dry mixes, stock cubes, and canned, processed, and some frozen meats. MSG does not change the flavor of the food, but acts on the tongue to heighten certain tastes in foods and minimize others—that is, masking unpleasant tastes and enhancing more agreeable flavors in the food. Susceptible people may often contract headaches from eating foods containing MSG, but recent research has shown that there may not be a problem with the MSG, but with other ingredients in Chinese foods, such as tyramine or histamine, which are often found in such foods as black beans and soy sauce.

Should you remove the seeds and central jelly from tomatoes before you cook them?

Many chefs advocate removing the seeds and central jelly—the mushy part of a tomato that usually contains the seeds—when making tomato sauces or other dishes, mainly to get rid of some of the liquid and seeds. But not everyone agrees, especially nutritionists: Recent research shows that the seeds and jelly actually contain three times the amount of flavor-enhancing glutamic acid (or glutamate) as the flesh (outside) of the tomato—and many of the fruit's nutrients.

Can doctors tell anything about your eating habits from your nails?

Yes, there are some fingernail conditions that can indicate certain eating habits. For example, some nail conditions can indicate a possible vitamin deficiency. An abnormally shaped fingernail (raised ridges and curved inward) can be a sign of iron-deficiency anemia, or lack of iron in your system. Or if you have certain depressed lines across the fingernail (called Beau's lines), it could be an indication that you are malnourished.

Can doctors tell if you have a nutritional deficiency by analyzing your hair?

Vitamin and mineral deficiencies can be determined through hair analysis testing, but there is a major problem: It's not possible to tell if the concentrations in the hair are the same in other tissues of the body. For example, a deficit in zinc in the hair may not mean your body truly has a zinc deficiency. In addition, hair testing often results in false readings. For example, hair treated with chemicals (especially perms and certain shampoos)—and hair washed in "hard" (mineral-rich) water—can give erroneous results. What scientists usually use hair analysis for is to check exposure to toxic levels of heavy metals (such as arsenic or lead), which is also confirmed by blood and urine testing. Another more familiar hair test is for drug use—in fact, there is an advantage to using hair analysis over urine drug testing: it can find drug use dating back several months, while urine testing can detect only recent drug use.

What famous emperor's hair has been studied to determine how he died?

One of the most famous hair analyses has been that of the French emperor Napoleon Bonaparte. Over 150 years after his death, researchers meticulously examined his hair and discovered that the assumption that Napoleon's guards had poisoned him with arsenic in Saint Helena was wrong. Hairs were placed in capsules and inserted in the core of a small nuclear reactor. Using a technique that gives very precise results on samples with a small mass—like hair—the researchers looked at samples taken during various periods of Napoleon Bonaparte's life, and also from the King of Rome (Napoleon's son), and the Empress Josephine. They found that *all* the hair samples had some traces of arsenic—at least 100 times greater than the average arsenic detected in samples from people today (the emperor's hair had an average arsenic level of about ten parts per million; the levels taken from contemporary people is about one tenth of a part per one million). The researchers concluded that people in the early 1800s somehow ingested arsenic in quantities that are now considered dangerous. This included the emperor, who probably did not die from his guards poisoning him, but as a result of continually ingesting—and thus, the constant absorption of—arsenic. (For more about arsenic in modern-day food and water, see the chapter "Nutrition in Eating and Drinking Choices.")

Does chicken soup really help lessen the effects of a cold or the flu?

Yes, if you're not a vegetarian, chicken soup may help to shorten your cold or flu, mainly because it contains cystine, a compound from the chicken that often thins the mucus in your sinuses and throat, thus relieving congestion. It is also good because the liquid in the soup keeps you hydrated—you may have a fever with a cold or flu and become dehydrated. And if you like spicy foods, you may want to add some to the soup: The capsaicin in such foods as hot peppers will help to break up sinus congestion.

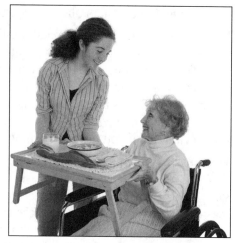

It's true! Chicken soup really *can* help relieve cold symptoms.

Are brown eggs more nutritious than white eggs?

No, brown eggs are not any more nutritious than white eggs—either in quality, flavor, or nutrient value. It merely means the brown eggs (or even blue or tan) were laid by different breeds of hens. Brown eggs are often thought of as "more natural," because many organic farmers pick breeds that are easier to raise—and that includes those chickens who lay eggshells of various colors. (For more about the nutrition of eggs, see the chapter "Nutrition in Eating and Drinking Choices.")

Does that Thanksgiving turkey really put me to sleep?

People who eat a great deal of turkey for Thanksgiving dinner often complain of feeling sleepy after the meal. For years, researchers blamed the tryptophan—a sleep-promoting compound found in turkey. But tryptophan actually works best if you take it on an empty stomach without any other protein—and turkey naturally has, of course, plenty of protein. It is thought that the real reason for your sleepiness after a Thanksgiving dinner are some of the other foods on the table, especially mashed potatoes and stuffing, two carbohydrates. They trigger a chain reaction, helping to concentrate the tryptophan at higher levels in your bloodstream; from there, it reaches your brain, and makes you sleepy. And of course, it doesn't help that people usually overeat at the Thanksgiving table—another factor that causes drowsiness.

Do potatoes cause arthritis?

This idea is based on an old folk legend: that potatoes or any other plants of the nightshade family, such as tomatoes, peppers, and eggplant, will cause or exacerbate arthritis in some people. But this is truly a myth: Some people may be allergic to these types of vegetables, but there is no epidemiological or any scientific evidence that such foods are connected to arthritis.

Is brown sugar better than white sugar?

Brown sugar is still "sugar," no matter what type (usually as light or dark). It either has molasses added to it to darken the color, or is not refined as much as white sugar, leaving in some of the molasses. Some advertising suggests that brown sugar has "more minerals" than refined white sugar; and although it does contain a minute amount of minerals, it is not enough to provide any real nutritional value.

Can some teas help you stay slimmer?

Although it is not a magic formula to stay or become slimmer—and more studies need to be done—some recent research indicates that many people who regularly drink caffeinated tea may have a tendency to be slimmer. The researchers attribute this slimness from white, green, and oolong teas to a combination of caffeine and catechins, both of which help to break down fat and give you energy (thus burning calories). The overall amount needed is not much, either—just two to three cups of tea per day may help you stay slimmer.

Does milk before bed help a person to sleep?

If a person doesn't have intolerance to milk, the beverage is often used before bedtime for a good night's sleep. For years, it was thought that the tryptophan in the milk made a person sleepy, but research now shows that the protein in milk actually blocks the tryptophan from working. Even though many people swear that it works, it may really be the comforting milk-at-bedtime ritual that is truly helping you sleep.

Does lack of sleep interfere with your health—and nutrition?

According to recent research, your "eight hours of sleep" is often important to your health—especially to help you maintain a good weight. One study found that when a person is groggy in the morning from lack of sleep (either because of insomnia or staying awake watching the late shows), he or she reports being hungrier in the morning. This usually translates to eating larger portions for breakfast and more snacks later. Researchers believe this may have to do with ghrelin, a hormone that stimulates your appetite: the lack of sleep causes a surge in the hormone. Another study showed that when we are sleep-deprived, our bodies release a molecule called 2-AG that causes us to be hungry. When participants had just over eight hours of sleep, the 2-AG levels were low; those who had just over four hours of sleep had higher levels that peaked in the afternoon—when snack cravings set in.

Do certain foods affect our sleep?

Yes, certain foods definitely can affect our sleep—and sleep patterns—preventing us from getting our usual, healthy (for most people) seven to nine hours of sleep each

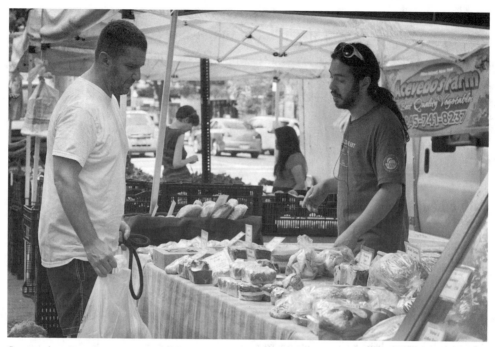

Grocery shopping on an empty stomach is never a good idea because it compels people to make impulse purchases. People tend to buy foods that are higher in calories when they are hungry.

night. Most of us know that if we eat too much before going to bed it can disrupt our sleep. This is because although we are trying to sleep, our digestive system is trying to digest our food. It is also why many people experience acid reflux or heartburn: a heavy meal (especially with plenty of fats) late at night delays the emptying of the stomach—and because you are lying down, gravity causes the acids and digestive juices to flow into your esophagus. In addition, for some people, drinking or eating foods with too much caffeine before bedtime can cause them to remain awake (although some people have no trouble sleeping after consuming large amounts of caffeine before bedtime).

Why does eating chocolate make some people feel good?

Chocolate contains over 300 known chemicals, some of which can alter mood, such as caffeine. But chocolate also contains a small amount of the chemical phenylethylamine (PEA), a stimulant to the nervous system that makes people feel more alert and gives them a sense of overall well-being.

Can strong bones be built only by eating dairy foods?

Although dairy products such as yogurt, milk, and cheese are known to contain a great deal of calcium for strong bones, there are also other nutrients that help to maintain your skeleton—especially if you can't or don't eat dairy products. For example, you also need vitamin D and protein for strong bones. You can get many of these nutrients from

Why shouldn't you shop for food when you're hungry?

Although we've all heard that we shouldn't shop for groceries when we're hungry, many people don't know why. But one recent study may have uncovered just why hunger causes us to load our carts with sugary sweets and calorie-rich foods. Using functional magnetic resonance imaging (FMRI) to record brain activity, the researchers first kept the participants' glucose levels normal—and the part of the brain (in the prefrontal cortex) that controls emotions and impulses was more active. But when the glucose levels were dropped, the deeper brain regions (hypothalamus, thalamus, and *nucleus accumbens*) became active—the parts that govern motivation, reward, and addiction. Although more studies need to be done, this may indicate that we are wired to crave very dense foods more when our stored energy reserves are perceived by the body (and brain) to be depleted—in other words, when we're hungry.

such foods as kale, broccoli, bok choy, tofu, and fortified foods, such as soymilk, some cereals, and orange juice. (But be aware, foods such as spinach and rhubarb are good sources of calcium, but are high in oxalates—a substance that decreases calcium absorption.) And as most nutritionists will mention, doing some weight-bearing exercise along with eating these nutrient-rich foods will also help your bones.

Can soy products lower my cholesterol?

Yes, it is thought that eating soy products helps to lower cholesterol, but the reasons why have changed somewhat: Researchers once thought the isoflavones in soy helped to lower cholesterol. But more recent research has shown that people who eat soy products (and eat more vegetarian meals) are essentially replacing meats, dairy, and other foods high in saturated fat and cholesterol. This drop in the ingestion of fats and cholesterol, of course, lowers your blood cholesterol—not the soy products.

Can food have cholesterol but no fat?

Yes, contrary to what most people think, you can have a food that has cholesterol but no fat—but it's not common. Foods with no fat, usually most fruits, vegetables, and grains, don't have cholesterol; you do find cholesterol—and fats—in animal products such as meat, eggs, milk, and cheese. So when it comes to "cholesterol but no fat" products, there are a very few, including nonfat yogurts and skim milk.

The opposite can also be true, with people being fooled about claims of no cholesterol, but then the food has a lot of fat in it. Thus, next time you buy a fat-ridden bag of potato chips to munch on, don't be fooled by the "no cholesterol" label. It may not have cholesterol because it's a potato product, but they are usually cooked in fats—and when eaten in excess, can make you gain weight.

HOW FOODS AFFECT YOU

How many calories do you expend, depending on which exercises you are doing?

According to the Mayo Clinic, there are many ways to exercise that will help a person expend calories. It recommends, as a general goal, to aim for at least 30 minutes of physical activity every day—plus, eating nutritious foods so you have the necessary energy to exercise!

The following chart shows the estimated number of calories burned while doing various exercises for one hour; this chart does not include all exercises, but many of the more popular ones. (*Note:* Each calorie burned varies widely depend-

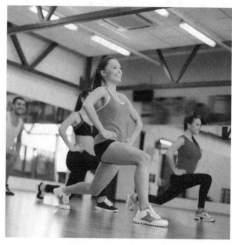

High-impact aerobics are one of the best ways to burn calories and lose weight.

ing on the exercise, intensity level, and your individual situation, such as health and any illnesses you may have that curtail your ability to do the exercise to completion.)

Calories Burned Based on Weight and Activity

Activity (1 hour)	Calories Burned per Weight		
	160 lb (73 kg)	200 lb (91 kg)	240 lb (109 kg)
Aerobics, high impact	533	664	796
Aerobics, low impact	365	455	545
Aerobics, water	402	501	600
Backpacking	511	637	763
Basketball game	584	728	872
Bicycling, <10 mph, for leisure	292	364	436
Bowling	219	273	327
Canoeing	256	319	382
Dancing, ballroom	219	273	327
Football, touch or flag	584	728	872
Golfing, carrying clubs	314	391	469
Hiking	438	546	654
Ice skating	511	637	763
Racquetball	511	637	763
Resistance (weight) training	365	455	545
Rollerblading	548	683	818
Rope jumping	861	1,074	1,286
Rowing, stationary	438	546	654

Calories Burned Based on Weight and Activity

Activity (1 hour)	Calories Burned per Weight		
	160 lb (73 kg)	200 lb (91 kg)	240 lb (109 kg)
Running, 5 mph	606	755	905
Running, 8 mph	861	1,074	1,286
Skiing, cross-country	496	619	741
Skiing, downhill	314	391	469
Skiing, water	438	546	654
Softball or baseball	365	455	545
Stair treadmill	657	819	981
Swimming, laps	423	528	632
Tae kwon do	752	937	1,123
Tai chi	219	273	327
Tennis, singles	584	728	872
Volleyball	292	364	436
Walking, 2 mph	204	255	305
Walking, 3.5 mph	314	391	469

Adapted from the Mayo Clinic; they adapted the list from: B. E. Ainsworth et al., "2011 Compendium of Physical Activities: A Second Update of Codes and MET Values." *Medicine & Science in Sports & Exercise, 43* (2011) p. 1575.

What are some easily prepared foods that help fight fat?

For most people, it is true—today's world is filled with fast-paced jobs, travel, and everything in between. Because of this, many people eat foods that are low in nutritional value—foods that are easy to fix or buy and easy to eat fast—thus, they pack on weight they don't need. Many recent studies have shown that obesity has become a major problem in the United States and other Western countries—and this "fast-food" factor may be a major piece to the weight gain puzzle (for more about obesity, see the chapter "Nutrition and Allergies, Illnesses, and Diseases.")

But there are some foods that seem to help fight weight gain, while adding healthy nutrients to your diet—and most are easy to prepare. For example, to make an easy salad, dice up bell peppers (they contain vitamin C, a nutrient that may help a person lose weight), some romaine lettuce and beet greens (both are low in calories, but high in nutrients such as vitamins A, C, and K), and chunks of canned salmon (it gives you healthy omega-3 fatty acids; plus, the proteins in the salmon require more calories to digest and keep you feeling full faster and longer). And for dessert, have some dark chocolate chips; because of their small size and intense flavor, you will eat fewer—in other words, a small handful will do, not the entire bag!

Do foods affect us when we are under stress?

Yes, and anyone who has reached for a candy bar at certain times in his or her life can verify that food does affect us mentally, especially in times of stress. Most nutritionists warn people against eating in response to stress or when they are depressed or worried, as most of the foods we choose are void of nutrients, minerals, and healthy fats. Instead, such foods are usually filled with sugars that raise our serotonin levels (the "feel good" hormone), salt, and bad fats that make us only *think* we feel better. For example, many people think soft drinks perk up their mood—and they are right, but the mood lasts only a short time. What really happens is that the sugar makes us feel good during the first rush of the "sugar high," but then our mood quickly plummets (all while the sugar turns to fat in our systems).

How does stress affect our eating habits?

Not only do foods affect us when we are under stress—but how we respond to food is also affected by the craziness in our lives. For example, stress often can shut down our appetites; this is because the part of our brain called the hypothalamus releases a corticotrophin hormone that suppresses our appetite in times of stress. The brain also sends out messages to the adrenal glands, causing them to pump out adrenaline (also called the hormone epinephrine), making us even less likely to want any food. This can eventually change if the stress keeps going, because the adrenal glands release yet another hormone called cortisol that increases our appetite.

Do some foods make us moody?

It's definitely been shown by many researchers that certain foods make us moody—either happy or grumpy. People who are not happy often reach for chocolate for a reason: This food triggers the release of endorphins, the morphine-like natural painkillers our brains secrete that create a sense of emotional well-being (they are usually mentioned in conjunction with exercise). Other positive mood-enhancing foods include milk, chicken, bananas, and leafy green vegetables, as they all trigger the release of the neurotransmitter dopamine from the brain. Foods that contain tryptophan—an amino acid that the body uses to make serotonin, the neurotransmitter that slows down your nerves so your brain isn't working so hard—can make you happy, too, and include dairy products, leafy greens, Greek yogurt, seafood, poultry, whole grains, beans, rice, and even eggs.

There are also some foods that can pull our moods down. They include most high-fat and high-sugar meals or snacks, all of which can first make you happy for a short time, but then make you feel bad. Foods that contain hydrogenated fats or corn syrup (or any type of processed sugar) can make you moody. And for some people, eating foods with artificial flavorings, colors, or sweeteners can have the same (bad) effects.

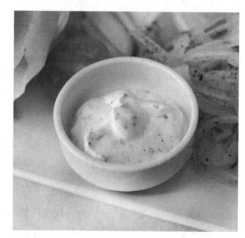

Eating Greek yogurt along with leafy greens is a terrific way to elevate your mood because these foods contain tryptophan.

Can certain nutritious foods help regulate our moods?

Yes, there are plenty of nutritious foods that can help regulate our moods. For example, a simple baked sweet potato (without any added sugar or butter) is loaded with beta-carotene, the precursor to vitamin A; this vitamin helps the enzyme activity that helps release mood-regulating neurotransmitters such as dopamine (a natural hormone that makes us feel better). Foods that are high in omega-3 fatty acids, such as wild-caught salmon, also help to boost our mood; and even organic eggs contain mood-enhancing B-vitamins, zinc, and iodine. And nuts such as walnuts (with omega-3s), almonds (with vitamin E), and Brazil nuts (with selenium) can also make you feel better.

Do processed foods affect our moods?

Yes, it is thought that people who eat diets packed with processed foods—especially meats, fried foods, snacks, and deserts—have more depressed feelings than those who eat more good-mood foods, such as fresh fruits and vegetables. In one study, it was found that the risk for depression in men and women rose by about 60 percent if they ate too many processed foods in their diet. In another study, it was shown that such processed foods, many with an overload of saturated and trans fats, were linked to low moods and even irritability and aggression.

YOU, NUTRITION, AND THE INTERNET

Are there any "good" resources about food and nutrition on the Internet?

Many researchers—and doctors, nurses, and other health practitioners—have found that the Internet is a boon, but also a bane when it comes to the general public's awareness of nutrition. Appendix 1 in the back of this book includes some of the "better" food safety and nutrition sites—many that have plenty of information available to the public—that are often noted by many nutritionists and health-care professionals (websites change over time; we apologize for any inconvenience caused by an incorrect Internet link).

Can a person lose weight by skipping meals?

Yes, of course, a person can lose weight by skipping meals—but it's really not a good idea if you want to lose some pounds. In particular, skipping meals can actually make you feel hungrier, and you will eat more at your next meal. According to the National Institutes of Health, several studies have shown that there is a definite link between skipping breakfast and obesity. For the average healthy person, one of the best ways to lose weight—besides eating healthier and less calorie-dense foods—is to eat several small meals during the day. Not only will this help melt away some pounds, but it will stabilize your blood sugar—and you won't crave as much food (especially sugary and fatty foods) at each meal.

Why is chronic dieting bad for most people?

Chronic dieting (also called yo-yo dieting or weight cycling) occurs when a person goes on and off diets—losing a significant amount of weight but eventually gaining it all back. This type of on-and-off dieting can result in several health problems. For instance, for those who want to conceive a child, some research shows that chronic dieting often leads to infertility. In addition, when your daily caloric intake becomes extremely low, your body tends to digest your muscle cells—and less muscle mass causes your metabolism to slow down. Other research indicates that weight cycling can increase the risk for certain health problems, such as high blood pressure and cholesterol, some types of cancer, and even gallbladder disease.

What are "diet pills"?

Diet pills (or dietary aids or supplements) are just as the name implies—pills you take when you want to diet and lose weight. But according to most experts, the majority of diet pills have not been proven effective—and some may be very dangerous to your health. One of the problems comes from the claims made by advertisers: many of them are just not accurate. This is because dietary supplements and weight-loss aids are not subject to the same rigorous standards as are prescription drugs—so they can be sold with limited (or no) proof of effectiveness or safety. But according to the FDA, once a diet product is on the market, it monitors it for safety, and can immediately take action to ban or recall a potentially dangerous one.

The government also monitors the diet pills on the market, giving the public an idea of potential problems with a product. For example, according to the USDA's Natural Medicines Comprehensive Database (2011), diet pills touting chromium claimed to decrease the appetite and increase the calories burned; but it was found that that the pills were probably ineffective, and had the potential to cause headache, insomnia, irritability, mood changes, and cognitive dysfunction. Another example is that of diet pills with green tea extract that the companies claimed would decrease appetite and increase calorie and fat metabolism; government studies found that there was insufficient evidence to substantiate the claim, and the product had the potential to cause dizziness, insomnia, agitation, nausea, vomiting, bloating, gas, and diarrhea. (Other studies have also shown such supplements may cause liver damage; in fact, it is estimated that dietary supplements account for about 20 percent of drug-related liver injuries that necessitate hospital care—an increase of about 7 percent in one decade.)

Why do some people seem to eat whatever they want and still lose or maintain their weight?

This question has plagued many people for years—especially those who want or need to lose weight. And yes, there are people who seem to eat anything they want, and still lose or maintain their current weight. In order to lose weight, you have to burn more calories than you eat or drink. For some people, that means exercise and cutting back on

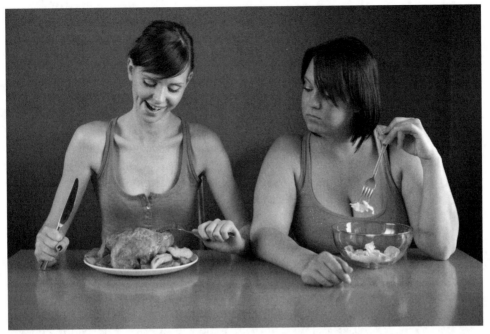

Don't you hate people who eat whatever they want and stay slim? Yes, one reason might be genetics, but other causes include whether a person has an active lifestyle or takes certain medication.

some calories. But for people who seem to be able to eat anything, they actually use more energy than they take in through food and drink. This can be for a number of reasons, including a person's age, medicines they take, what type of diet they are on, their lifestyle (such as how much they exercise or if their job entails sitting or physical work)—and of course, genetics. One of the best ways to lose weight is to talk to your health-care provider, who understands all the factors that may affect your weight.

Are some "fad" diets controversial?

There are plenty of "fad" diets out there—and some are very controversial. Most are thought to be more harmful than helpful, mainly because they do not provide all the nutrients your body needs to stay healthy. According to the National Institutes of Health, low-calorie diets—especially those based on fewer than 800 calories a day—can affect your heart. Other diets do not help you truly lose weight, but because you can lose water weight quickly, they give the *illusion* of weight loss.

But the real controversy comes from what a person learns (or doesn't learn) from the diet: Most fad diets do not teach a person how to eat well and keep the weight off—but are just a "quick fix." And when a person goes back to his or her usual eating routine—often because the fad diet becomes boring or too hard to follow—the dieter usually regains any weight lost. (For more about the various types of diets, see "Appendix 3: Comparing Diets.")

327

What are some interesting "fad" diets?

There are numerous "fad" diets, with each year bringing out more even amazing suggestions about what to eat to lose weight and/or eat healthier. The following list gives some of the more interesting—and some outrageous—diets that are in the diet literature. *Note:* It's not up to us to judge; if you decide to go on one of these diets, it's your choice, but we urge you to first contact your doctor in order to find out if there are other, healthier ways to eat better! (For more about fad diets, see "Appendix 3: Comparing Diets.")

Alcorexia or Drunkorexia Diet—Usually associated with college students, this very harmful diet takes its toll mentally and physically. The main idea is to eat very little in terms of calories so you can indulge in a great deal of alcohol, which contains calories. Not only is this damaging to the brain and overall diet, but excessive alcohol can cause liver and other organ problems, and even alcohol poisoning (for more about alcohol, see the chapter "Nutrition in Eating and Drinking Choices"). For a person who is on such a "diet," there will also be behavioral problems, as the lack of nutrients or healthy foods will make him or her feel weak, tired, and irritable.

Aztec Diet—This diet has one key element: chia seeds. The tiny seeds fueled the Aztec and Mayan empires, eating these seeds can help many people in terms of nutrition—they are low in calories and high in fiber, along with niacin, magnesium, and antioxidants—but they are not the answer to lowering a person's weight. (For more about chia seeds, see the chapter "The Basics of Nutrition: Macronutrients and Nonnutrients.")

Biotyping Diet—This diet involves using certain foods to change the body's hormonal balance. Like the Blood Type Diet, it is based on the five key blood types, but goes into much more details about the blood, all determined by genetic markers that tell our biological types: A1, A2, B, O, AB, and the Rh-negative subtype. Based on this, the diet determines safe and harmful foods for a person to eat, what food allergies, and even diseases, are related to each type; the diets are also said to be from various ecosystems where certain biotypes evolved and adapted to specific foods. Proponents believe a person using the Biotype Diet will have fewer food allergies, inflammation, and autoimmune diseases, no matter what age or sex.

Blood Type Diet—Everyone has a certain blood type—either O, A, B, or AB. The blood type diet is based on how your blood type reacts chemically with certain foods. For example, people with type O blood are advised to eat a diet heavy with lean poultry, meat, fish, and vegetables, but fewer amounts of grains, beans, and dairy. Type A should have a meat-free diet, with plenty of fruits, vegetables, beans, and whole grains—all fresh and organic, if possible, since the proposers of this diet say type A's have a sensitive immune system.

Breatharian Diet—People who are on this diet do not eat or drink at all—but live off of "air and sunlight alone." Contrary to what most Breatharians believe, humans are not plants. Vegetation survives such conditions because they undergo photosynthesis, a way of converting sunlight and air into energy in order for the plant to survive—humans cannot. The "rich and famous" seem to like this diet—maybe because they can afford different air? And if you live and breathe in a pollution-ridden city, will you be "ingesting" too many toxins and heavy metals?

Cabbage Soup Diet—You can really drop weight fast with this diet, as it is low-fat and low-calorie. But because it lacks the nutrients present in other vegetables, just eating cabbage can actually be detrimental to your body's overall chemical balance. There are other foods you can add, but the main push is for cabbage three meals a day. Again, this is not a long-term fix to a person's weight problem—just a quick fix.

Cookie Diet—This diet was obviously invented by a youngster who loves cookies. Yes, just as the name implies, the only thing you eat for breakfast, lunch, and snacks is cookies (for dinner, you can have something more sensible—hopefully not a doughnut!). But don't get excited—the "cookies" are actually made by the special companies that promote this diet, and most of them come at a high price; in general, the companies claim the high protein and fiber content of the special cookies keeps hunger at bay. But overall, there is a lack of healthy and fresh vegetables and fruits that are much better for health (and much less boring than cookies all the time). And although a person on this diet loses weight initially, he or she usually regains all the weight and more after going off the diet.

Grapefruit Diet—This diet has been around since the 1930s (yes, there were fad diets even back in "the old days"), and is based on the idea that grapefruit contains certain enzymes that can burn off fat—if you eat it before you eat other foods. The details can vary, depending on which grapefruit diet you choose, but overall, most say the regime lasts for about a week and a half. By then, you can lose about 10 pounds—but in reality, you gain the weight back fast. The reason seems to be that the water in the grapefruit makes you feel fuller, so you don't eat as much at a meal, but this fruit has no "fat-burner" enzymes.

Raw Foods Diet—This diet is primarily made up of unprocessed vegan foods—uncooked, unprocessed, mostly organic foods including raw fruits, vegetables, nuts, seeds, and spouted grains—that have not been heated any higher than 115 degrees Fahrenheit (46 degrees Celsius). It is mainly eaten by people who believe (and for some foods, this is true, including vitamins B and C) that heating foods at any higher temperature makes the food lose a significant amount of nutrients and important enzymes. They also believe that cooking at higher temperatures can create changes in the food that can harm our health. The problem with this diet is making sure you get enough protein, iron, calcium, and other vitamins and minerals that are not always present in raw foods; for example, cooking can boost the beta-carotene in certain foods. And note: Pregnant women, young children, elderly, and people with compromised immune systems should be careful about this diet—as there is a risk for foodborne illnesses if the raw foods are not washed thoroughly and carefully.

Zone Diet—This diet is actually a balancing act—a balance of fat, carbohydrates and protein, all a certain percent at each meal. To do this, you eat three meals and two snacks a day, each being a mix of low-fat protein (30 percent; such as skinless chicken), carbohydrates (40 percent; such as most fruits and vegetables), and some good fats (30 percent; such as olive oil, almonds, or avocados). You can still eat such carbohydrates as pasta and bread, but they should be thought of as just side dishes to the main meal. Plus, there are certain vegetables and fruits that are not favored because of their high sugar content, such as carrots, corn, bananas, and raisins; and fats such as those from red meat and egg yolk are also rejected in this diet. Calories also matter—around 1,200 for women and 1,500 for men; other rules include eating a meal within an hour of waking, never allowing more than five hours to go by without eating, and always having a snack before you go to bed. This diet does not cause a major, immediate weight loss, but rather a gradual loss of weight; the proponents of this diet also say that you will lose fat, but not muscle or water (so you tone up and slim down, making your clothes fit better, but you don't see as much weight loss on the scales). On the down side, you have to stick to the percents of foodstuff at each meal.

What is the ORAC diet—otherwise known at the O2 diet?

The ORAC or O2 diet is based on the ORAC score, or the oxygen radical absorbance capacity scale, as measured in laboratory tests. The O2 diet has a thirty-two-day plan that centers on the scale, as the proponents of this diet believe that you will have more energy if the foods you eat have a higher ORAC score—in other words, more antioxidants. In this plan, you count your ORAC scores, not calories, and eat the foods that have the highest scores (healthy fruits and vegetables, such as blueberries and greens) and less of those with the lowest scores (such as baked goods, candy, and soda). The entire thirty-two-day plan has various stages—from a cleansing stage through three more stages until you are eating within the guidelines. Probably the biggest concerns about this diet are twofold: Not everyone should be on such a diet—and there is still a controversy over what the ORAC scores truly mean in terms of health. (For more about the ORAC score, see the chapter "The Basics of Nutrition: Micronutrients"; for the debates about ORAC, see the chapter "Controversies with Food, Beverages, and Nutrition.")

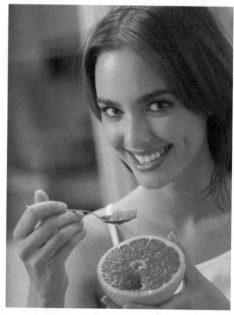

The grapefruit diet was started in the 1930s on the false notion that the fruit contains enzymes that help you lose weight.

How many vegans or vegetarians are there in the United States?

It is estimated that, in 2012, around 5 percent of adult Americans called themselves vegetarians, while around 2 percent considered themselves to be vegans.

Is there a difference between a vegetarian and vegan diet?

There is a definite difference between a vegetarian and vegan—although many people believe both types follow the same diets. In general, vegetarians eat mostly fruits, vegetables, whole grains, and no meat (including poultry and fish). But there are several "types" of vegetarians. For example, vegetarians who eat dairy, eggs, fruits, and vegetables, but no meat, are called lacto-ovo vegetarians; ovo vegetarians eat no meat or dairy, but will eat eggs; and lacto-vegetarians don't eat meat and eggs, but do eat dairy, such as milk, cheese, yogurt, and butter. There are also some vegetarians called pescetarians, who abstain from eating all meat with the exception of fish (mainly to obtain the fishes' abundant omega-3 fatty acids).

Vegans are those who do not eat meat of any kind, and no dairy, eggs, or any product or processed food derived from an animal. Some doctors have noted that patients who follow a vegan lifestyle are usually the healthiest—with lower incidences of diabetes, heart disease, and cancers. Some people choose to eat vegan for health reasons, while others do it for environmental or personal reasons, especially those who respect the rights of other animals on our planet. (For more about vegans and vegetarians, see the chapter "The Basics of Nutrition: Macronutrients and Non-nutrients.")

Do some studies show that eating a vegetarian diet is healthy for you?

According to the National Institutes of Health, for the average healthy person, research has shown that those who follow a vegetarian diet, on the average, often have lower levels of obesity, lower blood pressure, and a reduced risk for heart disease. In addition, the 35-year-long Harvard Nurses' Health study showed that dietary cholesterol intake (only from animal foods) was associated with living a significantly shorter life; while another study determined that vegetarians on the average live almost eight years longer than the general population.

These results are thought to be due to the types of low-fat foods eaten (mostly no animal fats, although some vegetarians eat dairy and eggs), and fewer calories consumed (most vegetables and fruits are low in calories). Vegetarians also tend to have a lower BMI (body mass index; for more about BMI, see this chapter) than people on other types of eating plans. But not all vegetarians are healthy—as with any diet plan, vegetarians, too, can make certain food choices that are high in fat and calories, and low in nutrients. (For more about this diet, see "Appendix 3: Comparing Diets.")

What is a macrobiotic diet?

A macrobiotic diet is really just a way to eat, not a true diet plan. In general, it includes unprocessed vegan foods, much like the raw foods diet (some people even call it a raw food diet), such as whole grains and vegetables and also, perhaps once a week, the occasional serving of fish, fruit, seeds, and nuts. Vegetables are often those found in Asian cuisine, including daikon and sea vegetables (such as the various types of seaweeds); also soybean and other bean foods (such as tofu and tempeh); and whole grains such as brown rice, barley, oats, rye, and buckwheat. But there are also several types of food to avoid; in particular, sugar, dairy, eggs, refined oils, and anything processed or with chemical additives are not used by most macrobiotic cooks. This diet is often cited as having some cardiovascular benefits, mainly because the diet is low in fats (especially saturated) and high in healthy vegetables, whole grains, and bean products.

APPENDIX 1:
FOOD SAFETY WEBSITES

- **Center for Food Safety and Applied Nutrition** (http://www.fda.gov/Food): provides information on the safety of products regulated by the FDA.

- **Centers for Disease Control and Prevention** (http://www.cdc.gov/foodsafety/): provides information on diseases and pathogens, environmental hazards, and surveillance illness data as well as emerging food safety and health issues.

- **Electronic Data Information Source** at University of Florida's Institute of Food and Agricultural Sciences (http://edis.ifas.ufl.edu): a comprehensive, single-source repository of all current UF/IFAS numbered peer-reviewed publications that provide research-based information on various topics including food safety, nutrition, and health. The website is equipped with a search engine to assist visitors with navigating the collection.

- **The Environmental Protection Agency** (http://www.epa.gov/): provides safety information related to environmental issues. This includes industrial chemicals and other man-made products.

- **European Food Safety Authority** (http://www.efsa.europa.eu/): provides science-based information on various food safety regulations and issues pertaining to the Europe Union.

- **FoodSafety.gov**: this is the gateway to all food safety information provided by federal and state government agencies for consumers, professionals, and others. This website also connects users to state agencies with a role in food safety such as the state department of health.

- **Food Safety and Inspection Service** (http://www.fsis.usda.gov/): This website of the United States Department of Agriculture (USDA) provides food safety information on meat, poultry, and egg products as well as seasonal food safety tips. The information generally is related to the products that are regulated under this program.

- **HomeFoodSafety.org**: This site belongs to the Academy of Nutrition and Dietetics (formerly the American Dietetic Association). It provides information on topics from home food safety to desktop dining

- **Institute of Food Technologies** (http://www.ift.org/knowledge-center/read-ift-publications.aspx): provides access to both members and the public on subjects related to food science, food technology, food safety, and nutrition.

- **International Association for Food Protection** (http://www.foodprotection.org/publications/): provides information specifically on food safety for both professionals and consumers.

- **Partnership for Food Education Safety** (http://www.fightbac.org/): provides educational materials related to safe food handling. It supplies materials for educators, media, and consumers.

- **World Health Organization**'s food safety page (http://www.who.int/foodsafety/en/): provides information related to food, nutrition, food safety, and health. The organization also provides publications on issues that are relevant to both the underdeveloped and developed world.

APPENDIX 2: NUTRITION WEBSITES

- **Academy of Nutrition and Dietetics** (http://www.eatright.org): (formerly the American Dietetic Association); this site provides science-based information related to nutrition, health, and well-being.

- **American Cancer Society** (http://www.cancer.org): provides information on types of cancers, statistics, current research, how to stay healthy, and various resources for support and treatment.

- **American Diabetes Association** (http://www.diabetes.org): provides information about diabetes research, prevention, and other helpful information for persons with diabetes, health professionals, and the general public.

- **American Heart Association** (http://www.americanheart.org): provides information on heart diseases and conditions, including heart attack and stroke warning signs, healthy lifestyles, publications, and resources available to the public.

- **American Institute for Cancer Research** (http://www.aicr.org): educates the public about cancer, the results of current research on cancer prevention, and strategies for reducing cancer risk.

- **Center for Nutrition Policy and Promotion** (http://www.cnpp.usda.gov/): This USDA site is a resource for educational materials, including those for MyPlate. Here you can find educational materials and information related to the Dietary Guidelines for Americans, the interactive Healthy Eating Index, and many other resources for adults and children. You also can link to the USDA's other program websites, such as Women, Infants and Children (WIC), the School Lunch Program, the Supplemental Nutrition Assistance Program or SNAP (formerly Food Stamps), etc.

- **Food and Nutrition Information Center** (http://www.nal.usda.gov/fnic): This USDA site is a reliable resources for consumers, nutrition and health professionals, and educators. The site includes downloadable educational materials, government reports, research articles, and more.

- **National Center for Health Statistics** (http://www.cdc.gov/nchs): Just about any health statistic can be found at this CDC website.

- **National Heart, Lung, and Blood Institute** (http://www.nhlbi.nih.gov): The site for the National Institutes of Health gives consumers and professionals free health information related to a variety of health conditions. It also includes information about clinical trials.

- **National Nutrient Database for Standard Reference** (http://www.nal.usda.gov/fnic/food comp/search/): This search page to the USDA database provides users a way to look up the nutrient content of over 7,000 different foods.

- **Nutrition.gov:** Dubbed *Smart Nutrition Starts Here*, Nutrition.gov is the federal government's gateway to reliable information on nutrition, healthy eating, physical activity, and food safety for consumers, educators, and health professionals.

APPENDIX 3: COMPARING DIETS

THE DIETS

These are *not* all the diets available in the lifestyle and healthy eating literature. Some are considered weight-loss diets; others are thought to be "lifestyle" diets—or ones that can help you maintain your health over a long time as opposed to just loosing weight in the short term. There are many more, but these represent some of the more well-known weight-loss diet plans, lifestyle plans, and overall ways of eating—and, if applicable, can help you nutritionally (for more details about several of these diets, see the chapter "Nutrition and You").

For those of you who have been on some of the more "questionable" diets and have lost weight, we applaud you! We are not here to argue about which diet is best, but to give you information about many of the diets available. But remember, it's not only about losing weight when it comes to diet; it's also about a lifestyle choice, keeping your weight at a healthy level for your body size, gender, and age, and eating well-balanced, nutritious meals—all while understanding your health needs (for example, if you are a diabetic, or have celiac disease).

And, as always, before you start any diet program, consult your doctor or health care professional, especially if you have any health restrictions or are pregnant or breast feeding.

GENERAL DIETS

FLEXITARIAN/SEMI-VEGETARIAN

Emphasis of the Plan—This is not so much a plan as it is a way of eating. In particular, people who like to eat vegetarian, but will occasionally eat meat, poultry, and fish (in moderation), are called flexitarians or semi-vegetarians.

Pros and Cons of the Diet
Pros: As long as you eat a balanced diet, you will get plenty of nutritious food. Research also indicates that, similar to vegetarian and vegan diets, you may experience less of a risk for heart disease, certain cancers, and allergies.

Cons: Many people will have a hard time on this Diet. Culturally in America, there is a bias toward meats (which is why there is the phrase, "He/She is a meat-and-potato person," meaning they like to eat meat at every meal). In addition, you can't consider eating more baked goods, fatty foods, and sweets as "eating vegetarian." No matter what the diet, if you're trying to lose weight, watching how much you eat—and what is in that food in terms of fats—is important.

Does It Work?—For people who like to eat vegetarian meals—but still like the taste of an occasional salmon or turkey burger—this is an easy diet to follow. Because the emphasis is on fresh fruits, vegetables, and whole grains, a person will ingest plenty of nutrients that are needed for good health; in fact, some research indicates that flexitarians weigh 15 percent less than their carnivorous counterparts and have a lower risk for heart disease, diabetes, and cancers.

GLUTEN FREE

Emphasis of the Plan—As with flexitarians, this is not so much a plan as it is a way of eating. It is primarily for people who have been diagnosed with celiac disease, or those who believe they have some type of gluten intolerance—or even wheat allergies.

Pros and Cons of the Diet

Pros: As long as you eat a balanced diet, you will get plenty of nutritious food—but you won't be able to eat products that contain wheat, barley, or rye. It can also be a very nutritious diet, as fruits, vegetables, and fresh meats do not have gluten (just be aware of gluten if the foods are processed or have a coating).

Cons: Many people will have a hard time on this diet, as there are many products that have gluten. One of the more difficult problems with this type of diet is looking for processed foods that do not contain any wheat; many times, if the amount is low enough, it can still be added to the product. The best way to minimize your chances of ingesting gluten in products is to check the labels—and note if the facility that processes the product also produces gluten products.

Does It Work?—For people who cannot tolerate gluten, and especially those with celiac disease, this is the best diet to eliminate or reduce gastrointestinal discomfort. Because the emphasis is on fresh fruits and vegetables, a person will ingest plenty of nutrients that are needed for good health; in fact, this diet will not only help you to eat better (because your gastrointestinal tract won't be irritated), but it also means you will have a lower risk for heart disease, diabetes, and cancers.

GLYCEMIC-INDEX

Emphasis of the Plan—This is another lifestyle choice, not a diet *per se.* It is often used by people who have been diagnosed with diabetes or are pre-diabetic to improve blood sugar levels; and it is often the basis for diets that emphasize blood sugar levels. (Also see the Nutrisystem and Zone diets below.) In general, the diet is based on ranking foods and drinks that contain carbohydrates because such foods have the biggest effect on the person's blood sugar.

Pros and Cons of the Diet

Pros: Glycemic index diets are good for many people who want to control blood sugar spikes; this is because proponents believe foods with a high glycemic index score are quickly digested by your body, causing blood sugar to also rise quickly (followed by a energy crash). Whereas foods with a low glycemic index score go into your system much slower, raising your blood sugar more gradually; this is not only good for your system, but keeping your sugar balanced can help reduce the risk for insulin resistance.

Cons: Because this diet is based on "food scores" that range from 0 to 100, it may be difficult to follow for people who do not have access to these food numbers—or for people to keep track of all the numbers. In addition, such a diet may be less healthy because it still contains large amounts of calories, sugars, and fats under the guise of being a "low glycemic index."

Does It Work?—In some ways, yes, but there are many restrictions. For example, there are hidden carbohydrates in certain processed foods, and foods the person has "no control over," such as meals eaten at restaurants. In addition, while lower glycemic index foods may have a low number to help blood sugar balance, eating the fattier, sugar-laden foods with low indexes can cause other health problems such as obesity.

MACROBIOTIC

Emphasis of the Plan—For most people who consume macrobiotic foods, there is a philosophical aspect to eating this way, maintaining balance in your life, physically, spiritually, and mentally. In general, this way of eating includes unprocessed vegan (or vegetarian) foods somewhat similar to the raw foods diet. It includes whole grains (the majority of the food eaten, between 40 to 60 percent per day, including brown rice, barley, oats, rye, and buckwheat); and vegetables (about 20 to 30 percent of food eaten per day, but not all vegetables—they frown on certain ones such as spinach, eggplant, tomatoes, and zucchini). The diet also emphasizes soups made from vegetables, especially those found in Asian cuisine, including daikon, and sea vegetables (such as the various types of seaweeds), and soybean and other bean foods (such as tofu and tempeh). It also includes, perhaps once a week, the occasional fish, fruit, seeds, and nuts. But there are several types of food to avoid: in particular, sugar, dairy, eggs, refined oils, meats, tropical fruits and drinks, and anything processed or with chemical additives are not used (or eaten) by macrobiotic cooks. Finally, most alcoholic, coffee, and soda beverages are also avoided.

Pros and Cons of the Diet

Pros: This diet is often cited as having some cardiovascular benefits, mainly because the diet is low in fats (especially saturated) and high in healthy, organic (if possible) vegetables, whole grains, and bean products.

Cons: This type of eating takes a great deal of time to prepare, since much of it is cooked from scratch; plus, there are other "rules," including chewing each mouthful at least fifty times before swallowing, and you are asked to stop eating before you are full. As for the foods a person can eat, there are some major questions about the lack of certain nutrients because of the foods that cannot be eaten—or if the diet is not followed correctly or is not planned properly.

Does It Work?—Initially, when the first macrobiotic diet was introduced, it emphasized mostly grains, which caused a great many health problems because of nutrient deficiencies. But more recent macrobiotic diets emphasize a more balanced diet of healthy foods—and if you're willing to pay very close attention to nutrient content (and follow certain rules), it can be a healthy diet for many people. According to some studies, though, it may not be for everyone, especially young children, pregnant or breastfeeding women, and the elderly, since this way of eating minimizes certain needed nutrients for those specific life stages.

MEDITERRANEAN

Emphasis of the Plan—The Mediterranean diet is not a true plan but a way of eating. It is based on the traditional cooking style of countries that border the Mediterranean Sea—diets high in fruits, vegetables, fish, and whole grains, while limiting certain fats and adding other more healthy fats. This diet doesn't use much salt, instead using herbs and spices to flavor the food.

Pros and Cons of the Diet

Pros: Most research shows that the traditional Mediterranean diet can reduce the risk for heart disease, cancer, and even, some say, the incidence of Parkinson's and Alzheimer's diseases. It has been connected to brain health and diabetes prevention and control—and it has been shown to reduce blood pressure and "bad" LDL cholesterol.

Cons: It is often difficult not to overindulge in the rich foods of the Mediterranean; thus, many people find it hard to stick to a lower amount of calories if they are beginning (or maintaining) this diet.

Does It Work?—Overall, it is an easy diet to follow and is high in healthy, nutrient-rich foods, "good" fats (such as mono- and polyunsaturated), fish (rich with omega-3 fatty acids) and whole grains (for example, in breads—not drenched in butter, but plain or dipped in olive oil). But if you don't keep track of your calories, it's possible to gain weight. So whether a person stays healthy—and maintains or loses weight—with this diet is up to the individual.

VEGETARIAN

Emphasis of the Plan—Most vegetarians consider this a "lifestyle" choice, sometimes connecting it with the idea that eating animals is not only unhealthy but also morally wrong. Vegetarians eat fruits, vegetables, whole grains, and no meat; there are also several "types" of vegetarians, including those who are okay with eating eggs and dairy, or those who still eat fish now and then. (For more about the types of vegetarians, see the chapter "Nutrition and You.")

Pros and Cons of the Diet

Pros: There are many studies conducted on vegetarians (and vegans; see below)—and most have been positive for healthy adults (there are some caveats for pregnant women and children; see the chapter "Nutrition throughout Life"). There are studies of how eating vegetarian can reduce heart disease and even cancers of the stomach, lungs, pancreas, and large intestines.

Cons: One of the most mentioned "problems" with a vegetarian diet is that you have to maintain a good balance of nutrients; some people find it difficult to plan such meals, especially in this world of everything "fast"—including fast foods. And although "vitamin B-12 deficiency" is often listed as a problem with vegetarians (and vegans), you can either take supplements or get the vitamin from fortified soy products and some breakfast cereals.

Does It Work?—Research conducted on the vegetarian lifestyle has been positive in terms of health—too many to mention here. But overall, there have been many studies that connect this diet with decreasing the risk for heart disease, strokes, and some cancers, while also increasing longevity.

VEGAN

Emphasis of the Plan—As with vegetarians, this is considered a "lifestyle." Vegans exclude meats such as beef, poultry, and fish; unlike vegetarians, they are much more strict about also excluding eggs, dairy products, and any other foods that are derived from animals.

Pros and Cons of the Diet

Pros: Because this diet means you don't ingest many foods that contain fats, many people lose weight when they go on a vegan diet. They also have a lower body mass index than most of their meat-eating counterparts. Like the vegetarian diet, there are benefits in terms of less risk for heart disease, certain cancers, and diabetes.

Cons: Like all diets, you have to pay attention to the amount of nutrients in your daily meals—and it often takes a great deal of planning and creativity. But if you have a health condition or are pregnant or lactating, before you "go vegan" it would be best to check with your doctor.

Does It Work?—Like the vegetarian diet, a great deal of research indicates that the vegan diet is a healthy diet—as long as you eat a variety of nutrient-rich foods.

INSTITUTION–SPONSORED DIET PLANS

DASH

Emphasis of the Plan—DASH stands for Dietary Approaches to Stop Hypertension, and it was partially developed by the National Heart, Lung, and Blood Institute. This diet concentrates on portion size, eating a variety of different foods, and balancing nutrients from that food. The main focus, as the acronym suggests, is to lower your blood pressure and help you maintain a healthy weight. This is done by eating vegetables, fruits, and low-fat dairy products, along with moderate amounts of nuts, whole grains, poultry, and fish, and very small amounts of beef, sweets, and fats.

Pros and Cons of the Diet

Pros: This diet has the potential to lower your blood pressure, not only by lowering your intake of salt, but also by increasing nutrients such as calcium, magnesium, and potassium.

Cons: This may not work for some people who have other diseases (and medications) that may raise their blood pressure. Thus, if you have a health condition contact your doctor before trying this diet plan.

Does It Work?—Proponents of this diet point out that this is not a weight-loss program but rather a way to potentially lower blood pressure and eat healthier (which means lowering your risk for heart disease, cancers, and diabetes). They offer several guidelines based on the calories you should eat for your age and activity level. But you also have to be aware of which DASH diet is truly best for you in terms of sodium intake, as there are two versions based on your health needs: the standard DASH diet (you can consume up to 2,300 milligrams of sodium per day), and the lower sodium DASH diet (you can consume up to 1,500 milligrams of sodium per day). To compare, it is estimated that a typical American diet has as much as 3,500 milligrams of sodium per day.

MAYO CLINIC

Emphasis of the Plan—The Mayo Clinic diet proposes to be a weight-loss—and also a lifestyle—program. It was developed by medical experts at the Mayo Clinic in Wisconsin and is based on their unique food pyramid (called the Mayo Clinic Healthy Weight Pyramid; it differs from the USDA food pyramid). If followed properly, the proponents claim that a person can lose six to ten pounds in two weeks, and then lose one to two pounds weekly until he or she reaches a weight goal—all why recalibrating eating habits to eat healthier and more balanced afterward.

Pros and Cons of the Diet

Pros: The Mayo Clinic, especially on its website, has an excellent guide that focuses on fifteen different key habits—the habits to keep and those to throw away—and it offers support for people who chose this diet plan. Its food pyramid focuses on more healthy foods, especially fruits and vegetables, with fewer calories. It also shows you how to estimate the best portion sizes and meal plans for your specific needs.

Cons: The weight-loss phase of the plan can be difficult for many people, as it is often a major change in eating habits for people. After the initial weight loss, many people say it gets easier to follow.

Does It Work?—Several studies show that if you follow the plan you will probably lose weight, and for some it can help maintain the desired weight. Like all weight loss plans, it is up to the individual to follow the diet's suggestions.

ORNISH

Emphasis of the Plan—This is not so much of a plan, as a way of eating. It is primarily for people interested in possibly reversing heart disease. It was developed by Dean Ornish and is a very low-fat, high-fiber, vegetarian diet, with ten percent of the calories coming from fats. But it does not allow dairy or meat products, oils, or fats.

Pros and Cons of the Diet
Pros: For many people, this diet has shown to reverse heart disease; not only does it emphasize eating well, but it calls for reducing stress and when it comes to getting regular exercise. Besides fighting heart disease, some research has shown that people who have to restrict their carbohydrates get some of the best benefits from this diet.

Cons: Although the dietary guidelines are straightforward, it is often difficult for people to follow such a restricted vegetarian diet, especially when it comes to getting portions correct. In addition, it may be difficult to find a support system to help with stress; and some people with heart problems will have to start slow in the exercise program that is suggested by this diet.

Does It Work?—This diet has a great following, especially for those who have experienced heart disease or have reversed their heart disease from following this plan. But it is often difficult to follow all the restrictions in foods for some people, especially those who have other health problems.

TLC

Emphasis of the Plan—This diet plan is not designed to help people lose weight; rather, its main focus is to cut high cholesterol, especially lowering the "bad" LDL cholesterol levels. It was created by the National Institutes of Health's National Cholesterol Education Program, and stands for Therapeutic Lifestyle Changes (TLC) diet. In order to lower cholesterol, the diet emphasizes cutting back sharply on all fats—in particular, saturated fats—or those from fatty meat, fried foods, and whole milk (and associated whole-milk products).

Pros and Cons of the Diet

Pros: This diet is endorsed by the American Heart Association, so, of course, it is considered a heart-healthy eating plan that can help reduce the risk for cardiovascular disease. You have a good deal of control when it comes to lowering your LDL, since you pick a target daily calorie level. The TLC diet also suggests one should eat more poly- and monounsaturated fats instead of saturated fats, and cut saturated fats to less than seven percent of those calories (no more than 200 milligrams of dietary cholesterol; for example, about two ounces of cheese).

Cons: Many people will have a hard time getting their correct percentages of daily foods based on the guidelines offered. In addition, contrary to what most people think when they see the word "diet," this was not developed for weight loss but to improve cholesterol levels.

Does It Work?—For people who want to lower their "bad" LDL cholesterol, and perhaps raise their "good" HDL cholesterol, this diet can help most people. And although it is said that it is primarily a cholesterol-lowering diet, the "fringe" benefit for many people is losing excess weight by lowering saturated fat intake and eating more fruits, vegetables, and whole grains, while eliminating fatty and fried foods and whole-milk products.

VOLUMETRICS

Emphasis of the Plan—Volumetrics is based on the idea that people tend to eat the same amount of food each day no matter how many calories are in that food. The idea of this diet is to determine a food's "energy density": cut back on foods offering too much energy density, and make choices that make you still feel full after a meal.

Pros and Cons of the Diet

Pros: The diet offers four food categories, each one based on the energy density of the food—from very low density to high density. It emphasizes more foods in the first two categories, to watch portion sizes of category three, and to keep foods in category four to a minimum. It is a slow way to loose weight, which, according to many experts, is the best approach. It is also heavy on fruits, vegetables, and whole grains, and light on saturated fats and salts.

Cons: Many people may have a hard time switching to lower energy foods on this diet, especially if they have been eating most foods from the highest energy category for a long time.

Does It Work?—For people who are determined to lose weight slowly, it seems to work, especially since there are so many low-energy density foods that are considered heart healthy. In addition, the daily menus that the proponents offer are designed to be filling, meaning you might more easily stick to the diet because you have fewer food cravings (especially for foods in category four).

POPULAR CULTURE DIET PLANS

ACID–ALKALINE

Emphasis of the Plan—This diet is based on the theory that our Western diet carries too many foods that produce acids, thus driving our body's pH down (meaning more acidic), and that, in turn, causes heart disease, cancers, obesity, and even such diseases as chronic fatigue syndrome.

Pros and Cons of the Diet

Pros: This is a very healthy diet because you eat plenty of plant-based foods; plus, it advocates limiting some foods that doctors often recommend to watch out for: sweets, caffeine, alcohol, and processed foods.

Cons: But, on the other hand, there is no scientific basis that you truly need to balance the acidity in the body, since we all have mechanisms that take on that task, especially your kidneys and lungs, which help maintain a steady pH no matter what you eat. The diet also cuts out some of the more healthy foods, claiming they are more "acidic," such as navy beans, whole eggs, and peanuts.

Does It Work?—You may feel better because you're cutting out some major calorific foods and eating more vegetables, but there is no scientific proof backing up the diet's premise. (One caveat: This diet may help prevent kidney stones because what you eat affects the pH of your urine; more acidic urine means your risk for stones increases.)

ATKINS

Emphasis of the Plan—The Atkins diet (formerly called the Atkins Nutritional Approach) is one of the more well-known "popular" diets and has been around since the early 1970s. Its proponents claim the diet helps you lose and keep weight off through a lifelong dieting approach. The main emphasis is on cutting back carbohydrates, especially sugar, white flour, and other refined carbohydrates, and eating more proteins and natural fats. It is broken into four phases, including induction, ongoing weight loss, pre-maintenance, and lifetime maintenance.

Pros and Cons of the Diet

Pros: Some people do lose weight during the first stages of the diet. Although highly debated, some research claims it may help lower blood lipids and increase the "good" HDL cholesterol. There are "Atkins Diet" products available so you don't have to cook all the time.

Cons: Although the diet proponents claim a weight loss of up to fifteen pounds the first two weeks of phase 1, they also note that this is not a typical result. The diet includes working out numbers of grams, net carbohydrates, etc. to eat each day, which many people often find difficult and time-consuming.

Does It Work?—For people who want to lose weight fast, it can work, but there are caveats: Many nutritionists believe cutting back drastically in carbohydrates can cause nutrition or fiber deficiencies in some people, and there can also be side effects from the early phases of the diet (such as headache, weakness, or constipation). It is also not appropriate for everyone, especially those with kidney disease, or who are pregnant or breast feeding.

BIGGEST LOSER

Emphasis of the Plan—This diet is based on the popular reality show *The Biggest Loser* in which the contestants eat healthy food and work out for about six weeks to lose weight. Thus, the diet is based on two simple concepts: calorie restriction and exercise. You eat small, frequent meals that are considered to be heart-healthy—including vegetables, fruits, whole grains, lean protein, and light on sugar and saturated fats—and you exercise. There is also a "pyramid" involved called the Biggest Loser's 4-3-2-1 Pyramid: four servings of fruits and vegetables, three of lean protein, two of whole grains, and 200 calories of "extras" per day.

Pros and Cons of the Diet

Pros: With restricting the amount of calories you eat, along with exercise (and sticking to it), most people will lose weight. The contestants—most of them very obese—lowered their "bad" LDL cholesterol, blood pressure, and triglycerides. The foods eaten are balanced and healthy.

Cons: Many people will have a hard time sticking to the diet—the incentive for the contestants was more "appealing" than for most people who take on this diet and exercise program! It's hard work, and this is a major change of diet for most people.

Does It Work?—This diet and exercise program is considered to be healthy, as it is similar to some of the other "lifestyle" diets mentioned above—especially those that emphasize a healthy diet of fruits, vegetables, lean meats, and whole grains.

DUKAN

Emphasis of the Plan—This is a low-carbohydrate, high-protein diet, offering the dieter four phases—attack, cruise, consolidation, and permanent stabilization. This might sound like a military strategy, since the diet has many rules and regulations (and proponents stress that any slip-up can throw off your diet plan). During certain phases of the diet, you cannot eat any carbohydrates, except small amounts of oat bran, and no vegetables or fruits, and there are major restrictions on fats.

Pros and Cons of the Diet

Pros: The proponents claim you can lose up to ten pounds in the first week if you follow the directions to the letter.

Cons: During certain phases of this diet, some research has shown that you will not be getting enough of certain nutrients. In addition, the rules are very restrictive, and with no true long-term studies of the Dukan, it is not known if this diet is good for the heart, brain, or other organs of the body. During the attack and cruise phases, certain recommended daily servings of nutrients, fats, and carbohydrates accepted by the government are not met.

Does It Work?—Some people who have tried this diet have lost weight in the first week, but it is not known if it is water weight or fat. And some research shows that eliminating entire food groups (for example, grains and fruits) may put a person at risk for nutritional deficiencies.

FLAT BELLY

Emphasis of the Plan—The Flat Belly diet promises what it says: a flat belly (lose several inches worth—and the claim is you can do it without exercise) and a drop in weight of about 15 pounds in 32 days. This is all based on monounsaturated fats (MUFAs, or monounsaturated fatty acids), which allegedly target and destroy belly fat, cause us to feel full after eating, and prevent us from overeating. The MUFAs are often found in nuts, seeds, chocolate, avocados, and olive oils; the rest of the diet is somewhat similar to the Mediterranean diet (see above), with the main ingredients being fruits, vegetables, legumes, whole grains, olive oil, and fish.

Pros and Cons of the Diet
Pros: This diet has many of the healthy foods nutritionists recommend. It can also be tailored to fit your gender, age, and activity level (although many people say its followers are mostly women). The dietary offering (available as a book and on the Internet) comes with guidelines and shopping lists.

Cons: There are some "fees" involved—it's from the editor of *Prevention* magazine—including buying the book and an online membership, so it's not completely self-contained. In addition, many experts say that it's more of a short-term weight-loss diet, not as much of a long term lifestyle change; in addition, it focuses on just one aspect of our foods—the MUFAs.

Does It Work?—For people who want a short term weight loss, it seems to work, mainly because, along with the MUFAs, the diet consists of fruits, vegetables, fish, legumes, and whole grains.

JENNY CRAIG

Emphasis of the Plan—Like many of the popular diet plans, the Jenny Craig diet tries to make it easier for a person to lose weight by offering support, a meal delivery service, and exercises that are tailored to the person. There are weekly phone consultations, and a diet advisor who helps you to determine why you gained weight and, as you are on the diet, helps you change your bad eating habits. It's not a fast weight-loss program, but is designed to help you lose one to two pounds per week.

Pros and Cons of the Diet

Pros: For people who can't—or don't want to—find the time to develop their own diet plans, the Jenny Craig may help. This is because almost everything is done for you, from all the meals and snacks being portion-controlled to delivery at your door.

Cons: Many people will not be able to pay for such a service. In addition, the meals don't contain fruit, vegetables, or dairy products, but those can be added for an additional fee. In addition, if you don't like the Jenny Craig foods, this diet truly won't work.

Does It Work?—For people who are really busy, this may be one choice to lose weight. And many people say this diet program is one of the more expensive ones offered. But overall, most experts agree, eating nutrient-rich, balanced meals that you prepare yourself is a better way to lose weight than having someone do it for you.

NUTRISYSTEM

Emphasis of the Plan—Similar to many popular plans, the Nutrisystem diet relies on making your meal choices for you—from determining the proportions based on your diet needs to preparing and delivering the meals and telling you what to eat and when. It is used mostly for a gradual or steady weight loss of about one to two pounds per week.

Pros and Cons of the Diet

Pros: Most of the foods you eat for this diet are prepared for you, although you still have to go to the grocery store to buy some of the other foods to "fill in" what you're not sent (for example, fruits, vegetables, meats, and dairy products—and they will tell you what to buy to supplement the packaged meals). There are also plans that are specifically for people with certain dietary differences, such as for people with diabetes, seniors, or even vegetarians.

Cons: The foods and plans may be expensive for many people. Because you don't count calories, and everything is sent to you, there is a chance that you won't learn how to eat healthy, so your weight will come back after you stop the program (although they do offer resources and recipes that will help to wean you off the Nutrisystem diet). In addition, you may not like the taste of the foods they offer.

Does It Work?—For people who don't want to think about their meals and still want to lose weight, this diet may work. But it may be expensive for many people. And many experts agree it is best to learn how to prepare your own meals.

PALEO

Emphasis of the Plan—This diet is based on the premise that if our ancestors of about 10,000 years ago ate this way then it is more natural for us to do so, too. The diet includes meat, fish, poultry, fruits, and vegetables (preferably wild-caught meats, or anything our ancestors hunted, gathered, or fished), but it eliminates refined sugars, dairy, legumes (beans or peas), and grains—foods eaten before our ancient ancestors learned about agriculture. The diet hasn't been around for long, and thus there have been few studies done on it, so nothing is really known about the diet's true effectiveness.

Pros and Cons of the Diet

Pros: Eating fewer processed foods, carbohydrates, and junk foods, and emphasizing more healthy, lean meats and plant-based food, is definitely good for your overall health.

Cons: This diet has been out such a short time that there are few studies that prove whether it is really good or bad for your health. It may also be hard for people to give up carbohydrates, or even their daily yogurt. Plus, no one truly knows what our ancient ancestors ate, as most of what we know about the diet of Stone Age peoples is based on educated guesses.

Does It Work?—Although there are few studies on this diet, there are some. For example, one stated that the Paleo diet is better than some "highly recommended" diets, such as the Mediterranean or diabetic diets, especially in terms of weight loss, energy levels, and risk factors that can cause cardiovascular disease or diabetes. Another finds the diet too restrictive, including the problem of eliminating nutrient-rich foods such as beans and grains; plus, it's not easy finding some of the foods, including "wild game" and wild plants—ours meats are domesticated, and most plant foods are cultivated.

PRITKIN

Emphasis of the Plan—This diet is close to a vegetarian diet (see above). It allows the dieter to have several ounces of fish or chicken and a small amount of low-fat dairy foods per day, but most of the diet emphasizes high-fiber fruits, vegetables, and whole grains.

Pros and Cons of the Diet

Pros: Because it emphasizes low fat and lean foods, as well as exercise, this diet usually helps people lose weight. Proponents also mention that it can possibly help reverse heart disease in many people, as most of the foods you eat are nutrient-rich fruits, vegetables, and whole grains.

Cons: Many people may have a hard time changing to such a diet.

Does It Work?—For many people, this diet may help—and may be healthy since it follows a combination of vegetarian diets and small amounts of lean meats and low-fat dairy foods.

SLIM-FAST

Emphasis of the Plan—Slim-Fast was mostly developed as a low-calorie meal replacement for people who have a body mass index (BMI; see the chapter "Nutrition and You" for more details about BMI) of 25 or more. Many Americans know about Slim-Fast meal replacement beverages, bars, and some meals; these all can be used to lose weight, and you can stay on the diet (found through their literature or on their website) as long as you want, depending on your weight loss goal.

Pros and Cons of the Diet

Pros: This diet has been effective in helping people lose weight and keep it off in many cases. The plans and meal replacement products makes it easy to follow.

Cons: Like many "pre-planned" diet products, this diet does not really teach people how to eat healthy foods in order to keep off weight, but makes them rely on the diet's product offerings, which means some people may gain back the weight they lost if they go off the diet. In addition, some people do not like the taste of the various products available.

Does It Work?—For people who want an "easier" way of losing weight, and don't mind eating what is actually processed foods, this diet may help, especially in the short term.

SOUTH BEACH

Emphasis of the Plan—This diet has been around since 2003 and is based on the book *The South Beach Diet: The Delicious, Doctor-Designed Foolproof Plan for Fast and Healthy Weight Loss*. Its main feature is to change the overall balance of the foods you eat to help you lose weight and have a healthy lifestyle—all by eating fewer carbohydrates and more lean proteins and healthy fats. There are three phases to the diet; the promise, like many popular diets, is to lose weight in the first phase (two weeks); then the next two phases focus on lifestyle and maintenance.

Pros and Cons of the Diet

Pros: Although it is debated, many people consider this diet a good way to lose weight in the short term, but some researchers believe there is little cardiovascular benefit to it. This diet also chooses "good carbs and fats" and includes healthy vegetables, fish, eggs, low-fat dairy, lean proteins, whole grains, and nuts.

Cons: Many people will not be able to change their eating habits to follow this restrictive diet, especially during the first phase; it is less restrictive in the last two phases. In addition, although it is not as carbohydrate-restrictive as some diets, there may be problems with the side effects of consuming so few carbohydrates (such as in the Atkins diet), but such problems are usually minor.

Does It Work?—For people who want to stick to a lower-carbohydrate diet and lose weight fast in the first two weeks (although that may just be water weight), this may help. But it may not be useful or easy to follow in the long term.

WEIGHTWATCHERS

Emphasis of the Plan—WeightWatchers has been around for many years; it is based on the ProPoints system, which is about giving a value to foods and beverages based on their protein, carbohydrates, fats, and fiber contents. It is mostly a calorie-controlled diet, with each person having a daily ProPoint allowance of foods. The exceptions are fruits and vegetables—you can eat as much as you like of either. In some towns and cities, there are Weight Watcher groups—places where everyone gets weighed each week, gets moral support from other members, and shares eating and health information.

Pros and Cons of the Diet

Pros: As long as you eat within your allotted ProPoint allowance per day, you can eat and drink what you want. It's also good to have the support system found in most towns and cities; plus, it is less restrictive than most diet plans. And on the Weight-Watchers' website, there are more than 40,000 foods with their point values listed—so you do have choices.

Cons: Many people will have a hard time counting the calories in order to keep track of allowances. Some people also claim that there is often marketing pressure to buy the WeightWatchers' brand of foods.

Does It Work?—For people who do learn how to change their eating habits for the better—and for the long term, if possible—this plan may work. In addition, the support groups can keep people motivated enough to stay on the diet and lose weight. But there are many people who have a hard time keeping up with the ProPoint system in the long term.

Further Reading

This is only a very small listing of general nutrition books on the market. If you're interested in more details about what you read in this book, just enter such keywords as "nutrition," or even more specific words, such as "vegetarian," into a search engine or your favorite online bookstores.

America's Test Kitchen and Guy Crosby, *The Science of Good Cooking,* Cook's Illustrated Cookbooks, 2012.

Barnes-Svarney, Patricia, and Thomas E. Svarney, *The Handy Biology Answer Book,* Visible Ink Press, second edition, 2015.

Blake, Joan Salge, Kathy D. Munoz, and Stella Volpe, *Nutrition: From Science to You,* second edition, Benjamin Cummings, 2013.

Bowden, Jonny, *The 150 Healthiest Foods on Earth,* Fair Winds Press, 2007.

Bown, Stephen R., *Scurvy: How a Surgeon, a Mariner, and a Gentleman Solved the Greatest Medical Mystery of the Age of Sail,* St. Martin's Griffin, 2005.

Campbell, T. Colin, *Whole: Rethinking the Science of Nutrition,* BenBella Books, 2014.

Duyff, Roberta Larson, *American Dietetic Association Complete Food and Nutrition Guide,* fourth edition, Houghton Mifflin Harcourt, 2012.

Evers, Connie L. *How to Teach Nutrition to Kids,* fourth edition, Carrot Press, 2012.

Gardeners and Farmers of Centre Terre Vivante, *Preserving Food without Freezing or Canning: Traditional Techniques Using Salt, Oil, Sugar, Alcohol, Vinegar, Drying, Cold Storage, and Lactic Fermentation,* Chelsea Green Publishing Company, 2007.

Gratzer, Walter, *Terror of the Table: The Curious History of Nutrition,* Oxford University Press, 2007.

Kingry, Judi, and Lauren Devin, *Ball Complete Book of Home Preserving,* Robert Rose, 2006.

Kobuszewski, Anita, *Food, Field to Fork: How to Grow Sustainably, Shop Wisely, Cook Nutritionally, and Eat Deliciously,* AnitaBeHealthy Publishing, 2012.

Librairie Larousse, *Larousse Gastronomique: The World's Greatest Culinary Encyclopedia,* Clarkson Potter, 2009.

Marcus, Jacqueline, *Culinary Nutrition: The Science and Practice of Healthy Cooking,* Prentice, 2013.

Margen, Sheldon, *The Wellness Encyclopedia of Food and Nutrition,* Random House, 1992.

Margen, Sheldon, *Wellness Foods A to Z: An Indispensable Guide for Health-Conscious Food Lovers,* Rebus, 2002.

McWilliams, Margaret, *Illustrated Guide to Food Preparation,* Prentice Hall, 2012.

Mullin, Gerald, *The Inside Tract: Your Good Gut Guide to Great Digestive Health,* Rodale Books, 2011.

Nestle, Marion, *What to Eat,* North Point Press, 2007.

Norman, Jill, *Herbs & Spices: The Cook's Reference,* DK Publishing, 2002.

Pollan, Michael, *The Omnivore's Dilemma: A Natural History of Four Meals,* Penguin, 2007.

Sears, William, and Martha Sears, *The Family Nutrition Book,* Little, Brown and Company, 1999.

Shield, Jodie, *Healthy Eating, Healthy Weight for Kids and Teens,* Academy of Nutrition and Dietetics, 2012.

Sizer, Frances, *Nutrition: Concepts and Controversies,* thirteenth edition, Cengage Learning, 2013.

Stollman, Lisa, *The Teen Eating Manifesto: The Ten Essential Steps to Losing Weight, Looking Great and Getting Healthy,* Nirvana Press, 2012.

Stone, Gene, ed., *Forks Over Knives: The Plant-Based Way to Health,* The Experiment, 2011.

Thompson, Janice J., Melinda Manore, and Linda Vaughan, *The Science of Nutrition,* third edition, Benjamin Cummings, 2013.

Ward, Elizabeth M., *MyPlate for Moms: How to Feed Yourself and Your Family Better,* Loughlin Press, 2011.

Willett, Walter C., *Eat, Drink, and Be Healthy: The Harvard Medical School Guide to Healthy Eating,* Free Press, 2005.

Wood, Rebecca, *The New Whole Foods Encyclopedia: A Comprehensive Resource for Healthy Eating,* revised edition, Penguin Books, 2010.

Glossary

aerobic—Aerobic most often refers to organisms that require oxygen in order to exist, such as humans.

allicin—A natural chemical in garlic that is purported to help lower LDL cholesterol (the "bad" one, versus HDL) and is said to have antibacterial qualities. It is responsible for the pungent, sulfur-like smell when you cut or crush garlic.

amino acids—Amino acids are considered the building blocks of our proteins. There are twenty amino acids the body needs to survive and function. Nine (some say eight) are considered essential and usually come from our food; the body produces the other eleven when they are needed.

anaerobic—Most often refers to organisms that need little or no oxygen in order to survive, in particular, it is in reference to bacteria, such as those found in the human gastrointestinal tract.

anthocyanidins—A class of plant pigments; a certain reaction on the anthocyanidins (by the addition of sugar) results in the formation of anthocyanins.

anthocyanins—Plant pigments derived from anthocyanidins through a certain reaction (adding a sugar).

antioxidants—Almost all antioxidants are derived from the foods we eat. They are molecules that carry a positive charge that potentially neutralize negatively charged, free radicals—a process that is thought to help mitigate damage by carcinogens, smoke, and pollutants that can create health problems. They are often classified as nutrient antioxidants, such as vitamins and minerals that act like antioxidants or are considered to be antioxidants, such as vitamins C and E, and non-nutrient antioxidants, such as carotenoids and phytochemicals.

arteriosclerosis—The hardening and stiffening of the arteries most often caused by plaque buildup within the vessels over time. It is frequently associated with unhealthy eating habits (especially foods high in fat) and obesity.

artificial sweetener—A synthetically produced, non-nutritive, sweet substance; each varies in sweetness and, in most cases, tastes sweeter than table sugar.

ascorbic acid—The chemical name for vitamin C.

B-complex vitamins—The B-complex vitamins—to date, there are eight—give the body energy by converting carbohydrates to glucose and help metabolize fats and proteins. They also are necessary for the nervous and digestive systems, among many other functions, depending on the vitamin.

bioavailable —The rate that a substance is absorbed into an organism's system; for example, when a drug is administered intravenously (through or within a vein), the drug is totally bioavailable to the organism's body.

bioflavonoids—Bioflavonoids, or flavonoids (sometimes called vitamin P, although they are not true vitamins), are a naturally occurring group of phytochemicals thought to function as antioxidants. There are several classes of bioflavonoids, including flavanols, flavones, and isoflavones.

Body Mass Index—A statistical way to determine the body's mass, based on the weight and height of a person.

botulism—An illness caused by the bacterium *Clostridium botulinum*, which produces a deadly toxin called botulinum. It is most often associated with foods that are not properly canned.

butter —A dairy product defined by federal regulations as having eighty percent butterfat. It is graded as to flavor, texture, color, and body, with the rated highest to lowest grades being U.S. Grade AA, A, B, and finally C. AA and A are most commonly found in supermarkets.

buttermilk—The liquid left over after churning butter, but few people obtain their buttermilk from this time-consuming process today, preferring to buy the liquid in stores. Thus, most buttermilk found in supermarkets is only a simulated version made from skim milk and flecks of butter.

caffeine—Caffeine is a stimulant with a bitter taste and is found in coffees, certain teas and soft drinks, chocolate, and some medicines. It affects both the body's metabolism and the nervous system and can have an adverse health effect, especially when ingested in excess.

calorie—In terms of nutrition, calories are the measure of energy produced after a person digests and metabolizes food. It is often listed by nutritionists as a measure of how much energy is within each type of nutrient.

carbohydrate—Carbohydrates are made up of carbon, hydrogen, and oxygen—all of which are "burned" by our bodies for energy. They are one of the three major macronutrients that the body needs for energy; they are often divided into monosaccharides, disaccharides, and polysaccharides.

caramelize—To caramelize means to heat sugar until it melts and turns a golden brown; the term is also used to define how to cook and bring out the sweetness in some vegetables, particularly such foods as carrots and onions.

carotenoids—Non-nutrient antioxidants that help destroy free-radical-causing agents; they include beta carotene, lutein, and lycopene.

celiac disease—A disease caused by a severe intolerance to gluten products. It usually results in severe gastrointestinal problems, such as diarrhea, bloating, and constipation.

cholecalciferol—A form of vitamin D$_3$; it is produced by our bodies in the intestines and converted to vitamin D by the sun's ultraviolet B radiation.

collagen—The fibers made of protein that hold our cells and tissues together are called collagen; as we age, the amount of collagen decreases and our skin loses its elasticity.

complementary proteins—When a person's meal contains foods in which the proteins lack one of more of the essential amino acids (called incomplete proteins), they can often obtain the missing amino acids though other foods in order to create a complete protein. One classic example is eating grains and beans together because both lack an amino acid that the other one has.

Crohn disease—A chronic inflammation of the digestive tract.

d-alpha-tocopherol—Vitamin E is most often found in supplement form as d-alpha-tocopherol or d-alpha tocopheryl acetate.

deficiency—When discussing nutrition, deficiency is usually used to describe health problems and conditions caused by the lack of a specific nutrient or nutrients. For example, a person may bruise easily if they are deficient in vitamin D, a nutrient that has natural blood-clotting properties.

diabetes—A metabolic disorder caused by the decreased ability of the body to use ingested carbohydrates. There are two forms: type 1 and type 2; and, more recently, borderline diabetes is often referred to by doctors as pre-diabetes.

Dietary Reference Intake —The U. S. government's Dietary Reference Intake (DRI) is the standard for nutrient intakes in the United States; it is based on the recommendations for energy, vitamins, minerals, proteins, amino acids, carbohydrates, fats, water, and electrolytes for specific genders and stage of life.

diverticulitis—Diverticulitis occurs when deep pockets (diverticula) form in the large intestines, causing food to collect; this, in turn, often leads to the pouches becoming infected or inflamed, resulting in pain in those regions.

DNA—The abbreviation for Deoxyribonucleic acid, the molecule represented by a double helix structure. It is a nucleic acid that is formed from the repetition of nucleotides, of which there are five types: adenine, thymine, guanine, cytosine, and uracil. It is necessary to our cells for reproduction and for all our life processes.

electrolytes—In the human body, electrolytes are needed for nerve and muscle function, for maintaining the body's fluid balance, and for the acid-basic balance of our cells. An electrolyte imbalance can occur if the body is not taking in enough liquids, sodium, potassium, or chloride; one classic example is runners who lose so much liquid while running—especially in hot weather—that their body's liquid-electrolyte levels become unbalanced. The result can mean fatigue and confusion.

enzyme—Enzymes—the human body has about 75,000—are actually proteins that act as biological catalysts; without them we would not be able to obtain energy and nutrients from our foods.

ergocalciferol—The synthetic form of vitamin D_2, usually obtained from supplements and fortified foods.

essential nutrient—Nutrients that can't be synthesized by the body or in enough quantity to maintain good health, so they are generally obtained by eating certain foods or supplements that contain the nutrient. The term is also used in reference to the six necessities for the human body: carbohydrates, fats, proteins, vitamins, minerals, and water.

fats—Fats are lipids that help us to maintain normal growth and development, cushion our organs, and provide better taste to many thing we eat. But fats—the wrong types that we consume—can also be bad for us, adding unhealthy calories and clogging arteries.

fat-soluble—Usually in reference to vitamins (such as vitamins A,D, E, and K) that are soluble only in fats. In the human body, fat-soluble vitamins are usually stored in our fatty tissues and liver to be used when needed.

fatty acids—Fatty acids are the fats and oils found in our foods—what are often referred to as saturated and unsaturated (monounsaturated and polyunsaturated) fats.

fermentation—A process that converts sugars to certain acids, gases, and/or alcohol; the process is carried out mostly by bacteria or fungi (such as yeast).

fiber—Also called fibrous carbohydrates or dietary fiber, fiber comes in two main forms: soluble, or those foods in which the fibers dissolve in water and stick together (such as oatmeal), and insoluble, or those foods in which the fibers do not dissolve in water, including wheat bran and brown rice. In general, dietary fiber is defined as the part of a plant that a human's digestive system cannot readily digest.

flatulence—A process that many organisms experience as methane gas escaping out the anus; in most cases, it is caused by intestinal bacteria that ferment the remains of eaten foods.

flavonoids—See bioflavonoids.

food—Food is a difficult term to clearly define, but in general, it means anything we eat that has (or sometimes doesn't have) a nutritious value—most often something that helps maintain good health.

free radicals—A person's metabolic activity uses oxygen, which produces unstable, highly reactive molecules called free radicals (it can also happen when a person is exposed to environmental pollutants, such as cigarette smoke). Free radicals are why people age as the molecules damage cells; the best solution is to eat more antioxidants and bioflavonoids that will help counteract the free radicals.

functional food—A term most often used to describe certain foods that provide benefits beyond our basic nutritional needs for good health.

genetically modified organisms—GMOs are organisms in which there is a change in the code or organization of genetic material. There continues to be concerns with GMOs, as there is no proof whether they are safe or not for humans; there is a concern about cross-pollination of GMO and organic plants.

gluten—A substance most often found in wheat, although other flours, such as rye and barley, carry smaller amounts. Gluten is one reason why bread rises. When the flour and yeast are mixed with a liquid, the gluten proteins absorb the liquid, making the dough elastic. From there, the gases given off by the yeast are trapped; this makes the bread lighter because of the holes the gases make.

gluten intolerance—People with gluten intolerance often react to certain cereal grain products, and they usually experience a slight to moderate gastrointestinal reaction.

glycemic index—The numerical ranking of foods based on the rate of their conversion to glucose in the body.

glycemic load—The body's response to a food based on the glycemic index and the amount of carbohydrates consumed.

glycogen—This is a form of glucose stored in the liver and muscles in the human body. When a person needs energy, the stored glycogen is then converted back to glucose for the body to use.

gout—Gout is caused by high levels of uric acid in the blood, which causes crystals to form around joints, causing pain. It is considered a form of arthritis.

high acid foods—Food that contains sufficient acid (either naturally, or as in canning, added as an ingredient) that has a pH lower than 4.6. This includes fruits, fruit juices, tomatoes, jams and jellies, and soft spreads; added acid, usually in the form of vinegar or citric acid, lowers the pH in foods not normally high in acid, making them high-acid foods; examples include pickles, relishes, and salsas.

hydrogenation—The process in which liquid oils are made solid. Most nutritionists say that a person should limit the intake of hydrogenated oils, as they are thought to raise LDL ("bad") cholesterol and lower the HDL ("good") cholesterol, which can increase the risk for cardiovascular disease.

inflammatory bowel disease—IBD is a gastrointestinal disorder. It is usually chronic, and includes Crohn disease and ulcerative colitis.

insulin—A natural hormone in the body that helps to regulate the metabolism of carbohydrates. (Diabetes can occur when the body cannot correctly balance the insulin in the blood.)

iron-deficiency anemia—One of the most common types of anemia, it is caused by a nutritional deficiency of iron in the blood.

irritable bowel syndrome—IBS is a gastrointestinal disease that has symptoms similar to inflammatory bowel disease, except there is no destructive intestinal inflammation.

lactic acid —The acid produced during fermentation.

legume—A family of plants that are rich in proteins, including beans, peas, lentils, and peanuts.

linoleic acid—One of the omega-6 essential fatty acids.

linolenic acid—One of the omega-3 essential fatty acids.

lipids—Lipids are, in general, fats, oils, waxes, and certain sterols and esters—all of which can be dissolved in alcohol, but not in water. They are also the main constituents of all organisms' cells and are an important food source for the cells.

low-acid foods—Those foods—including some meats, poultry, seafood, and certain vegetables—that contain little natural acid; they have a pH higher than 4.6.

macronutrient—A macronutrient (*macro* is Greek for "large" or " big") is a larger nutrient—molecule-wise—that humans need, usually in large quantities, for the body to exist and function. They include carbohydrates, fats, and proteins.

359

meat—Meat is most commonly defined as flesh from animals. It has several other definitions, including being the flesh from mammals (especially those raised for human consumption), but not fish and sea creatures, poultry, or certain other organisms.

metabolism —The chemical and physical processes that allow all cells, organs, and vessels to support functions in the human body. One of the most important functions includes metabolizing our foods to obtain nutrients.

micronutrient—A micronutrient (*micro* is Greek for "small") is a nutrient that humans (and other organisms) need in small quantities for the body to exist and function; they are just as important at macronutrients.

microorganism—A living plant or animal that is microscopic in size, including molds, yeast, and bacteria.

milk sugar—Sugar that comes from milk, or lactose.

minerals—In terms of nutrition, minerals are elements that are necessary for human health. They are generally classified as macrominerals, trace (or micro) minerals, and electrolytes.

mold—Microscopic fungi that look like fuzz growing on foods; they thrive on acids and often produce mycotoxins, a form of poison. They can easily be destroyed (especially in canning) in temperatures between 140 to 190 degrees Fahrenheit (60 to 88 degrees Celsius).

non-nutrients—Non-nutrients are just as important to our health as nutrients; this list includes non-nutrient antioxidants, bioflavonoids, and even water.

nutrients—Nutrients are considered to be any chemicals that any organism needs in order to survive. They allow organisms to grow, help sustain body organs, tissues, and cells, and allow the organisms to gain energy for all body functions.

omega-3—A polyunsaturated fat that is considered an essential fatty acid. They are thought to benefit the body in many ways, such as helping to prevent blood clotting and lowering triglyceride levels.

omega-6—A polyunsaturated fat that is found in plant sources, such as corn and sunflower oils. Although there is disagreement, many researchers believe that a balance of omega-6 and omega-3 have certain health benefits.

omega-9—A monounsaturated fatty acid; because our body can make some of its own omega-9 from the foods we eat, it is not considered as essential as omega-3 and omega-6 fatty acids.

ORAC (Oxygen Radical Absorbance Capacity)—Certain nutritionists often turn to the ORAC score of a food, or the total antioxidant power of foods and chemicals. The higher the number, the more the antioxidant value.

oral allergy syndrome—A food allergy that occurs when a food-sensitive person eats—and sometimes even touches—a certain fruit, vegetable, nut, or spice that results in an allergic reaction.

oxidation—In terms of the human body, oxidation is the chemical process in which food reacts with oxygen in order to release energy in our system. It is also responsible for the release of free radicals.

PAH (polycyclic aromatic hydrocarbons)—Research has shown that PAHs are cancer-causing substances that can form when meats are cooked at a high heat. They are also present in cigarette smoke and car exhaust.

partially hydrogenated oils—Oils created when hydrogen is added to a liquid vegetable oil through a mechanical process, making it solid. This type of process may extend the shelf life of the oil, but it can also, especially in excess, have a damaging effect on human health.

peristalsis—This is the body's way of pushing our ingested food and drink through the digestive tract—mainly by specialized muscle contractions.

pH—A chemical term that stands for "potential of hydrogen." It is used to determine the acidity (or alkalinity) of a substance. For example, in canning there are low-acid and high-acid foods with their acidity (or lack of) determined by their pH.

photosynthesis—The process by which plants use energy from sunlight to manufacture food molecules from carbon dioxide and water.

phytochemicals—Phytochemicals (or phytonutrients) are chemicals that act like non-nutrient antioxidants; they include polyphenols and bioflavonoids, and are found in such foods as soybeans, tomatoes, garlic, and onions.

pica—An eating disorder in which a person has an addiction for nonfood substances, such as dirt, clay, or paint.

plasma—Plasma makes up about 55 percent of our blood. This yellowish fluid carries cells, platelets, and important nutrients throughout the body.

polyphenols—Polyphenols are considered to be non-nutrient antioxidants—or specific types of phytochemicals that have antioxidant properties. They are found naturally in plants, and many appear to have antioxidant, anti-inflammatory, and/or anticarcinogenic effects.

polyunsaturated fats—Polyunsaturated fats, or polyunsaturated fatty acids, or PUFAs, are unsaturated fats that are thought to be helpful to human health. The two most helpful types—when both are balanced in our systems—are thought to be the essential fatty acids called omega-3 and omega-6, both of which we must obtain from our diet since our bodies cannot produce them.

probiotics—Probiotics are organisms that help us stay healthy and balanced, and which are often called our "friendly bacteria," especially in reference to our digestive tracts.

protein—Proteins allow life to exist; they are made up of amino acids—or a carbon atom attached to a hydrogen atom, an amino acid and acid group, and a side chain—all in different amounts that result in different proteins. The various proteins are used in the body for a multitude of functions.

provitamin—A substance that the body can convert into a vitamin, such as beta carotene converted to vitamin A in the liver.

Recommended Dietary Allowance (RDA)—A listing from the U.S. government that conveys the best amounts and most nutritious foods to eat to stay healthy—often broken down by gender, age, and health.

retinol—Retinol is also called retinal or retinolic acid. The word is most often used to indicate the amount of usable vitamin A that has already been broken down and is now in the body's bloodstream, and is thus available to be used by tissues and cells.

RNA—Ribonucleic acid—the molecule represented by a single chain of nucleotides—is a nucleic acid that is formed from the repetition of the nucleotides, of which there are five types: adenine, thymine, guanine, cytosine, and uracil. It is necessary to our cells for reproduction and for all our life processes.

salt—There are many forms of the mineral salt, such as sodium chloride (table salt) and sodium bicarbonate. In addition, salt is the most common source of sodium humans consume. For most people, ingesting salt (in moderation) aids several critical body functions, such as maintaining our fluid balance and helping our muscles move.

saturated fatty acids—Saturated fatty acids, or saturated fats, are fats that are solid at room temperature (with a few exceptions, such as palm and coconut oils), and they are also associated with most animal fats (for example, eggs, meat, and some dairy).

scurvy—Disease caused mainly by a dietary deficiency of vitamin C; it is not as prevalent today as it was centuries ago—especially on ocean-going vessels—thanks to access to plenty of foods containing the vitamin.

sodium—A chemical element and occurs naturally in many of our foods. One of the most common sources of sodium that humans consume is sodium chloride, or table salt.

soy sauce—A salty, brown sauce extracted from lightly fermented soybeans.

sugar—Sugar is most often from sugar cane and sugar beets; there are various types from different sources, including sucrose (the refined crystallized white sugar we use in sugar bowls), dextrose (pure glucose), and lactose (milk sugar). It is often divided into intrinsic (or the sugar we taste in fruits and some vegetables) and extrinsic sugars (or sugar added to food before, during, or while being consumed).

sugar-alcohols—Sugar-alcohols, or polyols, are often referred to as sugar substitutes, such as sorbitol and maltitol. These reduced-calorie sweeteners are often used in sugar-free gums, candy, ice cream, and some baked goods.

superfood—A somewhat trendy term used to define foods that have a relatively high level of vitamins, minerals, and other non-nutrient substances—all of which are said to have a very positive effect on some aspect of our overall health.

tofu—Tofu is made from pureed soybeans; it is often called soybean curd and can come as soft or extra firm varieties. It is often used by vegetarians and vegans as a source of protein and calcium; it also readily absorbs flavors and spices and so can be made to taste like meat, for example.

toxin—Any substance that can enter into our bodies and cause an adverse effect, ranging from illness to even death.

trans fatty acid—Trans fatty acids, or trans fats, are created through an industrial process, with small amounts found naturally in some meats and dairy products. They are thought to have no real health benefit; in fact, most research has shown that trans fats can raise a person's "bad" LDL cholesterol, possibly contributing to heart disease.

triglyceride—Triglycerides are a type of lipid found in fats and oils. They are natural fats from plants or animals composed of three fatty acid molecules bound to a glycerol molecule (a type of alcohol).

tryptophan—This is an essential amino acid that is converted by the body into the B vitamin known as niacin. It is also thought to stimulate the production of serotonin, the natural "feel good" hormone in our bodies.

ulcer—Ulcers usually occur when stomach acids have reached the stomach tissues below the protective layer of mucus. There are several types, including those from medications, heavy drinking, smoking, heredity, and surgery (often called gastric ulcers); another is caused by the bacteria *Helicobacter pylori*, called duodenal ulcers.

ulcerative colitis—Ulcerative colitis involves the gastrointestinal tract and is limited to the top layers of the body's colon.

umami—Umami is chemically a glutamate (a type of amino acid) that produces what is called a savory taste. It was only recently discovered that our tongues have receptors for umami (in addition to sweet, salty, bitter, and sour receptors), and thus, umami is considered our fifth basic taste.

unsaturated fats—Unsaturated fats come in the forms of polyunsaturated and monounsaturated fats—both considered helpful to human health when eaten in moderation.

vinegar—There are two major types of vinegar. Cider vinegar, in which the liquid is derived from apples, has a golden color and a tart fruit flavor. The second kind is distilled white vinegar in which the liquid is derived from grain alcohol; it has a sharp, pungent flavor. There are other vinegars, too, including malt vinegar, and white and red wine vinegar.

vitamins—Vitamins are classified as micronutrients—either water- or fat-soluble—that all organisms need. To date, there are thought to be thirteen essential vitamins for human health, although many studies indicate there may be even more.

vitamin C—Vitamin C, or ascorbic acid, is one of the more well-known and important vitamins humans need for health. It is thought to be a major antioxidant, helping all our cells to function, and for some people is often associated with helping to lessen the effects of the common cold.

vitamin D—One of the more important vitamins humans need for health, especially since it also plays an important role in the body's use of two minerals—calcium and phosphorus. For humans, it comes in two forms: one obtained from supplements and fortified foods, the other one from a reaction to sunlight on our skin.

water-soluble vitamins—Vitamins (such as vitamin C) that can be disolved in water. Because of this, they are not held in the body as long as fat-soluble vitamins, and thus foods with these vitamins have to be eaten more frequently. In addition, they are often excreted in the urine if the body ingests more then needed, which is why your urine is often a darker yellow if you take multivitamins.

wheat—Although there are nearly two dozen species of wheat, the most well-known are common wheat (*Triticum aestivum*), which accounts for ninety percent of all wheat grown worldwide, and durum wheat (*Triticum durum*).

whole grains—Whole grains are usually eaten whole, such as whole oats and bulgur. Although not a complete source of protein, whole grains are a good source of starchy carbohydrates and dietary fiber; they are also a good way to ingest many healthy nutrients because they keep both the germ and outer covering of the wheat, and thus retain nutrients.

yeasts—Yeasts are microscopic fungi that grow from spores during the fermentation process in various foods. They are inactive in frozen foods and are easily destroyed in temperatures above 212 degrees Fahrenheit (100 degrees Celsius), the boiling point of water.

yogurt—Yogurt forms from the fermentation of whole, low-fat, or fat-free milk, creating a thick, creamy curd. Plain yogurt is high in protein and calcium, and relatively low in calories, which is why many nutritionists suggest, if you are watching your calories and/or sugar intake, that you buy plain yogurt (not flavored) and add your own ingredients, such as fresh fruit.

Index

Note: (ill.) indicates photos and illustrations.